Stefano Carpani has assembled an incredible nur
Jungians" in this two-volume anthology, presentin;
on contemporary clinical and theoretical classi.
The New Ancestors will no doubt become a high.
anthology for the Jungian community and will most likely be found in the librar-
ies of most Jungian institutes and societies as well as on the shelves of scholars
and practitioners.

Misser Berg, *Jungian Analyst, Denmark, President-Elect of the IAAP*

In acknowledging Jungian voices from which we are all descended, Stefano
Carpani has put together this marvelous two-volume anthology on theoretical,
clinical and applied depth psychology that will be essential reading for generations of neo-Jungians to come. From orthodox, post-classical and contemporary
perspectives, these seminal analysts and academics offer a rich compendium of
novel ideas that are harbingers for the future of analytical psychology.

Jon Mills, *Faculty, Postgraduate Programs in Psychoanalysis &*
Psychotherapy, Adelphi University

The *Oxford Dictionary* defines evolution as the appearance or presentation of
events in due succession. This innovative book project sets for itself the rather
challenging goal of exploring the evolution of analytical psychology from its
roots and foundations in the formulations of the founding figures of C. G. Jung,
Marie-Louise von Franz, Jolanda Jacobi etc., to the following generation of
post-Jungians (till the mid 1980's), in order to reflect on the future direction and
evolution of these notions and concepts from the perspective of contemporary
neo-Jungians (recent graduates of analytic training programs). Rather than perpet-
uating conceptual splits from different schools of analytic thought, this younger
generation of analytical psychologists or neo-Jungians favors trans-disciplinarian
inclusiveness and recognizes the value, indeed the necessity, of integrating ideas
and concepts from different psychoanalytical schools of thought and perspectives
with regard to the very nature of the analytic relationship, and to the transference
and counter-transference as an interactive field in order to broaden and deepen
our understanding of psyche and psychic process. This expanded perspective also
includes the body as a channel for expression of psyche and makes allowance
for the exploration of evolving notions of sexuality and sexual identity. This perspective includes the psychosocial level as well and gives credence to and recognition of the very real impact of socio-economic conditions on psychological
development.

The goal of this novel and innovative undertaking is to explore what the current
notions and ideas of the authors in this anthology might portent for the evolution
and future development in our understanding of the mysteries of psyche and of
the individuation process. Each author is a recognized authority in their field of
interest and together they represent perspectives from different training orientations and different cultures, including Europe, North America, South America and
South Africa.

This anthology would be of great interest to analytical psychologists as well as to the candidates in analytical training programs around the world. In addition, I strongly believe that the inquisitive openness to and novel exploration of the notions presented will also appeal to and help build bridges to psychoanalysts and psychotherapists from different schools of thought and orientation as well as to academics interested in further exploring the underlying notions, concepts and theory. I also believe the chapters in this anthology will respond to the curiosity of a large lay audience that has a profound and devoted interest in Jung and in the mysterious and often convoluted process of individuation.

In light of the fact that this anthology seeks to broaden our perspective and to explore avenues for the future development of our understanding of psychological development and of the mystery of the individuation process, it seems very likely that it would rapidly become an essential resource for further discussion among future generations of analysts and therapists of every orientation as well as of academics and students.

Tom Kelly, *Past President, IAAP*

Anthology of Contemporary Clinical Classics in Analytical Psychology

This anthology of contemporary classics in analytical psychology brings together academic, scholarly and clinical writings by contributors who constitute the "post-Jungian" generation.

Carpani brings together important contributions from the Jungian world to establish the "new ancestors" in this field, in order to serve future generations of Jungian analysts, scholars, historians and students. This generation of clinicians and scholars has shaped the contemporary Jungian landscape, and their work continues to inspire discussions on key topics including archetypes, race, gender, trauma and complexes. Each contributor has selected a piece of their work which they feel best represents their research and clinical interests, each aiding the expansion of current discussions on Jung and contemporary analytical psychology studies.

Spanning two volumes, which are also accessible as standalone books, this essential collection will be of interest to Jungian analysts and therapists, as well as to academics and students of Jungian and post-Jungian studies.

Stefano Carpani, M.A., M.Phil., is an Italian sociologist (post-graduate of the University of Cambridge) and psychoanalyst trained at the C.G. Jung Institute, Zürich, accredited analyst CGJI-Z/IAAP and a Ph.D. candidate in the Department of Psychosocial and Psychoanalytical Studies from the University of Essex. He works in private practice in Berlin (DE) in English, Italian and Spanish. He is the initiator of the YouTube interview series *Breakfast at Küsnacht*, which aims to capture the voices of senior Jungians. Since 2017, he has collected more than 70 interviews. He is among the initiators of *Psychosocial Wednesdays*, a digital salon molded on those Freud's Wednesdays meetings in Vienna and on Jung's meetings at the Psychological Club, and feature speakers from various psychoanalytic traditions, schools and associated fields. He is the author of numerous papers and edited books, including *Breakfast at Küsnacht: Conversations on C. G. Jung and Beyond* (Chiron, 2020—IAJS book award finalist, for "Best Edited Book"); *The Plural Turn in Jungian and Post-Jungian Studies: The Work of Andrew Samuels* (Routledge, 2021); *Individuation and Liberty in a Globalized World: Psychosocial Perspectives on Freedom after Freedom* (Routledge, in print, June 2022); *Lockdown Therapy: Jungian Perspectives on How the Pandemic Changed Psychoanalysis* (Routledge, in print, July 2022).

Anthology of Contemporary Clinical Classics in Analytical Psychology

The New Ancestors

Edited by Stefano Carpani

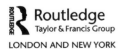

Routledge
Taylor & Francis Group

LONDON AND NEW YORK

Carla Indipendente, cover illustrator

First published 2022
by Routledge
4 Park Square, Milton Park, Abingdon, Oxon OX14 4RN

and by Routledge
605 Third Avenue, New York, NY 10158

Routledge is an imprint of the Taylor & Francis Group, an informa business

British Library Cataloguing-in-Publication Data
A catalogue record for this book is available from the British Library

Library of Congress Cataloging-in-Publication Data
Names: Carpani, Stefano, editor.
Title: Anthology of contemporary clinical classics in analytical
    psychology: the new ancestors / edited by Stefano Carpani
Description: Milton Park, Abingdon, Oxon; New York, NY :
    Routledge, 2022.| Includes bibliographical references and index. |
Identifiers: LCCN 2021047813 | ISBN 9780367710170
    (paperback) | ISBN 9780367710163 (hardback) |
    ISBN 9781003148968 (ebook)
Subjects: LCSH: Jungian psychology. | Psychoanalysis.
Classification: LCC BF173. A677 2022 | DDC 150.19/54—dc23/
    eng/20211001
LC record available at https://lccn.loc.gov/2021047813

ISBN: 978-0-367-71016-3 (hbk)
ISBN: 978-0-367-71017-0 (pbk)
ISBN: 978-1-003-14896-8 (ebk)

DOI: 10.4324/9781003148968

Typeset in Times New Roman
by Apex CoVantage, LLC

To my ancestors
And to Manuela, who enabled *To Wish Impossible Things*,
This book is dedicated.

Contents

Epigraphs

Two objects of the same logical form are
—apart from their external properties—
only differentiated from one another in that they are different.
Ludwig Wittgenstein (Tractatus Logico-Philosophicus)

Nel mezzo del cammin di nostra vita
mi ritrovai per una selva oscura,
ché la diritta via era smarrita.
. . .
Io non so ben ridir com'i' v'intrai,
tant'era pien di sonno a quel punto
che la verace via abbandonai.
Dante Alighieri, "Divina Commedia", Inferno, Canto I, vv.1/3–10/12

Acknowledgements

I want to thank all contributors who generously accepted my request to contribute to this anthology. I would like to express my gratitude to Routledge, who supported my idea to create such a book.

Introduction

The New Ancestors and the "Agenda 2050" for Analytical Psychology

Stefano Carpani

"Who exactly are today's Jungian ancestors?" asked Andrew Samuels, when endorsing my book titled *Breakfast at Küsnacht* (Carpani, 2020). "Not really Jung, von Franz, Wolff, Neumann, Jacobi, Hillman, Fordham, etc., etc.," he answered, and continued: "well, of course we all read them, but ancestors change. The analysts who studied under those giants are, if not today's giants, at least already ancestors in their own right."

This is the basis from which I developed the idea for this book,[1] and I asked myself, "Who are the (new) ancestors for my generation of newly certified analysts?" Of course, "ancestors" is a controversial term, and maybe we have to distinguish between mentors and ancestors. I propose that mentors are personal, and that the mentor and the mentored mutually attract each other and benefit from the relationship. Without this precondition, there is no mentor-mentored relationship: take, for example, Plato and Socrates, and Jung and Freud (which was certainly a mentoring relationship while it lasted and became for Jung an ancestral relationship only after Freud's death).

Therefore, ancestors—I propose—are collective and belong to the whole community (family). You cannot choose an ancestor; they are there! But when talking about ancestors, we have to be careful, because if we follow the *Cambridge Dictionary*, we find that an ancestor is "a person related to you who lived a long time ago."[2] I prefer the version from the *Collins Dictionary*: "Your ancestors are the people from whom you are descended,"[3] and there is no doubt that—although our daily lives are so different from those of our ancestors—we could trace our ancestors back a few hundred years. This is exactly what I am trying to do with this book! Synonymous to this are the concepts of forefather and -mother, predecessor, precursor and forerunner; someone who was there before you and had an influence on you and who you have become.

I propose that the ancestors mentioned previously by Samuels[4] are the ancestors of the previous generation [his generation: the post-Jungians (Samuels, 1985)]. Therefore, the question is, who are the ancestors of *my* generation [the neo-Jungians[5] (Carpani, 2021)] and the next generation(s)? Who are the *new* ancestors? This book tries to answer those questions. And hopefully this book will serve as

DOI: 10.4324/9781003148968-1

a guidebook for those venturing into this field, looking for the "new ancestors" as well as to serve future generations of Jungian analysts, scholars, historians and students.

The importance of this book to the Jungian community lies in the overall impact of the work of the individuals contributing to it. The book also plays a role in expanding current discussions on Jung, the post-Jungians and contemporary analytical psychology studies, and some of the important issues addressed by them. Furthermore, the book constitutes a recognition of the generation of post-Jungians who shaped analytical psychology.

Another important consideration, which helped me to advance and shape the idea of an anthology of contemporary classics in analytical psychology, is that fact that, despite the many differences [as Verena Kast underlined in the preface to my book *Breakfast at Küsnacht* (Chiron, 2020)], we should reflect deeper on the figure and symbolism of the "the Jungian analyst" and that, if and when we do so, we can "feel and discern a common basic attitude." I believe there is a truth in what Kast stated. Therefore, there is "a common basic attitude" as well as heterogeneous one. It is also important to underline that Jung should not be taken as a *Messiah* (who already said everything there is to say) and that the *Jungians* are not a cult! This would arm our field.

How were the ancestors included in this anthology chosen? I conducted an informal (international) survey of candidates and colleagues in 2019. I asked them, "Who exactly are today's Jungian ancestors?"

I asked colleagues to name their own "new ancestors" among those analysts and scholars (living) active in analytical psychology from the 1980s onward. This was to avoid confusion with the first generation of Jungians [i.e. the *classical school* as Andrew Samuels (1985) put it, or—as I call them—"the orthodox Jungians"]. Out of this survey, 48 names were suggested. I contacted all 48 suggested contributors via email. Only 29 agreed to take part in the project. One dismissed my invitation with contempt, saying that they did not wish to join a mass grave with those with whom they had lifelong acrimony; all others did not respond.

When contacting each of the contributors, I asked them to provide the following: "a chapter which you feel represents yourself, your work, and your intellectual and/or clinical trajectory" and "a detailed and *poetical biography* (written in first person), including as much information about you as you are willing to share." Therefore, I did not choose which chapters to publish; they decided! They also decided how much personal information to share about themselves. And we know how little personal information confident analysts are willing to share.

This book, of course, is full of biases. The first bias is that fundamental authors at least as seminal as those included are missing. This is because, for instance, I was not able to include those who were no longer alive by the time I knew I would be doing this book. Some living analysts who influenced my generation, on the other hand, are no doubt not yet ready to regard themselves as "ancestors." And I may not have realised that I should have contacted others. Perhaps a third volume can be published in the future (if a colleague wants to take over this from me) that covers work in analytical psychology as applied mainly in the arts and humanities in the academy and others omitted here.

Right now, a bias can be seen in the balance (or imbalance) of clinical versus academic contributors. There is a reason for this. In thinking of analytical psychology as a clinical field, the people whom I asked to recommend those who they thought of ancestors and who had shaped their understanding of analytical psychology were all accredited analysts and candidates in training. If I had asked the same question of academic scholars, the names supplied would likely have been different.

Apart from celebrating new ancestors within analytical psychology, this book aims to bring a (finalistic) look at the future and ask, "what is the task of my generation?" "What is the 'agenda 2050' for analytical psychology?" I feel the answers lie in the following steps:

1   A Jungian psychosocial-relational model
2   *Kulturkritik*: social critics as much as personal therapists
3   The neo-Jungians
4   Time for extraversion
5   Medicine contra *the soul*

Jungian Psychosocial-Relational Model

Let's look at psychosocial studies and relational psychoanalysis—which have been the models within which psychoanalysis has moved (adapted) in the past few decades—and try to link them with our field.

Jung and the Psychosocial

In my Ph.D. work (unpublished), which employs the pioneering survey of the reach of analytical psychology offered by Progoff (1955: 161), I show the first element that makes Jung a pioneer of psychosocial studies and, thereby, the fact that Jung perceived that "the human psyche cannot function without a culture, and no individual is possible without society." Moreover, Jung "makes it his principle that all analysis must start from the primary fact of the social nature of man" (Progoff, 1955: 161). In the development of analytical psychology, Redman's claim (2014, cited in Frosh, 2014) is that what can be called Jungian psychosocial studies

> have . . . an equal concern for the depth and range of *social* processes that are in play and help constitute the context or phenomenon in question . . . this implies a concern for phenomena over and above those arising from social interaction to include those belonging to large groups and social system and structure.

On this basis, I would claim that Jung's work is by its very nature psychosocial and vice versa. I claim this because Frosh (2014: 161)—when discussing which books would be published as part of Palgrave's *Studies in the Psychosocial*—underlines that "books in the series will generally pass beyond their points of origin to generate concepts, understanding and forms of investigation that are distinctively psychosocial in character" and that "transdisciplinary objects of knowledge are continually invented in ways that demand the blurring of previously disciplinary boundaries" (Frosh, 2014: 167). This is certainly Jung's approach: from medicine to psychiatry to occult phenomena (Ph.D. thesis) to alchemy (beyond drive theory) to myth (collective unconscious) and physics (synchronicity).

This is also confirmed by Redman (cited by Frosh, 2014: 166), who stated that "seeking to investigate how the social is implicated in the psychological, psychosocial studies necessarily pay close attention to psychosocial and emotional states and view these states as lively and consequential, for psychological and social life as well."

Furthermore, Frosh emphasises that psychosocial studies "draw[s] heavily on psychoanalytic studies, but also on various models of social and political theory." In this attitude, I frame Jungians such as Progoff, Samuels and Watkins as well as non-Jungians such as Craib, Orbach and Layton. All of these authors share the common characteristic of transdisciplinarity. In fact, Frosch developed his theory from the core premises of depth psychology, which he linked to different areas of investigation, sometimes giving the impression that his work was about religion or anthropology, ethnology, philosophy, etc., rather than psychology.

Interestingly, both contemporary psychosocial studies and Jung's method of cross-disciplinary survey dovetail with what Freud suggested in 1926 in *The Question of Lay Analysis*, that in

> a college of psycho-analysis, much would have to be taught in it which is also taught by the medical faculty [alongside] branches of knowledge which are remote from medicine . . . the history of civilization, mythology, the psychology of religion and the science of literature.

If we add ethnology, anthropology and alchemy (among Jung's other interests), and take Jung's view that all of these apply to analytical psychology, we will describe the usual curriculum of the C.G. Jung Institute in Zürich since 1948.

Jung and the Relational

As noted by Aron and Mitchell (1999: xii), relational psychoanalysis emerged in the context of early 1980s' American psychoanalysis and now "operates as a shared subculture" that "has stuck deep, common, chords among current clinical practitioners and theorists." Relational psychoanalysis developed thanks to the pioneering effort of psychoanalyst Stephan Mitchell, supported by Robert Stolorow, Jay Greenberg and Aron himself (Aron and Mitchell, 1999: x). The factors contributing to its development were as follows (Aron and Mitchell, 1999: x): (a) the influence of the interpersonal psychoanalysis of Harry Stack Sullivan,

Erich Fromm and Clara Thompson from the 1930s and 1940s; (b) object relations theory and the works of Fairbairn, Winnicott and Bowlby from the 1970s; (c) Kohut's "self-psychology" of the late 1970s; and (d) American psychoanalytic feminism and feminist psychoanalysis, including the work of Jessica Benjamin, and social criticism of the late 1970s and early 1980s.

It was in this landscape that, as Aron and Mitchell (1999: xi–xii) noted, Greenberg and Mitchell coined the term "relational" in 1983 to bridge the various strands of psychoanalysis current at that time, which included interpersonal *relations*, object *relations*, self-psychology, social constructivism, psychoanalytic hermeneutics and gender theorisation.[6] From these standpoints, Greenberg and Mitchell worked on a model (Aron and Mitchell, 1999: xiii–xv) that would do the following:

1 Provide an alternative understanding (to classical drive theory)
2 Generate a new understanding of precisely the phenomena that drive theorists have traditionally regarded as foundational: the body, sexuality, pleasure, aggression, constructionality, the patient's free association
3 Argue that mind occurs in "me-you patterns" (see Sullivan) and that the analyst is merely a "participant-observer . . . embedded in the transference-countertransference matrix" (Aron and Mitchell, 1999: xv)
4 Build on Winnicott's (1960: 39n, cited in Aron and Mitchell, 1999: xi) statement that "there is no such a thing as an infant—only the infant-mother unit"
5 Emphasise the emergence of what Ogden calls "the intersubjective Analytic-third" when speaking of "two-person psychology" (Aron and Mitchell, 1999)

Del Loewenthal and Samuels (2014: 4) recently highlighted the "widespread realization that the therapy relationship runs in both directions, is mutual, and involves the whole person of the practitioner," adding that "the 'relational' is most apparent in . . . Freud, Klein and object relations theories as well as Jung." Thus, he (Ibid., 2014: 4–5) reminds us of the mounting research evidence that the analytic relationship is the crucial factor in successful psychological therapy, and in asking why this is the case, he refers to Hargaden and Schwartz's (2007) description of relational psychoanalysis:

6   Emphasise the centrality of the relationship
7   Emphasise that therapy involves a bi-directional process
8   Emphasise that therapy involves both the vulnerability of therapist and client[1]
9   Emphasise the use of countertransference in thoughtful disclosure and collaborative dialogue
10 Emphasise the co-construction and multiplicity of meaning

---

1 I do not like to refer to those coming into analysis with me as "clients." I prefer to refer to them as "patients" (from latin *patiens -entis*), which means to suffer and to bear. In fact, patients, come to us because they suffer emotionally.

As noted by Andrew Samuels (2012, unpublished), Jung asserted that because analysis was "dialectical," involving mutual transformation through the therapeutic relationship, its method was necessarily dialogic and would have to include "emotionally charged interactions" between therapist and patient. Samuels (2012, unpublished) notes that analysis, according to Jung, is "an encounter . . . between two psychic wholes in which knowledge is used only as a tool" (points 3 and 4 presented earlier). Therefore, with Sullivan's idea "that mind always emerges and develops contextually, in the interpersonal field" (Aron and Mitchell, 1999: xv) and with Greenberg and Mitchell's assertion that "[t]here is not such a thing as either the patient or the analyst—only the patient-analyst unit" (Aron and Mitchell, 1999: xv).

Additional reasons why Jung should be considered a relational *ante litteram* (points 1 and 2) include that Jung (together with Adler) realised the need to move beyond Freud's drive theory and sought an alternative in which Freud's drive theory and sexuality, Adler's inferiority and compensation, and Jung's symbolic life and spirituality could coexist. Such an approach would, as Aron underlines, examine "issues of sex and gender" (Aron and Mitchell, 1999: xi), which in drive theory, with its fixed attitudes toward sexuality and aggression, are obscured with regard to how they take in meaning in the relational context (Aron and Mitchell, 1999: xvi). I think most of the analysts who contributed chapters to these two volumes would agree with this view.

I should mention here that my own Jungian relational-psychosocial model is based on the following pillars:

1   It connects theory and clinical work (therefore helping to prove the accuracy and efficacy of analytical work with patients)
2   It is transdisciplinary
3   It is pluralistic (Samuels, 1989) and demonstrates an attitude of inclusion (to replace the split and separation typical of the history of psychoanalysis)
4   It "starts from the premise that the individual is born into a set of social and psychological circumstances" (Orbach, 2014: 16)
5   It "investigate[s] the ways in which psychic and social processes demand to be understood as always implicated in each other" (Frosh, 2014: 161)
6   It has an "emphasis on affect, the irrational and unconscious process, often, but not necessarily, understood psychoanalytically" (Frosh, 2014: 161)
7   It offers a conflict-relational approach (Orbach, 2014) and stresses the need for continuous adaptation in the process of people becoming who they authentically are
8   Becoming (who people authentically are) is seen as a liberation (Watkins, 2003)
9   Analysis is framed as "accompaniment" (Watkins, 2013) based on "the co-construction and multiplicity of meaning" (Hargaden and Schwartz, 2007)

All of these points are developed in pioneering form in the chapters included in this book. They contextualise the "agenda 2050" for a Jungian relational-psychosocial model that knows how not to disturb the deep process of individuation which is the task of my generation to continue to protect, following the guidelines laid down by our newest ancestors.

Kulturkritik: Social Critics as Much as Personal Therapists

Samuels suggests that within both the microcosm of an individual and the macrocosm of the global village, "we are flooded by psychological themes" and that "politics embodies the psyche of a people" (Samuels, 2001: 5). Thus, he reminds us that "the founders [of psychoanalysis] felt themselves to be social critics as much as personal therapists" (Samuels, 2001: 6), and in this respect, he recalls Freud, Jung, Maslow, Rogers, Perls, the Frankfurt School, Reich and Fromm. He also notes that, in the 1990s, psychoanalysts such as Orbach, Kulkarni and Frosch began to consider society once more, but notes that although "the project of linking therapy and the world is clearly not a new one . . . very little progress seems to have been made."

Thus, he stresses that today "more therapists than ever want psychotherapy to realize the social and political potential that its founders perceived in it" but is aware of the "large gap between wish and actuality" (Samuels, 2001: 7). I argue that the Jungian relational-psychosocial model might fill this gap.

In contrast to Hillman, Samuels actively demonstrated "how useful and effective perspectives derived from psychotherapy might be in the formation of policy, in new ways of thinking about the political process and in the resolution of conflict" (Samuels, 2001: xi), and he claimed that "our inner worlds and our private lives reel from the impact of policy decisions and the existing political culture." In considering why policy committees do not include psychotherapists, Samuels notes that "you would expect to find therapists having views to offer on social issues that involve personal relations" (Samuels, 2001: 2). This is Samuels' most innovative proposition: to see psychoanalysts (as well as individuals) as activists with a fundamental role to play within society.

I propose that we should work both inside and outside the consulting room as successful consultants for politicians, organisations, activist groups, etc., and also work to regain the *quid*—which we inherited, although did not enact—of the founders of psychoanalysis (social critics and personal therapists). Becoming again and anew *Kulturkritik*, we might be able to continue to play (or to play anew!) a role in the development of 21st-century societies.

The Neo-Jungians

The neo-Jungians are the third generation of Jungians [the first generation (1961–1985) being initially called the Zürich School[2] or "the orthodox Jungians" (by me), and the second generation (1985–2011) being called "the post-Jungians" by Samuels].

---

2 Also called Classical School by Samuels

The *neo-Jungians*[7](Carpani, 2020) employ Jung (in a new fashion) along with other schools and traditions of psychoanalysis (and beyond psychoanalysis) that mutually contaminate and enrich each other. The neo-Jungians, encompassing eclecticism and integration, aim to restore and enhance Jung's work and analytical psychology at the core of depth psychology by studying the psyche as plural. This new approach is constituted by

> a heterogeneous, international, and multicultural group of scholars who on the one hand base their work on the teachings of Jung (and the post-Jungians), while on the other hand have opened their investigations beyond analytical psychology. Therefore, the *neo-Jungians* are able to balance the teachings of Jung and the post-Jungians with those teachings coming from other schools and traditions (both within and beyond psychoanalysis) in a mutual and plural, enriching exchange. In fact, contemporary *neo-Jungians* can be linked (although not limited) to relational (and post-relational) psychoanalysis, feminist psychoanalysis, the intersubjective approach, psychosocial studies, and cultural studies, to name a few.
>
> (Carpani, 2020)

The *neo-Jungians* find their frame of reference in the aforementioned Jungian psychosocial-relational model. Thus, there are many ways to be Jungian (or to be a Jungian), and this is very good news. It signifies that analytical psychology is alive and reflects the continuing interest in, as well as perhaps even rejuvenation of, Jung's theories at the beginning of the 21st century.

The task of the neo-Jungians is to look at the future and, first,—to honour and preserve the work of the first and second generations of Jungians.

Extraversion Is Not Superficial

Jungians mainly stress introversion in their clinical writings. And this has not always been helpful outside our circle. I hope that, in the next 30 years, some of us (the most extraverted ones perhaps!) will be able to influence society as *Kulturkritik* (outside of our usual circles), by presenting our work at non-Jungian and non-psychoanalytic conferences and talking about our approach (with pride and courage and without inferiority) with different media outlets, policymakers and institutions of different sorts.

Becoming extraverted would be the most innovative aspect. Therefore, to follow Samuels would mean to see psychoanalysts (as well as individuals) as activists with a fundamental role to play within society.

Medicine Contra *the Soul*

Another point, which is of fundamental importance, concerns training analysis, who is to be admitted to train within Jungian Institutes around the world, and how this will be conducted.

Hillman (2010: 156) underlines that "it is up to each individual involved in the analysis to defend their own experience—the symptoms, the sufferings, the neuroses, and also the invisible positive results—in front of a world that gives no credit to these things." And he continues, "the soul can return to being a reality only if it has the courage to take it as the reality before its life, to take sides with it instead of just 'believing' in its existence."

As such, this appears to support the model carried forward by the C.G. Jung Institute in Zürich, where—by tradition—non-MDs and non-psychologists can participate in the training. I am convinced that this approach is the best and that it must be implemented globally. It follows that the title of medical doctor or psychologist should be removed as a criterion for admission. This is because the approaches of medicine and psychology, as Hillman suggests, have nothing to do with working with the soul, while the analysis aims to "facilitate the flow and to reconnect the symbolic fragments in a mythical configuration" (Hillman, 2010: 156). And it is no coincidence that among the best analysts are non-MDs and non-psychologists (e.g. Riedel, Samuels and Zoja).

Mine, like Hillman's (2010: 159), is a campaign in favour of analysis, as "modern medicine imposes a split between doctor and his soul" and as it is fundamental that "the practice of psychotherapy, must leave the medical background behind to proceed independently."

Freud wrote on the subject as early as 1926. Freud intervened in defence of Theodor Reik (an Austrian psychoanalyst and collaborator of the same who, in 1924, was accused of abusing the medical profession because he practised psychoanalysis, but had a degree in philosophy) and helped to exonerate him by defending the legitimacy of the use of psychoanalysis by lay people. Freud, in a letter addressed to Julius Tandler (an influential anatomist and Viennese politician), asserted the legitimacy of practitioners like Reik by writing that "psychoanalysis, whether it is considered a science or a technique, is not a purely matter medical" and, second, "it is not taught to medical students at university."[8]
Hillman observes that

> Freud soon realized that it was necessary to partially abandon medicine because the analyst does not physically examine his patient, does not prescribe him medicine, for organic disorders he refers it to others; in the analyst's office there are no medical devices; you don't see white coats and black briefcases.
>
> (2010: 161)

Then Hillman points out that "Freud's fears have come true: Freudian analysis has become the handmaid of psychiatry" and that "Freudian therapy becomes acceptable by medicine" as a natural science (2010: 163). In fact, most MDs, psychiatrists and psychologists have not been analysed. They have never undergone training analysis.

So, I propose that a degree in medicine or psychology should not be the prerequisite to access psychoanalytic training; instead, the criteria used at the C.G. Jung

Institute in Zürich should be adopted: write a ten-page autobiography, go through six interviews with accredited analysts, complete 300 hours of training analysis in parallel with (during the second half of the training) individual and group supervision and—as enantiodromia—internship at a psychiatric institution.

Last, following Andrew Samuels' proposal at the 4th Analysis and Activism Conference San Francisco (online) 2020, I agree that, to be truly egalitarian, training should not require a master's degree (or even a bachelor's degree). Candidates should be interviewed and accepted on the basis of their fulfilment of the aforementioned requirements (see those in the preceding paragraph used by the C.G. Jung Institute Zürich) and their willingness to train (learning the theoretical aspects of this profession) and to undergo self-analysis to become a Jungian psychoanalyst.

"Structure of the Book"

The book consists of 15 chapters introduced by a poetical autobiography written by the new ancestor who wrote the chapter in question. These speak for themselves and need no further introduction here. But this is what the new ancestors have said to me about their individual chapters.

John Beebe: "The Trickster in the Arts"

The author, a psychiatrist and Jungian analyst, compares the effects of certain works of art in painting, film, fiction and song to the double binds that emerge in communications between psychotic patients and their families. These artistic effects reveal a trickster at play and illuminate some of the dynamics of the archetypal field between artist and audience, in which unambiguous communication is almost impossible and the artist's rage at being misunderstood must somehow be contained. The defensive strategy that is employed in creating a trickster work of art is connected to surreptitiously sustaining psychological values in communication with a world that may not wish to attend to them directly. The integration of the trickster's gift for irony and ambiguity into the anima's interest in making a sincere connection are important not only to the making of art that can endure, but to every psyche's ability to survive an often uncomprehending and unempathic world.

Astrid Berg: "Psychoanalysis and Primary Health Care"

Although the universal access to psychotherapy was an ideal that Freud already had in 1918, conservative psychoanalysis and primary health care have occupied opposite ends of the therapeutic spectrum. In South Africa, there is an ethical and moral imperative that mental health services be broadened to include all communities.

Many years of working in a Parent-Infant Mental Health Service have shown that it is used and appreciated in a so-called "township" community. Analysis of the patient demographics revealed that three-quarters of the caregivers returned for follow-up visits and/or followed the recommendations made. The active ingredients of this infant-parent psychotherapy were found to be similar to those described in the literature and follow basic psychoanalytic principles. In addition, and perhaps unique in this situation, were the "concept of the third" and "yielding control"—two theoretical constructs that were manifest by working with an interpreter who spoke the language and had the cultural knowledge of the caregivers living in that particular community. This kind of situation calls for an adaptation of psychoanalytic technique, which should not be regarded as a dilution of psychoanalysis, but rather as a deepening and widening of Freud's original ideal.

Pat Berry: "Rules of Thumb Toward an Archetypal Psychology Practice"

In this chapter, the author addresses "Rules of Thumb" for clinical practice within the discipline James Hillman called "Archetypal Psychology." These rules include attitudes such as "any Idea can be used defensively and will"; the danger of "sacred cows"; the importance of thinking poetically; the "connatural"; symbols "with" rather than symbols "of"; sticking to the image whatever image is; the importance of framing, observer and observed; contrasts; stealing tools; daimones and demons; true versus truth; Layard's rule with dream work.

Fanny Brewster: "The Racial Complex and the Dissociated Self"

One hundred years ago C.G. Jung began investigative work on the Unconscious and what he initially labelled the complexes. Following his psychological complex theory that he wrote about in A Review of the Complex Theory, Jung proceeded to minimally write about the "colour complex." The Racial Complex and the Dissociated Self re-visits Jung's earlier writing seeking to expand and deepen elements of a racial complex. Our 21st-century considerations of race, raciality and psychological complexes related to racism appear to require more understanding and connectedness to not just cultural groups but also self-reflection of the Self. How does this archetype exist in relationship to unconscious processes of the complexes and specifically a racial complex? This question is posed as are others that seek more clarity and creative imaginings as the work of joining ego to unconscious is discussed in this chapter.

Joseph Cambray: "Moments of Complexity and Enigmatic Action: A Jungian View of the Therapeutic Field"

The chapter looks at presenting clinical case material for a panel on archetypes and/or primal phantasies an initial discussion of archetypes as emergent phenomena organizing "moments of complexity" is given. The relationship of such moments to "moments of meeting" as developed by the Boston Change Process Study Group is commented on and explored within the context of the case. A condensed report of a multi-year analytic treatment of a bipolar patient having a severe trauma history is offered for discussion. Several unusual, enigmatic events are detailed to illustrate the occurrence of moments of complexity. Dreams high-lighting psychological transformation stemming from a changing relationship to emerging archetypal material related to a psychotic process in the patient are offered to further detailed moments of complexity.

Joan Chodorow: "The Body as Symbol: Dance/Movement in Analysis"

This chapter discusses the use of dance/movement as a form of active imagination in analysis. The history of this work emerges out of two traditions: depth psychology and dance therapy. The roots of both can be traced to earliest human history, when disease was seen as a loss of soul and dance was an intrinsic part of the healing ritual. The importance of bodily experience in depth psychology has not been fully recognized, despite Jung's interest in and experience of the body and his understanding of its relationship to the creative process. I will take up some of this material; look at the early development of dance movement therapy, with attention to Mary Starks Whitehouse and her contribution to the development of active imagination through movement; and explore the process of using dance/movement in analysis. This will lead to discussion of dance/movement as a bridge to early, preverbal stages of development.

Warren Colman: "Reflections on Knowledge and Experience"

As analysts become more experienced, theoretical knowledge becomes more integrated and implicit and is gradually transformed into the practical wisdom (phronesis) described by Aristotle. While this leads to greater freedom in ways of working, it remains conditional on the consistent disciplined practice represented by the analytic attitude. In the context of my own development as an analyst, I suggest that increasingly the analyst works from the self rather than the ego and link this with Fordham's account of "not knowing beforehand." Some implications for boundaries, enactment and the use of personal disclosure are discussed in relation to clinical material. I compare analysis with the wisdom traditions of religious practice and suggest that analysis is concerned with a way of living rooted in humane values of compassion and benevolence.

Lionel Corbet: "Varieties of Numinous Experience: The Experience of the Sacred in the Therapeutic Process"

The author describes the importance of numinous experience for Jung and presents a range of ways in which such experiences might appear. The examples include numinous dreams, visions, experiences in the natural world, through the body, and by means of entheogens. The chapter makes the point that whether these experiences are taken at face value or interpreted reductively depends on the psychotherapist's personal metaphysical commitments.

George B. Hogenson: "Comment on Synchronicity and Moments of Meeting"

The author considers the role of synchronicity in the establishment of meaning in analysis and links it to the notion of moments of meeting proposed by the Boston Process of Change Study Group. In so doing, the chapter proposed to view synchronicity as an element in developmental processes, wherein attributions of meaningfulness are made in relation to patterns of action that do not have intrinsic meaning, but which have evolved in an environment of meaning, thereby bootstrapping the infant into the world of meaning. Jung's paradigmatic example of synchronicity—the scarab beetle event—is examined in this context and the argument is made that the event was primarily meaningful for Jung and carried with it important countertransference implications that Jung did not consider. The chapter concludes with some suggestions for further investigation into the relationship between synchronicity and clinical practice.

Donald Kalsched: "Getting Your Own Pain: A Personal Account of Healing Dissociation With Help From the Film War Horse"

In this chapter the author describes a poignant emotional "moment" that occurred while watching the Steven Spielberg film War Horse. This moment and the dreams and relational process that followed it proved to be a *via regia* to an encapsulated trauma from his early childhood that 20 years of psychoanalysis had never penetrated and that had lain dormant and encapsulated inside a dissociated "cyst" in the psychic musculature of the deep unconscious. Not unlike a classical flashback, the triggering of this un-remembered "complex" brought intense vehement emotion into consciousness against the resistance of angry defences. The author relates this to the hermeneutics of true personhood—what it means to "become real" i.e., to have a personal autobiography—as opposed to a generic one; in other words, what it means to "get your own pain" as opposed to living inside a "story" about one's own suffering that isn't fully "true." Thus "individuation" is not so simple as realizing those potentials that lie dormant in oneself—what Jung called "becoming the person you were meant to be—" but involves recovering parts of the self that dissociative defences have banished from consciousness "forever." The process sometimes looks more like self-recovery than self-realization.

Eva Pattis Zoja: "Breathing—Physical, Symbolic, Spiritual and Social Aspects"

The chapter explores the symbolic meaning of breath in a variety of expressions from religious to social and from clinical to physical. In most religions, breathing is directly connected to the divinity. We know from clinical practices that breathing patterns are linked to specific mental states and generally to emotions. The Dutch therapist Cornelis Veening—after his encounter with Jung—has observed and studied how breathing and imagination are linked to each other. Today we have difficulties to breathe. Covid-19 is a respiratory illness: symbolically an illness between the inner word and the outside.

A specific breathing practice in Tibetan Buddhism, the Tonglen meditation, will be described and observed in its relation to imagination, to dreams and to the way we relate to shadow aspects of our existence, individually and on a collective level.

Andrew Samuels: "The "Activist Client": Social Responsibility, the Political Self, and Clinical Practice in Psychotherapy and Psychoanalysis"

The author discusses the idea of the "activist client," which is intended to be taken both literally and metaphorically—applying to some extent to a wider range of clients than actual activists. The chapter develops a set of ideas about a "political turn" in psychotherapy and psychoanalysis, using the tag "the inner politician." There is a focus on working directly with political material in the session, and the pros and cons of this practice are reviewed. Wider issues such as social responsibility and social spirituality are discussed, as well as an exploration of the limits of individual responsibility. Some specific topics covered in the chapter include the political roots of depression, difficulties with the concept of the therapeutic alliance from the point of view of democratic perspectives on clinical work, and a challenge to the unquestioned valuing of empathy (based on a reading of therapy though a Brechtian lens). There are numerous clinical examples.

Pia Skogemann: "The Daughter Archetype"

The author introduces the term the daughter archetype as a basic concept for the woman as a subject for herself, a concept for female agency that otherwise is lacking in analytical psychology. The phenomenology of the daughter archetype is represented at all levels of psychic functioning. The images range from ego-representations to goddess-like Self representations.

Skogemann's notion of the daughter archetype does not question our basic concepts, but it does question the use of binary-gendered properties as a metaphorical common denominator.

A presentation of the Sumerian Goddess Inanna will serve as an illustration of a very different archetypal Daughter-figure. Her title in the Sumerian-Akkadian era was "daughter of the gods." (Ishtar was her Akkadian name.) Skogemann amplifies the archetypal imagery with an example of a modern superstar, the American Madonna, who has staged herself in an Inanna-like way, with a typical mixture of sexual and spiritual elements.

The notion of the daughter archetype is not limited to the postmodern gender discussion as it is also represented in ancient times in ways that transcend the classical binary way of defining feminine and masculine properties.

Ursula Wirtz: "Traumatic Experiences and the Transformation of Consciousness"

Traumatic states are boundary experiences which have the power to destroy but are also capable of producing a radical transformation of consciousness. Trauma survivors often undergo altered states of consciousness after an encounter with the numinous mythopoetic structure of the unconscious. Chaotic processes of great emotional distress can initiate painful processes of change and open a door to deeper spaces of consciousness that were previously inaccessible.

Complementary conceptualizations of trauma are discussed with correspondences between contemporary neuroscientific research, the self-organizing features of complex adaptive systems and insights of the wisdom traditions. The spiritual dimension of Trauma is seen in the context of dying and becoming, the quest for meaning and the potential for trauma as a transcendent experience where the relationship to space and time is fundamentally altered. Changes from disorder to order are based on the concept of analytical psychology that even at the darkest point of the nigredo, archetypal energies can expand consciousness and bring about self-extension and self-transformation.

Polly Young-Eisendrath: "Projective Identification in a Famous Zen Case: Implications for Relationships With Spiritual Masters"

This chapter hypothesizes that projective identifications enter into scandals between idealized spiritual teachers and their students, in such a way that leads to unconsciously motivated ethical, sexual and financial misconduct, due to unrecognized and disavowed desires in both teachers and students. Opening with definitions, descriptions and examples of projective identifications, I then describe a "therapeutic impasse" as an opportunity for the two parties in the analytic dyad—if the therapy is to be effective—to engage in a special inquiry about their motivations and situation that are creating an obstacle. Such an impasse, if not taken as an opportunity for deepened inquiry, can lead to a premature ending or to other kinds of acting out. Then, I relate the Zen case of Emperor Wu and Bodhidharma, the famous story of their encounter that is often used as a koan, teaching about the nature of Zen. I describe their notorious impasse as a projective identification involving power, specialness and idealizing projections. Finally, I re-imagine their encounter as the beginning of analytic therapy with Dr. Bodhidharma as a therapist and Mr. Wu as the patient and what could have led to a different outcome.

Notes

1 This book is part of a two-volume collection (its twin is titled *Anthology of Contemporary Theoretical Classics in Analytical Psychology: The New Ancestors*).

2 https://dictionary.cambridge.org/dictionary/english/ancestor
3 https://www.collinsdictionary.com/dictionary/english/ancestor
4 Jung, von Franz, Wolf, Neumann, Jacobi, Hillman, Fordham.
5 The neo-Jungians are the third generation of Jungians [the first generation (1961–1985) initially was called the Zürich School and later the Classical School (Samuels, 1985), and the second generation (1985–2011) was called the post-Jungians (Samuels, 1985)].
6 It is also worth mentioning that relational psychoanalysis is linked to the rediscovery of Ferenczi's work and mutual analysis, but it is important to underline that Jung was the first to engage in mutual analysis (with Otto Gross in 1908), much earlier than Ferenczi. I, therefore, claim that Ferenczi built on Jung's legacy without recognizing it openly. The same can be said of Rank and his work on individuation.
7 Not to be confused with Robert Moore's *Neo-Jungian Mapping of the Psyche*: https://robertmoore-phd.com/index.cfm/product/122/a-neo-jungian-mapping-of-the-psyche-understanding-inner-geography--our-challenge-of-individuation.html
8 Letter from Sigmund Freud to Julius Tandler (8.3.1925), retrieved from https://www.psicolinea.it/lanalisi-laica-freud-e-il-caso-theodor-reik/

Bibliography

Aron, L., and Mitchell, S. A. (1999). *Relational Psychoanalysis, Volume 14: The Emergence of a Tradition*. New York and London: Routledge.
Carpani, S. (2020). *Breakfast at Küsnacht*. Asheville, NC: Chiron.
Carpani, S. (2021). *The Plural Turn in Jungian and Post-Jungian Studies: The Work of Andrew Samuels*. London and New York: Routledge.
Freud, S. (1926/1990). *The Question of Lay Analysis*. New York: Norton & Company.
Frosh, S. (2014). The nature of the psychosocial: Debates from studies in the psychosocial. *Journal of Psycho-Social Studies*, 8(1).
Hargaden and Schwartz's (2007), cited in Loewenthal, D., and Samuels, A. (2014). *Relational Psychotherapy, Psychoanalysis and Counselling: Appraisals and Reappraisals*. New York and London: Routledge.
Hillman, J. (2010). *Il Suicidio e l'anima*. Milano: Adelphi.
Loewenthal, D., and Samuels, A. (2014). *Relational Psychotherapy, Psychoanalysis and Counselling: Appraisals and Reappraisals*. New York and London: Routledge.
Orbach, S. (2014). Democratizing psychoanalysis. In D. Loewenthal and A. Samuels (Eds.), *Relational Psychotherapy, Psychoanalysis and Counselling: Appraisals and Reappraisals*. New York and London: Routledge.
Progoff, I. (2013 [1955]). *Jung's Psychology and its Social Meaning*. London: Routledge.
Redman, P., cited in Frosh, S. (2014). The nature of the psychosocial: Debates from studies in the psychosocial. *Journal of Psycho-Social Studies*, 8(1).
Samuels, A. (1985). *Jung and the Post-Jungians*. London: Routledge.
Samuels, A. (1989). *The Plural Psyche*. London: Routledge.
Samuels, A. (2001). *Politics on the Couch*. London: Profile Books.
Samuels, A. (2012). *Jung as a Pioneer of Relational Psychoanalysis*. Unpublished.
Watkins, M. (2003). Dialogue, development, and liberation. In I. Josephs (Ed.), *Dialogicality in Development*. Westport, CT: Greenwood.

Chapter 1

John Beebe

My engagement with the trickster began long before I came to look on it as an artistic relationship. For me, childhood demanded a paradoxical attitude: it seemed the only way I could survive a gorgeous, anima-woman mother who nearly mirrored me to death and a father whose ambitions required the kind of son who would serve as golf caddy to his ego. She, a Georgia Peach, was from Venus and he, a military officer from Eisenhower's Kansas, was from Mars. The only way I could keep from being drawn and quartered by their oppositions was to move in middle childhood to Mercury and keep my own counsel there.

That is where I stayed through my long adolescence, near enough to the brilliance of the Sun to be dauntingly intelligent and kept by that dry enough not to be seriously hurt by my peers' envy and suspicion. But I was forever going backward in my tracks, taking out more books that any 11-year-old could ever read from the Princeton University Library—which I could do since my mother had a typing job on campus after her divorce from my father—only to return most of them unread, a strategy that left me unsupervised to read the books on homosexuality down in the stacks. I stayed precocious, and by the age of 15 had learned to appreciate the syncopated irony of the great jazz singers all working in New York in the year of my birth, 1939: Mildred Bailey, Billie Holiday, Ethel Waters, and Lee Wiley. Later the sexual *doubles entendres* of Henry James in novels like *The Awkward Age*, which I encountered while majoring in English at Harvard, informed my own slow coming out, and by then I was in love with ambiguity. It took Jungian analysis to bring me down from the kind of sense of humor that kept everyone else a little bit afraid of me and that led me to explore the parallel universe of sincerity with an equally frightening intensity.

It was not until midlife that I could put these opposites in my adaptation together and become what Jung would have called fit for life. I'm grateful to this chapter for helping me survive a forty-first year that would otherwise have proved the crack in my own Golden Bowl, and to the great movie auteurs such as Hitchcock and Welles who knew how to mend their own most notorious splits with touches of evil that would make anyone not want to kill them. Being a film buff helped me, while I wrote about suicide in my earliest serious publications as a psychiatrist.

DOI: 10.4324/9781003148968-2

I was watching movies from the late 20s and early 30s and saw Garbo and Craw-
ford, in their late silents and early talkies, avoid the fate of Monroe and Garland
in the 60s. I come from a generation of Americans who too often died before they
turned 30 and am one of the few in my surviving cadre who did not end up on
antidepressants in midlife. The trickster saved me from all that by toughening up
my anima. I hope the essay I'm sharing is as empowering to readers now as it was
to me when it was published at the beginning of my forty-second year, which was
only my second as a Jungian analyst.

The Trickster in the Arts

Originally published in *The San Francisco Jung Institute Library Journal*
in 1981. Reprinted with permission.

What I want to discuss here are the effects of certain works of art. Particularly,
I have in mind works of art like *Hamlet* or the *Mona Lisa* which have a paradoxical, ironic, or ambiguous effect. Such works affect us rather in the manner of certain difficult people, who "get to us" with their unexpectedly unsettling impact.
These works of art perplex or madden us as we try to comprehend what is being
said or shown to us, yet all the while they appear to be pleading innocent of any
such confusing intention. They just go on being themselves.

One response to such a work is to go to some outside source for help in understanding it. Nowadays, it is the fashion to interview the creator of the work.

For instance,

When Gertrude Stein was lecturing at the University of Chicago a young
student in her seminar asked her for the meaning of "rose is a rose is a rose."
This was her reply:

Now listen. Can't you see that when the language was new—as it was
with Chaucer and Homer—the poet could use the name of a thing and the
thing was really there. He could say "O moon," "O sea," "O love," and
the moon and the sea and love were really there. And can't you see that
after hundreds of years had gone by and thousands of poems had been
written, he could call on those words and find that they were just worn out
literary words. The excitingness of pure being had withdrawn from them;
they were just rather stale literary words. Now the poet has to work in the
excitingness of pure being; he has to get back that intensity into the language. We all know that it's hard to write poetry in a late age; and we know
that you have to put some strangeness, as something unexpected, into the
structure of the sentence in order to bring vitality to the noun. Now it's not

enough to be bizarre; the strangeness in the sentence structure has to come from the poetic gift, too. That's why it's doubly hard to be a poet in a late age. Now you all have seen hundreds of poems about roses and you know in your bones that the rose is not there. All those songs that sopranos sing as encores about "I have a garden! Oh, what a garden!" Now I don't want to put too much emphasis on that line, because it's just one line in a longer poem. But I notice that you all know it; you make fun of it, but you know it. Now listen! I'm no fool. I know that in daily life we don't go around saying "... is a ... is a ... is a ..." Yes, I'm no fool; but I think that in that line the rose is red for the first time in English poetry for a hundred years.

(Meyerowitz, 1971, p. 7)

In this case, the young questioner struck gold. So did the person who asked the Belgian artist René Magritte about his well-known surrealist painting, *Ceci n'est pas une pipe*. In this piece, the larger than life-size, flat, commercial image of a curved briar pipe floats above an inscription in French which reads, "This is not a pipe."

Of this work, painted in 1928–9, Magritte told a 1966 interviewer: "The famous pipe. How people reproached me for it! And yet, could you stuff my pipe? No, it's

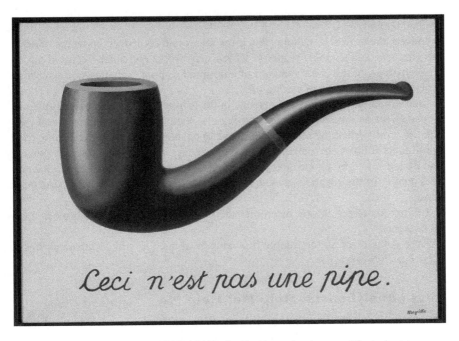

Figure 1.1 René Magritte (1898-1967). *La Trahison des images (Ceci n'est pas une pipe)*. [The Treachery of Images (This is Not a Pipe)]. 1929. Oil on canvas. Digital Image © 2021 Museum Associates / LACMA. Licensed by Art Resource, NY.

just a representation, is it not? So if I had written on my picture, 'This is a pipe,' I'd have been lying!" (Torczyner, 1977, p. 118). (See Foucault, 1973/2008 for the way the work itself makes this very statement.)

When the work of art is generally recognized as a masterpiece, one can also turn for help to a critic. But with the kind of work I have in mind, one is likely to be offered rather too much in the way of help from critics. *Hamlet* is our best example of that. James Kirsch quotes a *Hamlet* editor who remarked in 1907, "the literature on *Hamlet* was larger than the national literature of some of the smaller European nations." Writing in 1966, Dr. Kirsch could already add, "since 1907 the literature has probably doubled" (Kirsch, pp. 3–4). One shudders to think where it is now.

One can find this same sort of voluminous response around Leonardo's *Mona Lisa*, Herman Melville's *The Confidence-Man*, and Henry James's "The Turn of the Screw." Around each of these works a mountain of criticism has grown, even if not on quite the scale of the *Hamlet* mountain. If one digs into such critical mountains, one is likely to find, in addition to useful insights, critics bickering endlessly with each other about details, wrangling over interpretations, and competing with each other via complicated theories. From time to time, theories are offered which pretend to explain the other theories, as if their own deft sweep could finally circumambulate the work in question. Pursuing what has been said about a controversial work of art is like reading a series of interviews by analysts from different psychotherapeutic schools who were all asked to see the same celebrated patient.

Indeed, the critical mountains that grow up around controversial works of art—the immense and troubled response which such works engender—remind me, as a psychiatrist, of the chain reaction of emotional responses that certain psychotic individuals are capable of setting off.

I am thinking particularly of persons in the grip of a full-blown manic episode, whose effect on others resembles nothing else that one sees in the course of psychiatric work. When the diagnosis is going to be mania, a veritable trail of harried individuals follows the patient into the emergency room. They come in person, and by letter, and by phone, and their numbers, as well as the distraught, exasperated quality of their responses, testify to the demonic impact of the possession at hand.

I think this effect closely resembles the impact of a difficult masterpiece upon its audience.

Here is the brief, unforgettable first chapter of such a work, Nathanael West's *Miss Lonelyhearts*:

Miss Lonelyhearts, Help Me, Help Me

The Miss Lonelyhearts of the New York *Post-Dispatch* (Are you in trouble?—Do-you-need-advice?—Write-to-Miss-Lonelyhearts-and-she-will-help-you) sat at his desk and stared at a piece of white cardboard. On it a prayer had been printed by Shrike, the feature editor.

"Soul of Miss L glorify me.
Body of Miss L, nourish me.
Blood of Miss L intoxicate me.
Tears of Miss L wash me.
Oh good Miss L, excuse my plea,
And hide me in your heart,
And defend me from mine enemies.
Help me, Miss L, help me, help me.
In saecula saeculorum. Amen."

Although the deadline was less than a quarter of an hour away, he was still working on his leader. He had gone as far as: "Life *is* worth while, for it is full of dreams and peace, gentleness and ecstasy, and faith that burns like a clear white flame on a grim dark altar." But he found it impossible to continue. The letters were no longer funny. He could not go on finding the same joke funny thirty times a day for months on end. And on most days he received more than thirty letters, all of them alike, stamped from the dough of suffering with a heart-shaped cookie knife.

On his desk were piled those he had received this morning. He started through them again, searching for some clue to a sincere answer.

Dear Miss Lonelyhearts—
I am in such pain I dont know what to do sometimes I think I will kill myself my kidneys hurt so much. My husband thinks no woman can be a good catholic and not have children irregardless of the pain. I was married honorable from our church but I never knew what married life meant as I never was told about man and wife. My grandmother never told me and she was the only mother I had but made a big mistake by not telling me as it dont pay to be innocent and is only a big disappointment. I have 7 children in 12 yrs and ever since the last 2 I have been so sick. I was operated on twice and my husband promised no more children on the doctors advice as he said I might die but when I got back from the hospital he broke his promise and now I am going to have a baby and I don't think I can stand it my kidneys hurts so much. I am so sick and scared because I cant have an abortion on account of being a catholic and my husband so religious. I cry all the time it hurts so much and I dont know what to do.
                                                            Yours respectfully,
                                                            Sick-of-it-all

Miss Lonelyhearts threw the letter into an open drawer and lit a cigarette.

Dear Miss Lonelyhearts—
I am sixteen years old now and I dont know what to do and would appreciate it if you could tell me what to do. When I was a little girl it was not so bad because I got used to the kids on the block making fun of me, but now I would like to have boy friends like other girls and go out on Saturday nites, but no boy will take me

because I was born without a nose—although I am a good dancer and have a nice shape and my father buys me pretty clothes.

I sit and look at myself all day and cry. I have a big hole in the middle of my face that scares people even myself so I cant blame the boys for not wanting to take me out. My mother loves me, but she crys terrible when she looks at me.

What did I do to deserve such a terrible bad fate? Even if I did do some bad things I didnt do any before I was a year old and I was born this way. I asked Papa and he says he doesnt know, but that maybe I did something in the other world before I was born or that maybe I was being punished for his sins. I dont believe that because he is a very nice man. Ought I commit suicide?

Sincerely yours,
Desperate

The cigarette was imperfect and refused to draw. Miss Lonelyhearts took it out of his mouth and stared at it furiously. He fought himself quiet, then lit another one.

Dear Miss Lonelyhearts-

I am writing to you for my little sister Gracie because something awfull happened to her and I am afraid to tell mother about it. I am 15 years old and Gracie is 13 and we live in Brooklyn. Gracie is deaf and dumb and biger than me but not very smart on account of being deaf and dumb. She plays on the roof of our house and dont go to school except to deaf and dumb school twice a week on tuesdays and thursdays. Mother makes her play on the roof because we dont want her to get run over as she aint very smart. Last week a man came on the roof and did something dirty to her. She told me about it and I dont know what to do as I am afraid to tell mother on account of her being liable to beat Gracie up. I am afraid that Gracie is going to have a baby and I listened to her stomack last night for a long time to see if I could hear the baby but I couldn't. If I tell mother she will beat Gracie up awful because I am the only one who loves her and last time when she tore her dress they locked her in the closet for 2 days and if the boys on the block hear about it they will say dirty things like they did on Peewee Conors sister the time she got caught in the lots. So please what would you do if the same happened in your family.

Yours truly,
Harold S.

He stopped reading. Christ was the answer, but, if he did not want to get sick, he had to stay away from the Christ business. Besides, Christ was Shrike's particular joke. "Soul of Miss L, glorify me. Body of Miss L, save me. Blood of . . ." He turned to his typewriter.

Although his cheap clothes had too much style, he still looked like the son of a Baptist minister. A beard would become him, would accent his Old-Testament look. But even without a beard no one could fail to recognize the New England puritan. His forehead was high and narrow. His nose was long and fleshless. His bony chin was shaped and cleft like a hoof. On seeing him for the first time, Shrike had smiled and said, "The Susan Chesters, the Beatrice Fairfaxes and the Miss Lonelyhearts are the priests of twentieth-century America."

A copy boy came up to tell him that Shrike wanted to know if the stuff was ready. He bent over the typewriter and began pounding its keys.

But before he had written a dozen words, Shrike leaned over his shoulder. "The same old stuff," Shrike said. "Why don't you give them something new and hopeful? Tell them about art. Here, I'll dictate:

"Art is a Way Out.

"Do not let life overwhelm you. When the old paths are choked with the debris of failure, look for newer and fresher paths. Art is just such a path. Art is distilled from suffering. As Mr. Polnikoff exclaimed through his fine Russian beard, when, at the age of eighty-six, he gave up his business to learn Chinese, 'We are, as yet, only at the beginning. . .'

"Art Is One of Life's Richest Offerings.

"For those who have not the talent to create, there is appreciation. For those. . .

"Go on from there" (West, 1962, pp. 1–4). [By Nathanael West, from MISS LONELYHEARTS & THE DAY OF THE LOCUST, copyright ©1939 by Estate of Nathanael West. Reprinted by permission of New Directions Publishing Corp.]

I have written elsewhere that "on initial contact the therapist's only clue to the presence of mania may be the 'interpersonal havoc' that the acutely manic patient can create" (Beebe, 1975, p. 99).

An chapter in the psychiatric literature called "Playing the Manic Game" states,

> Possibly, no other psychiatric syndrome is characterized by as many disquieting and irritating qualities as that of the manic phase of manic-depressive psychosis. These characteristics seem specific to the acute attack. . .
>
> The acutely manic patient is often able to alienate himself from family, friends, and therapist alike. This knack is based on the facile use of maneuvers which place individuals relating to the manic in positions of embarrassment, decreased self-esteem, and anxious self-doubt.
>
> (Janowsky et al., 1970, pp. 252–261)

The authors of this chapter found that the manic patient uses five types of activity to induce discomfort in those around him:

1. Manipulation of the self-esteem of others: praising or deflating others as a way of exerting interpersonal leverage.
2. Perceptive exploitation of areas of vulnerability and conflict.
3. Projection of responsibility.
4. Progressive limit testing.
5. Alienating family members.

Now I think it is very sane of the British to call people who have such effects "mad," because one would have to be loaded with anger to be driven to do such things to other people.

We get our word mania from the Greek word that begins *The Iliad, mainis,* meaning wrath or rage. The remarkable thing is the ability the unfortunately *mainis*-possessed manic patient has for putting his wrath into other people, who are induced to act it out for him. Indeed, in that same textbook chapter I said:

> one way to recognize the manic patient is from the size and exasperation of his [concerned social system]. Many people will call the emergency room angry with the patient and with each other, each with a different idea of what must be done. The appearance of a *manipulated* [system of persons] at war with the patient and with each other is strong evidence of mania.
>
> (Beebe, 1975, p. 100, emphasis in original)

Now, to me, this sounds very much like the trickster at work, reducing those around him to a state of bewilderment and helpless outrage (Radin, 1956, pp. 4–7). Indeed, I have found it helpful to think of manic states as instances of possession by the archetypal trickster attitude. What interests me here, however, is the similar impact an ambiguous work of art may have upon its audience.

In using the analogy of a patient in a psychotic state to define the characteristic quality of a famous, but upsetting, work of art, I am trying to get across what Henry James famously called "the madness of art" (1893/1996, p. 354), art's liability to be mad, and to drive others mad who are trying to understand it. A work of art, too, may emanate the spirit of the trickster.

For those who expect art to soothe, illuminate, or please, this quality of art is hard to accept, and it is difficult to see what the artist's motive in producing such a provocative, unsettling work may have been.

In the case of the manic patient, depth psychologists have usually postulated that the patient is unconsciously expressing his rage by acting it out on others. In the family histories of such patients, researchers have found that the individual, as early as childhood, accepted adult responsibility, adopting a conscience-ridden, nose to the grindstone attitude quite prematurely in life, with all too considerate a response to the needs and feelings of others. Of course this can produce as a compensation a very large shadow of pent-up resentment, and it may be that the psychosis functions to allow this shadow its day.

Critics, too, have speculated that the perpetrator of a maddening work of art may have been in a state of rage at the time of its composition. Henry James, for instance, made his first notebook entry recording the germ of his idea for "The Turn of the Screw" just after the failure of years of conscientious efforts to get himself accepted as a dramatist. The opening night London audience was so hostile to James's play, *Guy Domville,* that the vengeful leading actor called the unsuspecting James onto the stage, to be booed and hissed by his public, certainly the worst moment of James's working life (Edel, 1978, p. 84). "The Turn of the

Screw," one of the most confusing, deceptive, and reader-manipulating stories ever written, may well be James's revenge upon that audience. Ironically, it has also turned out to be his most widely appreciated work.

I myself, during my secondary school years, belonged to a creative writing class, where I tried unsuccessfully week after week to get my classmates and teacher to accept an autobiographical story that I was writing. The rule in our class was that one could not go on to revise until the class had certified that the approach to the material was right, and each week my first draft would get struck down, even as other members were well into advanced drafts of their work. I kept ticking off the unconventional details of the faintly Bohemian apartment I shared with my mother, in a tone that reeked of self-pity. I recall one member of the class asking me please to leave the Simmons hide-a-bed that I slept on out of the next draft.

Eventually I fell ill with pneumonia, and as I lay in bed recovering, a great rage came over me regarding my bondage to my material and at the class's frustrating response to it. In this state of rage, I rewrote the story, shifting to a first-person narrative and casting the whole thing in the form of a ridiculously long personal letter to a middle-aged woman who had advertised for a young pen pal in *Modern Art Quarterly*. The narrator consistently bragged about the supposedly creative life he led with his mother.

My classmates split over the new approach. One said, "you're making fun of the whole thing." Another, from an authentically artistic family, recognized the satiric thrust and was amused.

The teacher asked us to identify the *tone* of my story. No one could. Eventually, he supplied us all with a new word: ironic. In my rage, I had stepped outside of my identification with my material and discovered irony: I had learned as well not only how to captivate an audience, but also how to split it into warring camps.

On the personal level, I had broken through to the latent tension in my story, which was really about the problem that a mother-bound youth faces if he has not yet discovered the trickster in himself. I discovered the trickster in anger, which meant that I could make fun of my own character in the story, and this was the beginning of my battle for deliverance from my mother. I got permission to finish the story, and when it was published in our school magazine, a novelist guest-reviewer called my piece a "fictional matricide." I had to hide it from my mother.

I wasn't satisfied with this literary solution to my problem, by the way, for I never turned that story into the ironic short novel it might have been. I got interested in psychiatry instead and went to medical school, eventually working on my rage analytically rather than through the madness of art. So I cannot write as an artist who has resolved the aesthetic dilemmas posed by autobiography in art. But my discovery of irony, and of the trickster approach to art, was an unforgettable experience for me, which has informed my whole later response to works of art. All through college, where I majored in English, I paid attention to the problem of tone in the works of art I studied, and I marveled at the ability of certain works to create paradoxical, even contradictory, emotions in an audience and between members of the same audience.

This much the working out of personal shadow material in a creative effort can accomplish. But I think that in a real masterpiece, the activation goes far deeper than the personal shadow, just as in a true psychosis the archetypal shadow is activated. One's personal shadow is just not skilled to so demonic a degree at upsetting people, nor is it so difficult to integrate as is the shadow that appears during a manic episode or from deep within the structure of an ambiguous masterpiece. A manic episode seems to be a centrifuge of archetypal shadow imagery (which is why it is so notoriously difficult to contain with psychotherapy alone), and so, too, does a great, dark work of art as it spins out its meanings (which explains why no single critical response is ever adequate to it).

In both cases, as I have been hinting, there is an activation of the trickster archetype. The only difference—but it is crucial—is the controlling ethical sense of the great artist who has unleashed the disturbance. This ethical sense does not seem to be present in the manic patient when he is out of control.

Except for the seriousness of purpose that is behind this ethical restraint, it would be acceptable (as many critics actually have done) to dismiss the works I have been talking about as aberrations of the creative spirit, or as harmless and amusing teases, undeserving of serious, sustained attention. But as soon as one looks into the effect of a book like *Miss Lonelyhearts*—the way it produces a confusion of feelings, not only through the manipulation of sympathy and ridicule but even, subtly, through misspelling and inconsistent punctuation, one gets the sensation that Sartre (1938/2013) described as the basic reaction to existence— nausea. One can resent the reaction, but one can't deny that *Miss Lonelyhearts* is a serious book.

In trying to understand the upsetting impact of such a work, I think we ought first to recognize that we are led by it into a region where simple, linear, feeling judgments about the subject matter do not hold, because the consistency of tone and unity of form and content within the work itself have apparently broken down. To be put into this ambiguous position by a work of art is something many people cannot stand, among them many critics.

In the world of film criticism, the sort of movie that may involve the viewer in marginal reflections about its creator's intentions has long been the basis of critical argument. Considerable controversy broke out, when, in the early 1960s, Andrew Sarris attempted to argue that the real purpose of many Hollywood movies was to express their directors' personalities and that this made them succeed in hitherto unsuspected ways as works of art. Sarris's vehicle for making this point was a defense of the French "*auteur* theory" of cinema, which had been advanced by Francois Truffaut to champion the work of certain directors over time against the prevailing production-oriented view that an individual film was either good or bad.

A director's theory, the "*auteur*" view tries to define the ways in which the film director is the "author" of a finished film, the one whose style controls the meaning of the film, whatever its actual content may be in terms of script, cinematography, and star acting. One way to see this is to follow a given director's work over time. Like a series of dreams from the same person, a series of films by the same director reveals an evolving pattern of meaning which is, for the *auteur* critic, the ultimate interest of cinema as art. Thus, Jean Renoir's least interesting film is more significant for Truffaut than an isolated good movie by an undistinguished "*auteur*."

The French critics applied this theory to Hollywood studio pictures filmed by directors they liked, like George Cukor, Vincente Minnelli, Alfred Hitchcock, and Howard Hawks, in whose work they found meaningful inner autobiography where only well-done formula comedies, musicals, mysteries, and Westerns had previously been apparent. It was this line of argument that Andrew Sarris was to develop in his Columbia University course, and later book, on the American cinema, and he provided in the process of doing so one of the clearest formulations of the trickster approach to making art.

As Sarris has observed, film direction is "a very strenuous form of contemplation" (1968, p. 37) by which a film's content is ordered, so that the way a director chooses to present the separate elements of a film, through his cutting, silent sequences, camera movements, degree of distance from the action, choreography of actors, framing of shots, and so on, becomes a sort of ongoing active imagination in which the real subject proves to be the development of the director's cinematic perspective.

For this reason, says the *auteur* theory, some of the greatest film directors have chosen to work within the Hollywood studio system, taking advantage of the motivational loopholes that formula stories like mysteries and Westerns provide, and using each loophole as an opportunity to fill in with material from their own inner lives. One may well ask, as did Pauline Kael, one of the leading critics of the *auteur* approach, whether this was not a cynical choice for these men, a compromise which made it possible for them to work in film at all, given the economics of their trade. Nevertheless, the theory champions the choice of popular material by a director for his creative medium because the handling of popular material provides so many avenues for the director's originality. The validity of such personal tampering with the intentions of a film script or production has been part of what has sparked the controversy which pursues the *auteur* theory: are such tamperings, even if interesting or fun, really art?

At the very least, the idea that the power of the film is wrought largely from the intrusion of the director's personal drama enables one better to appreciate directors like Vincente Minnelli, who has told the story of his own anima struggle with success through his musical and other dream sequences; Howard Hawks, who used actors like Bogart and Bacall to kid his own hero myth; and Alfred Hitchcock, who brought to detective and spy stories his satanic sense of the mysterious vicissitudes of the man-woman relationship. And it is evident that the ability of these men to insert emotional autobiography into formula material through tricks of tone or imagery inspired more somberly classical European artists like Bergman, Antonioni, and Fellini, working from art scripts, to begin to use their films as vehicles for frank imaginal autobiography.

Sarris sensed that this kind of creativity requires something other than the ability straightforwardly to render subject matter. As he put it, "the ultimate premise of the auteur theory is concerned with interior meaning, the ultimate glory of the cinema as an art. Interior meaning is extrapolated from the tension between a director's personality and his material" (Sarris, 1970, p. 133). Sarris seems not to have realized that he was providing the rationale for a perverse approach to cinema making, but other critics were quick to sense the implications and to take offense. Annoyed at the subjectivity of the *auteur* approach and its legitimation of forceful interventions of the director into the work, Pauline Kael replied:

> This is a remarkable formulation: it is the opposite of what we have always taken for granted in the arts, that the artist expresses himself in the unity of form and content. What Sarris believes to be "the ultimate glory of the cinema as an art" is what has generally been considered the frustrations of a man working against the given material.
>
> (1963, p. 302)

Clearly, Sarris and Kael were split over the degree to which an artist can work "against" his own material—that is, function as a trickster—and still turn out coherent work. Pauline Kael later went on to develop her own approach to witty popular movies (1971b) and apply it to at least one great film (1971a), and to champion outright trickster directors like Robert Altman and Brian de Palma, but at the time she wrote her famous reply to Sarris, she seemed incapable of appreciating the trickster approach to art as anything but a joke or a cynical compromise. Not content with repudiating the *auteur* theory, she seems to have insisted that all art must be made straightforwardly. This point of view, which has occurred repeatedly in the history of criticism ("The mind can only repose on the stability of truth," declared Samuel Johnson in his "Preface to Shakespeare," (1765/2004)), denies the trickster artist his right of way. The denial of the instability on which the trickster artist must make his stand may even lead to absurd failures of comprehension, like the one which inspired Nahum Tate to tack onto *King Lear* a happy ending, which was used in productions for two hundred years, or Kael herself to assume that the outbreak of nuclear conflict around the couple in Bergman's *Shame* made that picture an anti-war film rather than a portrait of an exploding marriage.

It was not only whimsy that made Hitchcock show up in a walk-on in each of the movies of his mature years, or Bergman put his own picture on the cover of the sentimental novel that the mother reads in *Autumn Sonata*. The trickster artist intrudes himself deliberately and outrageously into the work, in order to change its meaning. Any *auteur*, of course, wants his creative personality to make its appearance in the work, since the individuation of that personality is the real story he is interested in telling. The jokey self-insertions chosen by the most tricksterish of *auteurs* have, however, the effect of opening up for the most casual viewer that region between the lines of the script which is the trickster artist's favored lurking place. The tension between the director's personality and his material is exploited through humor. Archetypalists speak of a love for inhabiting spaces between psychosocial regions established by convention as "liminality," and liminality is a hallmark of the trickster. For example, Alfred Hitchcock overstepped the bounds of theatrical convention in *Psycho* when he got his star, Janet Leigh, killed off so early in the film. Liminality is considered to be a primary attribute of the Greek god Hermes, whose winged feet get him nimbly around the conventional regions supervised by the other gods, among whom he moves as messenger. And liminality is an attribute of Aphrodite, too, whose trickster aspect is actualized by the winged Eros, or Cupid, who tricks us with his darts into falling in love.

My Jungian colleague Murray Stein tells us in a precise definition, that liminality is "the idea, borrowed from von Gennep and elaborated by Victor Turner, of a cultural social psychological interstitial space between fixed identities and 'locations' which predominates during transitional periods in the life-cycle" (Stein, 1980, p. 21). Liminality also predominates during transitional periods in the history of art as when Hollywood genre pictures were developing into art forms. And liminality figures too in the history of an individual artist's work, as when the artist himself is undergoing a personal or aesthetic crisis. Of course, there are artists like Alfred Hitchcock, who are always tricksters, and therefore one finds liminality throughout their work.

In contrast to the outcast—the marginal, alienated man who has been extruded from conventional psychosocial regions and is unhappy about it—the trickster takes pleasure in his liminality. Nowhere is this better shown than in this passage from *Huckleberry Finn*, where Huck objects to the boundaried approach to mealtimes at the widow's house:

> The widow rung a bell for supper, and you had to come on time. When you got to the table you couldn't go right to eating, but you had to wait for the widow to tuck down her head and grumble a little over the victuals, though there warn't really anything the matter with them—that is, nothing only everything was cooked by itself. In a barrel of odds and ends it is different; things get mixed up and the juice kind of swaps around, and the things go better.
>
> (Twain, 1965, pp. 3–4; Warwick Wadlington points this passage out in his discussion of liminality in *The Confidence Game in American Literature* (1975, p. 20.))

It is just its liminality which makes Magritte's *This Is Not a Pipe* so outrageous. At first we find ourselves agreeing, "of course it's not a pipe, it's a *picture* of a pipe," and this admission locks us into the field of the picture. We are drawn into a dialogue with the artist about art, in which further reflections follow. If we like the interior life of painted things in art, we are likely to reflect, "of course it isn't a pipe, it isn't well enough painted to be anything," yet if we approach the work naturalistically, we have to concede, "of course it could be a pipe; it looks just like a pipe; it could serve as a sign over a tobacconist's shop and induce someone to long for a smoke." Whichever way we think, we are drawn into talking from that liminal space between art and life, and the conjunction we usually experience between them when we suspend disbelief and simply enjoy the work of art is broken down. Because we have been forced into that conceptual no-land that exists between things and their representations, everything we say back to the painting only reinforces our liminal entrapment. This makes the work itself a formidable trickster.

I have been engaging in some liminality of my own by discussing the trickster without giving a Jungian definition of him. Yet once one gets beyond the obvious definition, "one who tricks," the trickster becomes an elusive concept. Jung thought of the trickster as a personification of the archetypal shadow (Jung in Radin, 1956, pp. 195–211). As such, the trickster came up between Jane Wheelwright and her dying patient, Sally, in the therapy Wheelwright describes in her book, *Death of a Woman* (1981, pp. 223–224, 252). The trickster is important in the story because he emerges just as Sally begins to reach the limit-line between this existence and the unknowable Beyond; the author therefore provides a definition in the glossary:

> TRICKSTER Image of the archetype of mischievousness, unexpectedness, disorder, amorality, the trickster is an archetypal shadow figure that represents a primordial, dawning consciousness. Compensating rigid or overly righteous collective attitudes, it functions collectively as a cathartic safety-valve for pent-up social pressures, a reminder of humankind's primitive origins and the fallibility of its institutions. Frequently uniting the opposites itself, the trickster can have transformative powers as a transcendent symbol. Constellation of the archetype in an individual bogged down in the sterility of an excessively entrenched, well-ordered, or one-sided consciousness can provide access to creative possibilities in the collective unconscious, helping to restore psychic balance. Thwarting of conscious intentions, inner upheavals, outer mishaps, disrupted plans, are likely indicators that the trickster has been constellated.
>
> (Wheelwright, p. 286)

The concept of "constellation" deserves some explanation, since it is important to understand better why an archetype like the trickster comes up at all. When an archetype is "constellated," it shows up like the Big Dipper in the night sky, making its pattern apparent within the universe of the entity in which it appears. The archetypal constellation is even more like the star in the east which led the wise men to that place where an important new being lay. I accept Jung's idea that the archetype is constellated when it is needed, and not otherwise, and so it was in Jane Wheelwright's patient's life. The trickster showed up at the point of the patient's departure from life.

We see the trickster in another needed instance in the stage of infancy mothers know as the "terrible twos," when the developing toddler needs to test out the limits of its mother's authority. It is also importantly present in normal preadolescence, when the limits of socialization as learned in the family and at school are tested. Indeed, before the trickster concept had been formulated by Paul Radin, Jung used to speak of a side of himself he called the "enfant terrible," the terrible child.

Obviously, the trickster is important in adolescence; it's difficult to imagine anyone's becoming sexual without some experience of the trickster. And, he comes again during the midlife crisis, which, as so many recent movies have been showing us, is a time when the authority of spouse and career over one's life is apt to be challenged.

At each of these times, as often again before death, the trickster appears to give that extra bit of energy for stepping outside of one's frame and seeing one's life from a radically new perspective. He also provides that amount of treachery necessary to be disloyal to an old pattern and find one's way into a new one. It is clear that the trickster is a great strain on others who live around the developing individual at these times, and, worse, it is possible for a person to get stuck in a manifestation of the trickster and miss the purpose of the particular developmental stage. Such failures of integration of the trickster at these various stages play a large role in the development of borderline and sociopathic conditions, as well as in the psychological tangles that surface later in life. (I think this getting stuck in the trickster may be what occurs in manic-depressive psychosis. Lithium then seems to be required to get the trickster to release his stranglehold on the personality so that ongoing development may proceed without quite so much archetypal help.)

But even the strain produced by the trickster has its point, for each time the trickster appears, something about the individual and his social setting is revealed that wasn't apparent before. During adolescent turmoil, it is usual for both the parent and the child to learn something, so that Mark Twain's famous joke about his being impressed, after his own adolescence, with how much his father had learned, is as a comment double-edged, because it is very probably true. One may say that when the trickster appears, a bit of fate unfolds, so that no one involved is quite the same.

The trickster may also appear when one is forced to contend with an evil from outside of one's own nature. It is especially liable to be constellated when someone is in a state of disappointment that attends upon a loss, a failure, or a betrayal. *Hamlet* is thought to have been written after Shakespeare's only son, Hamnet, had died at the age of eleven. Melville experienced the commercial and critical failure, in turn, of his novels, *Moby Dick*, *Pierre*, and *Israel Potter* before he took up his pen to write *The Confidence-Man*, and this trickster work was to be the last piece of fiction he wrote for nearly thirty years. It may be that the turn to the trickster in art, like the turn to mania in life, is an alternative to feeling guilt over the rage that appears at such times of disappointment. The artist, like the patient, is provided a sulfuric alternative to leaden depression. For the artist, this alternative may be especially important if it keeps his creative fire from going out. But we cannot be sure that the trickster is merely a savior, for it is like the trickster to set up a personal or a creative disappointment in order to emerge. In Melville's phrase, the trickster is "knave, fool, and genius."

When a work of art involves the trickster archetype, I think it is likely both to have a trickster subject in it and to be a trickster itself in the way the total work makes its audience react. In Magritte's painting, the famous pipe is the trickster subject, but it is the total painting that provides the trickster effect. In *Hamlet*, the Prince becomes a trickster, but the play is the ultimate trickster. And so on with the sadistic feature editor, Shrike, and *Miss Lonelyhearts*; with the haunted governess and "The Turn of the Screw"; and with the enigmatically smiling subject and her painting, the *Mona Lisa*. In each case, the work is the concealed trickster, which tricks us into responding to the subject as well. I am concentrating in this discussion on the living trickster quality of the work itself, on all the ways in which the work works upon us, contriving to fascinate and upset us. Not least of these ways is the haunting anxiety that such a work can generate.

Jung points out that when we cannot evaluate an unconscious content with clarity, it tends to exert a fascinating quality. Often trickster individuals that we meet in life exert a similar fascination, because we can't decide how we feel about them. They behave exactly like unconscious contents of our own, and in a sense they are, because we are not conscious enough to know how to deal with them. The trickster work of art exerts a similar fascination.

Often its trick is to get us into a double bind, by making us think or feel two different things at once, all the while exerting a hypnotic fascination that makes us want to stay within this ambiguous field. This is the uncanny fascination of Billie Holiday's singing and of Greta Garbo's acting. These great trickster performers had the ability to project two contradictory emotions at the same time behind a mesmerizing facade. The effect of their art was both divine and satanic.

The double bind stems directly from the duplex aspect of the archetype itself. Jung stressed this duplicity in his discussions of Hermes's Roman descendant, "the wily Mercurius," who became the alchemical trickster. It is an unsettling ambivalence, a splitting into two minds, that the trickster work is able to accomplish. William Willeford said of the tricksterish Renaissance stage favorite, the Fool, that as we contemplate this figure "on the border" he introduces us to "the autonomy of the unknown," and "the center of our awareness may divide" (1969, p. 132). Containing opposite feelings is what makes being a trickster so difficult. Often the trickster artist is responding to some cultural double bind placed on him or her. That is why Gertrude Stein said, "it is *doubly* hard to be a poet in a late age."

The trickster kind of artist is inordinately concerned with the response of others to him, so that artists like Hitchcock, Garbo, and Billie Holiday often have enormously complicated relations to their publics, which involve elaborate strategies for winning and retaining the confidence of others in the face of numerous violations and betrayals of public expectations. Their publicity becomes part of their art. This phenomenon goes with the archetype. The trickster seems to love most to win the confidence of those who would have every reason not to trust him.

This is certainly the activity in which *Wakdjunkaga*, the tricky one, is engaged, when we first meet him in Paul Radin's book about him, *The Trickster*. Radin's account of this North American myth, found in the culture of the Winnebago Indians, first delineated fully the trickster archetype.

In the first scene of the narrative, we meet the tricky one, or trickster, as a chief preparing to go on the warpath, something that Winnebago tribal chiefs are traditionally forbidden to do. Nevertheless, the men of the tribe join his feast and partake of it, even though it is incorrectly prepared, and they wait for him to lead them into battle. Instead, the trickster disappears, and they find him cohabiting with a woman, a behavior also strictly taboo for any Winnebago about to go on the warpath. The men disperse.

And yet, the trickster gets them to come back a second and a third time to participate in the same charade. On a fourth summons, they decide he's merely talking about fighting, and the men come only for the pleasure of the feast. But this time the trickster actually does set out on the warpath, oddly enough giving his men encouragement that he will at least do as he seems to intend. Instead, he destroys his war bundle, another sacrilege, leaving them to conclude that he is in fact a wicked person (Radin, 1956, pp. 4–7).

As one can see, the trickster manipulates the other men to the point that even their lack of confidence in him is betrayed. Although it is entirely against tribal custom, they finally want him to go on the warpath without further stalling; and they resent it when he fails to do so by tearing up his war bundle. Even though tradition gives him no right at all to go to war, the ironic effect of his multiple sacrileges is to make the men feel that he ought to have done so. They have been tricked into taking up attitudes in opposition to their own traditions.

Exactly the same manipulation of confidence and of attitudes is practiced by a trickster artist upon his audience. Homer gives us an excellent image of this sort of manipulation when, at the beginning of the second book of his *Iliad*, he has his central divinity, Zeus, "father of gods and men," send a false dream to Agamemnon, urging in a spirit of wise counsel that the time is propitious for an attack upon the Trojans. To rouse his men to battle, Agamemnon in turn uses a ruse, telling them that they may go home instead, in the expectation that they will protest and want to fight. Agamemnon is doubly deceived: the Greeks are so sick of the war that they don't stage the protest he expected. Instead, they race madly to their ships, to head for home. It takes the cunning of Odysseus, stimulated by emissaries from the worried Zeus, to get the men to turn back to the trap that Zeus has laid for them.

Despite the usual emphasis in archetypal writings on Hermes as the pre-eminent trickster god among the Greeks, Zeus is very much a trickster here, and not the more or less good Victorian father we sometimes assume him to be. To have a trickster divinity at the very center of Homer's *Iliad* is important inasmuch as the *Iliad* is the fountainhead of Western art and poetry, and is to the later development of Western art like an initial dream to the development of an analysis. One can on one level see the *Iliad* as an early statement within the poetic tradition of the West about the archetypal energies that will inform its creative expressions. Thus the Zeus who sends the false dream personifies the trickster aspect of Western poetic rhetoric itself, which so often works through manipulation of an image in the reader's or hearer's mind. Such divine tricksterism, it would follow, is at the very heart of Western poetry.

The extent of the trickster aspect of our greatest poetry was exposed by William Empson's *Seven Types of Ambiguity* (1953), a classic of modern literary criticism, which abundantly demonstrates the tricks our great poets have employed to exploit the loopholes in language. The trickster gift of ambiguity, Empson argues, is intrinsic to serious poetry. And, since the protean *Iliad* is really poetry, drama, and fiction, we can expect to find the trickster prominently featured also in the later poetics of drama and fiction in the West.

It was Henry James who first worked out a systematic criticism of the novelist's relationship to his reader, through his careful studies of the way other novelists had handled the problem of narration. These studies preceded James's own great experiments with narration in the later 1890s which include "The Turn of the Screw" and which prefigure the trickster effects that abound in the modern novel. As a result of studying Anthony Trollope's narrative style, James had this to say about the linear approach of the great English realist:

> There was nothing in his theory of the storyteller's art that tended to convert the reader's or the writer's mind into a vessel for polluted things. He recognized the right of the vessel to protest, and would have regarded such a protest as conclusive. With a considerable turn for satire . . . he had as little as possible of the quality of irony. He never played with a subject, never juggled with the sympathies or the credulity of his reader, was never in the least paradoxical or mystifying. He sat down to his theme in a serious, businesslike way, with his elbows on the table and his eye occasionally wandering to the clock.
>
> (James, 1970, p. 103)

In other words, unlike Homer's Zeus, who was willing to send a false dream to get an effect, Trollope the realist did not implant misleading impressions for dramatic or ironic purposes. He was not a trickster, and I think James missed this quality in him, which James was later to cultivate in himself. In contrast, James speaks in another place with charmed fascination about the novelistic technique of a writer like Robert Louis Stevenson, a "romancer." Says James:

> The balloon of experience is in fact of course tied to the earth, and under that necessity we swing, thanks to a rope of remarkable length, in the more or less commodious car of the imagination; but it is by the rope we know where we are, and from the moment that cable is cut we are at large and unrelated: we only swing apart from the globe—though remaining as exhilarated, naturally as we like, especially when all goes well. The art of the romancer is "for the fun of it," insidiously to cut the cable, to cut it without our detecting him.
>
> (James, 1934, p. 34)

The romancer, therefore, is a trickster. James's remarks come from his preface to his novel, *The American*, in which the title character, Christopher Newman, deftly manages to escape a series of traps laid for him by Europeans.

It is appropriate that the trickster was named from a myth found on American soil, for despite the worldwide distribution of the trickster mythologem within figures as disparate as Loki and Krishna, it is in America that the trickster has become a more or less conscious part of the national character (Wadlington, 1975, pp. 9–23). This is clear not only in the tradition of Southwestern humor from which Mark Twain emerged (Lynn, 1959), but also in the Northeastern figure of the clever Yankee Peddler, Sam Slick, who was admired for his shrewd deceptions whenever they managed to make him a buck. In my own lifetime, trickster elements in Southwest and Northeast United States cultures came together in the durable irony Bob Dylan forged by channeling Woody Guthrie and Johnny Cash.

Although the methods of the trickster artist can certainly be found in Leonardo and Shakespeare, American artists have most consistently explored the possibilities of the trickster approach to art. We see this in our classic movies and jazz, as well as in our new wave of rock, but the trend is equally present within our classic and contemporary fiction. Our novelists fairly love to manipulate the reader through ambiguous and contradictory language, misleading narration, and other forms of deliberate mystification.

In his 1975 book, *The Confidence Game in American Literature*, Warwick Wadlington traces some of these experiments with tricksterish rhetoric back to our classic authors, who first engaged in storytelling which deliberately manipulates the confidence of the reader. Wadlington is the first critic systematically to explore the relationship of the trickster archetype to such insistent American rhetorical devices as (1) using frankly misleading narration; (2) emphasizing startling shifts of tone; and (3) casting the story in the form of a narrative shared by the author with someone else who is said to have heard or told or written it—a device creating an ironic "frame" qualifying the story's point of view. Wadlington explores the predominance of such effects in the work of Herman Melville, Mark Twain, and Nathanael West. A host of other critics have demonstrated the same effects in the work of Henry James.

In Herman Melville's *The Confidence-Man*, for example, tricky rhetoric is actually the basis for a whole series of confidence swindles enacted by a man who appears before the reader only in a succession of disguises, so that we never know what he really looks like. Nowhere do we have a stable point of reference from which to evaluate the many stories he tells in the course of getting some Mississippi riverboat passengers to swindle themselves, which he does by cleverly manipulating their instinctive mistrust of him. At one point, one of the swindler's own stories—about the circumstances of his supposed bereavement—is even about to be retold to him by a merchant he has already successfully swindled with it. To complicate the narrative further, Melville inserts himself at just this point to do the retelling for the swindled man, implying that as a writer he can probably narrate better. Thus the reader gets the story as a narrative within a narrative within a narrative, a device that Henry James was to employ later in "The Turn of the Screw." Such "framed" narrative is characteristic of trickster fiction. The framing of the story in this manner has the liminal effect of putting all points of view in the story under suspicion even as it enhances the reader's interest in the tale. When Melville finally tells the story, which is about the wife that the swindler is supposedly mourning, he employs an exceedingly peculiar rhetoric.

> Goneril was young, in person lithe and straight, too straight, indeed, for a woman, a complexion naturally rosy, and which would have been charmingly so, but for a certain hardness and bakedness, like that of the glazed colors on stone-ware. Her hair was of a deep, rich chestnut, but worn in close, short curls all round her head. Her Indian figure was not without its impairing effect upon her bust, while her mouth would have been pretty but for a trace of mustache. Upon the whole, aided by the resources of her toilet, her appearance at a distance was such, that some might have thought her, if anything, rather beautiful, though of a style of beauty rather peculiar and cactus-like.
>
> (Melville, 1964, p. 66)

As a perceptive critic, R. W. B. Lewis, has noted:

> The whole tone, purpose and strategy of *The Confidence-Man* are in those sentences, with their parade of notations and counter-notations, and the final flurry of phrases that modify, hesitantly contradict, and then utterly cancel one another out, leaving not a rack of positive statement behind. Goneril is in fact repellent: flat-chested, with a baked face and matted hair, heavily made-up, mustached and prickly-looking; *or is she?* As her physical actuality is blurred and dissolved by Melville's prose, we belatedly remember that Goneril probably does not even exist, but is simply an invention of the Confidence-Man himself in his guise as "the man with the weed."
>
> (Lewis, 1964, p. 265)

Elsewhere, Lewis calls this sort of rhetoric "self-erasing prose" (1964, p. 272). Elizabeth Renker says:

> In my estimate, *The Confidence-Man* is Melville's fully controlled novel, the one in which he is most in command of his craft. But the early reviews were right in an important sense: the book *is* unreadable. By "unreadable" I mean that it's aggressively resistant, not only to interpretation but also to even superficial comprehension.

In support of this view, she mentions "characters who are unnamed or whose names change without warning, long exchanges of dialogue between unidentified speakers, an almost plotless plot, and a narrator who fails to clear any of this up" (Renker, 1998, pp. 114–115).

Recalling Jung's classical philologist friend Karl Kerenyi's observation that where mythic materials are involved, "the narrator's words are themselves determined by the figure he wishes to evoke," (Kerenyi, cited in Radin, 1956, p. 173), I consider such "self-erasing" prose to be a hallmark of the trickster. An image that expresses this is found in the tale of the Winnebago trickster, when the trickster's left arm becomes impatient with the right arm, which is skinning a buffalo:

> suddenly his left arm grabbed the buffalo. "Give that back to me, it is mine! Stop that or I will use my knife on you!" So spoke the right arm. "I will cut you to pieces, that is what I will do to you," continued the right arm. Thereupon the left arm again grabbed hold of the right arm. This time it grabbed hold of his wrist just at the moment that the right arm had commenced to skin the buffalo. Again and again this was repeated. In this manner did Trickster make both his arms quarrel. That quarrel soon turned into a vicious fight and the left arm was badly cut up. "Oh, oh! Why did I do this? Why have I done this? I have made myself suffer!" The left arm was indeed bleeding profusely.
> (Radin, 1956, p. 8)

I am suggesting that when Trickster writes a novel, as when he skins a buffalo, it appears to the reader as if even within a single sentence his right and left arms are quarreling; the latent meaning of the piece seems to bleed upon the page a mess of feeling-confusion which upsets the reader. The motivation for adopting such a style is difficult to fathom. As Wadlington tells us, *The Confidence-Man* seems to be "stuffed with words"; Melville's prose bears an uncomfortable resemblance to the pressured speech, flight of ideas, irritability, and ambivalence displayed in the first stage of mania in a manic-depressive psychosis. This cloudy wordiness is another hallmark of the trickster.

We find an ability to originate effects within the reader or viewer's mind over and over again in trickster works. As one peruses "The Turn of the Screw," the governess's terrified quest for reliable information becomes the reader's. The longer one stares at the *Mona Lisa*, the more one takes on the state of ambivalent, tender amusement that seems to emanate from the subject. Such works deliver their impact by reworking the audience's mind in the image of their central characters. This is their tricksterish "originality," their capacity for originating tricksterish effects.

The "original" effect of *Hamlet* was recognized by the young T. S. Eliot, who in a celebrated essay remarked:

> Few critics have even admitted that *Hamlet* the play is the primary problem, and Hamlet the character only secondary . . . In several ways the play is puzzling, and disquieting as is none of the others. Of all the plays it is the longest and is possibly the one on which Shakespeare spent most pains; and yet he has left in it superfluous and inconsistent scenes which even hasty revision should have noticed. The versification is variable . . . Both workmanship and

thought are in an unstable position. We are surely justified in attributing the play, with that other profoundly interesting play of "intractable" material and astonishing versification, *Measure for Measure*, to a period of crisis, after which follow the tragic successes which culminate in *Coriolanus*. *Coriolanus* may not be as "interesting" as *Hamlet*, but it is, with *Antony and Cleopatra*, Shakespeare's most assured artistic success.

(Sacks and Whan (Eds.), 1960, p. 53)

Shakespeare's problem, according to Eliot, stemmed from the fact that he wanted to deal in *Hamlet* with the effect of a mother's guilt upon a son, and that the revenge drama he was reworking, Thomas Kyd's *The Spanish Tragedy*, simply was too "intractable" to accept this motive and be re-formed successfully. Thus "Shakespeare tackled a problem which proved too much for him," and to explain why he attempted it at all, "we should have to understand things which Shakespeare did not understand himself" (Eliot, 1960, pp. 55–6).

Following Eliot's lead, such psychoanalysts as Ernest Jones and Kurt Eissler have sought these "things which Shakespeare did not understand" in the Oedipal conflicts of the bard himself (see Eissler, 1971). I think it is a shame that in his youth Eliot had come such a long way from St. Louis, for if he had stayed closer to the boarding port of Melville's Confidence-Man, which is also near the birthplace of Mark Twain, he might have absorbed more of our own American confidence game and understood that it is the same game being played by Shakespeare's celebrated trickster drama.

I do think *Hamlet* is about a mother problem, for as an analyst I could not else explain the magnitude of the dilemma that is posed for Hamlet by the ghost of his father, who appears to demand revenge for his murder so that he may go to his grave in peace. I would describe this apparition psychologically as a constellation of the father archetype in the psychological field of a young man with a big, positive mother complex who has up to now managed to evade the father principle. The ghost of the father who bears his own name is therefore, as James Kirsch has pointed out, a Self figure for the younger Hamlet, who demands that the father archetype now be honored. For Hamlet, this means a break with the mother world, the sort of disloyal act or creative disobedience which usually requires some tricksterism to bring off.

The remarkable effect of this drama is to cause the audience to experience along with Hamlet a progressive integration of the trickster. As the play unfolds, the audience begins to experience the moral topsyturvydom, or challenge to accepted values, that the integration of archetypal shadow material always entails. With the development of the drama, we become mired in ambivalence and uncertainty, and any material dependence we may have on this work of art for consistency and reliability breaks down. I really think it is because the play does not behave like a good mother that the younger Eliot found it so distressing. It was that Eliot who turned for satisfaction to the Roman tragedies, where a strong maternal influence reigns. In his later years, an Eliot who had integrated the negative aspect of the mother archetype came to repudiate the *Hamlet* essay of his youth that we have been considering here.

Here are some of the many questions that have been raised by this confusing play:

1. Is Hamlet mad?
2. Is Hamlet callous?
3. Is Hamlet melancholic?
4. Is Hamlet an ideal hero. . .?
5. Does Hamlet vacillate [for good reason]?
6. Is Hamlet . . . a victim of excessive intellect?
7. Does Hamlet overhear Polonius and Claudius plotting in [Act] 2?
8. Is Hamlet's emotion in excess of the facts of the play?
9. Is Hamlet in love with Ophelia?
10. Is Gertrude . . . privy to the murder of . . . King Hamlet?
11. Is *Hamlet* a myth ritual celebration of the mystery of human life [rather than] a revenge tragedy?
12. What is an adequate explanation of *Hamlet*?

(Taken from Weitz, 1964, pp. 207–212)

That the play releases such a waterfall of aggrieved inquiry demonstrates how skillfully it disturbs anyone who engages with it. The play manages to induce in its audience the same ambivalent self-questioning that his soliloquies suggest is continually occurring within the skull of the Prince of Denmark. A contemporary familiar with Renaissance alchemy (and there were many in Shakespeare's England) would have recognized the "affective power of a state of irresolution or undecidability"(Chave, 1989, p. 181, quoted in Marlon, 2005, p. 87) as the mark of the *nigredo*, the ground of which, antimony, is "black, blacker than black" (Jung, 1968, p. 327).

To this darkness, Hamlet's certainty about his own moral position is lost as soon as he begins to adopt the trickster style of the court around him, yet this is the shadow he must incorporate if he is going to be able to get past the "good boy" stage of loyalty to an unworthy mother. He has to give up any semblance of filial piety toward her. This means for Hamlet a breakdown of the entire archetypal structure that has organized his existence. The confusion which Shakespeare forces us to experience alongside Hamlet belongs to a time "that is out of joint," an existence that has lost its moorings. We are once again in the liminal region of the trickster, who in this case provides the energy for the transition from the world of the mother to the world of the father.

As Hamlet begins to integrate this trickster, with its awesome potential for destructiveness, he sexually insults his girlfriend and his mother, kills his girlfriend's father, stages a trickster drama of his own to test his stepfather's conscience, and gets himself exiled from the kingdom. The audience watching all this finds itself torn between shock at the limits that Hamlet is transgressing and desire to see him go even further, to obey his father's ghost and kill the usurper, Claudius, whose own tricksterism had put the prince in a double bind. Worse, we experience an intensity of voyeuristic participation in it all which makes us co-conspirators with the unstable prince. This sort of voyeuristic participation is another feature of the trickster effect, similar to the plight of the Winnebago tribesmen who attended the fourth phony call to battle just to enjoy a feast and to see what the trickster was going to do next, and were thus themselves led to participate in the trickster's sacrilege of the tribal customs. In our own time, Alfred Hitchcock's great trickster movie *Psycho* has successfully turned millions of viewers into peeping toms, looking on with fascination as the last guilty drop of Janet Leigh's blood is washed down the motel shower drain. We take on the point of view of the shower-murderer himself as we look. It is this sort of participation in evil that occurs within the first three acts of *Hamlet*, as we are drawn into fascinated alliance with the mischief-making of the prince.

Just as the play within a play in *Hamlet* is "the mousetrap" which Hamlet constructs to "catch the conscience of the King," so *Hamlet* is the mousetrap Shakespeare has constructed to catch us (Aldus, 1977). We are put in the position of the girl in the Beatles' song, "Penny Lane," who, "though she feels as if she's in a play, she is anyway." As we are tricked into a genuine experience of the moral uncertainty that is at the heart of this ambiguous drama, its genius causes us to be deeply touched by the problem of evil, not just to watch it from outside. Seeing the play is thus an exercise for us in the integration of the trickster, as we are led into a far more complex attitude than was possible for us at the outset of the drama. Our sensibilities are shaped by the experience of the archetype, so that by the end of the gravedigger's scene, in which Hamlet and Laertes shockingly duel upon the dead Ophelia's grave, something sentimental in us has died, and we are ready for the nihilistic treachery of their confrontation in the play's last scene. By then, we have accepted the trickster element as the only way to dissolve this corrupt mother world. We are not utterly surprised when Hamlet dies because the fencing foil used against him has been poisoned. He succumbs; we in the audience, having for once been undeceived as to what happens in *Hamlet*, survive. Each time I have sat through a production of the play, I have experienced a sense of having survived and of having been returned to myself at the point that Fortinbras appears on stage to order Hamlet's funeral and to reorder the realm.

I do think the young T. S. Eliot's intuition was correct, when he said that the writing of *Hamlet* reflected a personal crisis for Shakespeare. At midlife, the task for the male is to integrate the trickster into his anima structure. By anima, I mean his working spontaneous sense of life: not just the sexual urgency or immediate feeling of well-being that signal falling in love, but also his gut emotional responses to any situation. This anima response may run from the sentimental and gullible to the cynical and "worldly." It is critical for the health of a man's instinctive, unreflected judgments that his anima structure include a healthy grasp of the shadow. The chastened quality which results is seen in certain of the speeches made by male characters who appear in the dramas Shakespeare wrote in the years following *Hamlet*. I'm particularly interested in statements by two of those figures, Kent in *Lear* and Prospero in *The Tempest*, because I feel they are Shake-speare's personal representatives, characters that Shakespeare the actor may even have played himself. When Lear asks Kent how old he is, Kent replies:

> Not so young, sir, to love a woman for singing, nor so old to dote on her for anything. I have years on my back forty-eight.
> (*King Lear*, Act I, Scene 4, lines 37–39 in Shakespeare, 1998, p. 638.)

And after Miranda, in *The Tempest*, exclaims:

> 0, wonder!
> How many goodly creatures are there here!
> How beauteous mankind is! O brave new world,
> That has such people in't!

Prospero says to her:

> 'Tis new to thee.
> (*The Tempest*, Act V, Scene 1, lines 181–184 in Shakespeare, 1998, p. 1091)

There is a cynical edge to these men's replies, but they are not "stuffed with words," nor do they have a confusing effect upon any hearer. Each registers the opinion of a mature anima that has experienced the trickster and reflected upon its effects.

What I have presented so far is from a male perspective, and it is presumptuous for me to assume that a woman integrates the trickster into her animus in a pre-cisely parallel way. Ricki Tannen (2007), however, has made a convincing case, examining female sleuths in American detective fiction, that the female trickster helps the animus of a woman develop the resilience, autonomy, and irony needed to avoid becoming the victim of patriarchal one-upmanship.

When a man's anima has failed to integrate the trickster, she tends to be at the trickster's mercy and to become paranoid when she must respond to the shadow side of others. This is the dilemma of the governess in Henry James's "The Turn of the Screw." I feel justified in reading this as an anima story in part because of the way this trickster classic is framed. The story is presented as a ghost story told to the person who introduces the tale. That person claims that he heard it from a man named Douglas, who had originally read it aloud to an assembled company "with a fine clearness that was like a rendering to the ear of the beauty of his author's hand" (1898, p. 15). This author is the governess, and it is her diary he is reading. This woman's story, read by a man, to produce a dramatic emotional effect, makes a good metaphor for an anima outpouring, and it is from this angle that the story has most to tell us.

The governess is described as an attractive young woman of the 1840s, who has come newly from a convent to an English country house to care for two orphaned children of latency age, whose angelic appearance belies a certain trickster quality that she senses about them. Indeed, the elder of the children, Miles, has been expelled from school for "saying things." It is to this governess, this Jane Eyre, that the celebrated ghosts appear. One is a man, the other a woman. After persistent inquiries, the governess learns that Miles had had a close relation to his father's valet, Peter Quint, now dead, but who in life was "always too free." The governess who preceded her, Miss Jessel, also had an association with Quint, and she, too, is now dead. Was she also "too free?" Did Miles learn bad words from Quint? Were he and his sister Flora privy to an illegitimate liaison between Miss Jessel and Quint? Above all, are the ghosts those of these people? The governess cannot get to the bottom of it. Nor can the reader, for James leaves everything in innuendo, in open-ended prose so ambiguously suggestive that the reader is led to guess what the dark secrets are. "Make him *think* the evil, make him think it for himself, and you are released from weak specifications," James writes in his preface (1934, p. 176). In other words, the reader is forced to project, and so the tale itself is a trickster. Just so, the unintegrated trickster archetype in the governess renders her peculiarly vulnerable to the normal tricksterism of these latency-age children.

As the governess continues to see the ghosts of Peter Quint and Miss Jessel, she begins to project evil all around her, growing ever more certain that the children are seeing these ghosts too, but not telling her. She determines to make an inquisition of the children which will continue until they admit that they have relations with these spirits. In her relentless attempt to "do right" by the children, which she says will require "but another turn of the screw of ordinary virtue" (James, 1898, p. 193), she turns her Victorian convent mentality into the ruthlessness of the Spanish Inquisition.

In the process, this would-be rescuer alienates the little girl and bullies the little boy into heart failure. As he finally gasps out Peter Quint's name, which to her proves that she has exorcised him, he dies in her arms.

Henry James was every bit as great a believer in consciousness as C. G. Jung, and almost as subtle a critic of forms of unconsciousness. This short novel, I feel, is James's bitterest attack on the sort of pseudo-consciousness that the anima can create when she has not integrated the trickster and must project and fear it. Since, as Jung tells us, the anima is the projection-making factor in a man, one could consider this story—written by a woman, but recounted by a man—a cautionary tale about the anima, demonstrating the dangers of living by her projections. But we can go a little further in understanding the psychological circumstances under which the anima makes her most dangerous projections by taking into account the characteristics of the tale itself along the lines I have been following in other works of art. For this tale is a trickster, which delivers its impact by drawing the reader into identification with the anima-figure governess. As Leon Edel says:

> In the charged account of the governess, with her phantoms, her "certitude," her suppositions, which she turns into "fact," her "facts" which are mere suppositions, we recognize the materials of the witch-burners and executioners

of old. Her narrative, with its consummate interweaving of paranoid fancy with circumstantial reality, is indeed capable of making readers pronounce the innocents guilty—as the testimony of Salem children long ago turned innocent men and women into sorcerers and magicians.

(1978, p. 205)

In the last scene of the story, when the governess insists that her charge Miles name the man, Peter Quint, whose ghost she believes is continuing to come onto the boy, perhaps sexually, as she believes he did in life, we are confronted with the stakes of the projection-making game. Trying to make sense of the confusing ending, in which the boy, exhausted by the governess, answers her, "Peter Quint," and then adds, "You devil," Edel claims with the authority of a close reading of the text:

> Miles never sees Quint. The boy is described as if he were a dumb trapped little animal seeking a way of escape from the smothering presence not of the ghost but of the intense and exigent governess. "No more, no more, no more," she shrieks thinking she has banished the phantom . . . When Miles, after guessing wrongly, dredges up the name she wants him to pronounce, that of Peter Quint, he is able in his frightened state to add the words "you devil!" A careless reader might think he is addressing the apparition. However throughout this scene Miles has his back to the window where the governess sees Quint hovering ominously. It is indeed the governess who has become the devil; and the subtlest twist of the story is that the demon she seeks to exorcise is the demon within herself. She rids herself of her private ghost; and in the process little Miles's heart is "dispossessed," and she is left "alone with the quiet day," with the dead boy in her arms—as in the medieval tales of possession. Her evil spirit has been driven out; but innocence has died.
>
> (Edel, p. 206)

This is a meticulous, and illuminating, reading of the way the scene is laid out, at least logically, and one with which I concur, but it does not put to rest the dark trickster cloud that hangs over the story and emerges whenever it is read again, because James's words, designed to make readers "think the evil" themselves, invite projections. Who after all *is* the "you" that the boy Miles calls a devil? Is it not possible that the governess, especially since she is persecutory, has convinced Miles that he is seeing Peter Quint again, so that the boy is having, and terrified by, a stress hallucination of Quint himself? Or even, terrified by what she seems to be seeing, a vision of Quint that Miles temporarily shares? James's brother William, who had lectured on "exceptional mental states" in 1896, would certainly not have refused the possibility that the governess had pushed the boy's consciousness "beyond the margin" (Taylor, 2011). The controversy as to whether Quint's specter makes its appearance at the end of the story continues, therefore, despite Edel, and the critical mountain grows, as it began to do as early as 1934, when Edmund

Wilson, in his essay "The Ambiguity of Henry James," first aroused a storm of controversy by suggesting, in a "Freudian" interpretation of the story, that the ghosts were nothing but the governess's projections. Reading this story, one's own consciousness becomes overrun by a state of opposed views of it. One often wonders whether the evil that the governess senses is not somehow present, and some critics have even argued that the governess acts with integrity because she is intuitive enough to have sensed the danger. I do not think they are right, but with its endless and unfathomable ambiguities, the story forces us to recognize the fallibility of our understanding in the face of the unknown. It is this fallibility which the governess herself tragically cannot accept, preferring the certainty of a paranoid solution which leaves the evil outside her. She substitutes her theory of what is going on for the dilemma of not being able to know. And the reader is shaken to realize, as he rereads the story, how much he too has filled in the blanks and gaps in his knowledge with suppositions. He is left with the uneasy feeling that he, too, might have tried too hard to save the child and has inadvertently but ruthlessly killed him.

For me, the governess, with her network of moods, opinions, and projections, makes a good image of the kind of anima which has failed to integrate the trickster, so that the trickster is perceived as a lurking danger from outside, requiring efforts at suppression. I believe James saw such a danger in the Victorian moral sense, which had been recently tested in English literary circles as to whether to sign a petition for Oscar Wilde's release from prison a year after he had been jailed for "gross indecency" (i.e. open homosexuality). James thought the petition would not have any effect and chose not to sign, but George Meredith flatly refused on principle, stating that literary men, as setters of standards, should not condone immorality that was also abnormal. T. S. Eliot once commented that Henry James was the most intelligent man of his generation, and that "he had a mind so fine that no idea could violate it" (1918). In "The Turn of the Screw," the governess's mind is violated by Victorian principles, and James's modernist moral fiction often demonstrates, with its tricksterish irony, the damage that such a violation can do.

The more such an anima resists, the more the unaccepted trickster is constellated and, in the end, overruns the psychological field. When the anima is overrun by the trickster, her instinctive responses are poisoned, and she becomes a dangerous trickster herself, capable of inducing paranoia. I feel that the reader manipulation exerted by the story expresses the power of the trickster that this kind of anima figure refuses to recognize. The strength of that power is the final impression that the tale leaves on its reader, when he or she is finally able to put the story aside.

What is the man's anima like when she has included, rather than projected, the problem of the trickster? I think Robert Frost gives us a picture:

> She is as in a field a silken tent
> At midday when a sunny summer breeze
> Has dried the dew and all its ropes relent,
> So that in guys it gently sways at ease,
> And its supporting central cedar pole,

That is its pinnacle to heavenward
And signifies the sureness of the soul,
Seems to owe naught to any single cord,
But strictly held by none, is loosely bound
By countless silken ties of love and thought
To everything on earth the compass round,
And only by one's going slightly taut
In the capriciousness of summer air
Is of the slightest bondage made aware.

(Robert Frost, 1961, p. 514)

In other words, the trickster currents that affect the mature anima seem to strengthen her alert relation to the world and to the ego-Self axis, so that the liminality of the trickster actually serves to keep the anima aware of what her true limits are. Presumably then her role will not so much be to project, insinuate, or poison, as when the trickster has not been integrated, but will be to guide and compensate. Indeed, the trickster around her compensates her in a mysteriously helpful way.

Here Frost is speaking of the personal aspect of an anima that has integrated the trickster. When we get to her archetypal aspect, we find that the trickster seems to be a living part of her. Within the bank of great pictures that continue to inform our culture, one creative image, pre-eminently, expresses what the anima looks like at this stage: Leonardo's *Mona Lisa*.

When the trickster has become a working part of the anima, the goal of the sort of work of art I have been referring to has been reached. Despite the containment, such a work as the *Mona Lisa* remains a free-roaming trickster, able to insinuate its own creative energy into the consciousness of a collective, just as the Winnebago trickster, Wakdjunkaga, could unroll his enormously long penis and slip it at a distance into the unsuspecting body of the Chief's daughter (Radin, pp. 19–20). A great trickster work of art, like Leonardo's masterpiece, wants to penetrate the level of our gut responses, just where we are most sentimental and vulnerable, and by disturbing us force us all to reconsider our complacency.

As we delight in the liminal transgression of the trickster's touch, we feel inside the limits of our most cherished values. The *Mona Lisa*, for example, is reflecting the limits of Renaissance humanism, expressed in all the ego portraits of upstanding and powerful men and women painted during that period; her irony permits her to transcend the genre and the psychology of mastery that it expresses (see Hillman, 1975, pp. 168–228).

We experience, through trickster works of art, the one-sidedness of whatever exists in us to threaten the ongoing development of consciousness, and we are forced into a duplex mode which challenges our basic suppositions. Particularly, we experience the limits of our own trusting upstandingness, when this favorable result of good mothering has begun to threaten our understanding. If in a work of art the trickster succeeds in shocking or confusing us out of our complacency, he does this that we may see anew and thereby manage to survive the world.

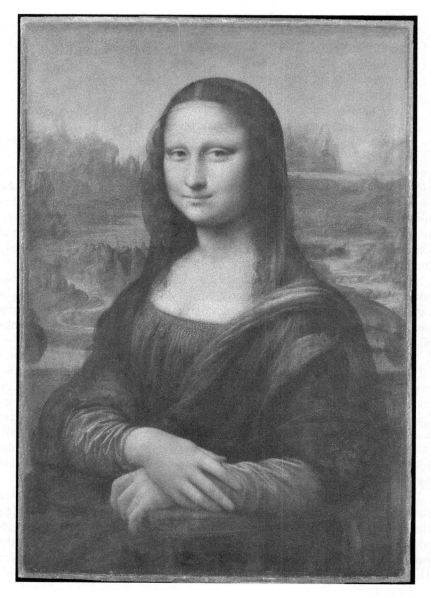

Figure 1.2 Leonardo da Vinci (1452–1519). Mona Lisa (La Gioconda). Oil on wood.

Photo: Michel Urtado 2011. © RMN-Grand Palais/Art Resource, NY.

References

Aldus, P. J. (1977). *Mousetrap: Structure and Meaning in Hamlet*. Buffalo: University of Toronto Press.

Beebe, J. (1975). Evaluation and treatment of the psychotic patient. In C. P. Rosenbaum and J. Beebe (Eds.), *Psychiatric Treatment: Crisis, Clinic, and Consultation*, pp. 82–114. New York: McGraw Hill.

Chave, A. C. (1989). *Mark Rothko: Subjects in Abstraction*. New Haven: Yale University Press.

Edel, L. (1978). *The Life of Henry James: The Treacherous Years: 1895–1901*. New York: Avon Discus Books.

Eissler, K. (1971). *Discourse on Hamlet and Hamlet: A Psychoanalytic Inquiry*. New York: International University Press.

Eliot, T. S. (1918). In memory of Henry James. *Egoist*, 5, 1–2.

Eliot, T. S. (1960). Hamlet and his problems. In Claire Sacks and Edgar Whan (Eds.), *Hamlet: Enter Critic*, pp. 53–58. New York: Appleton Century Crofts.

Empson, W. (1953). *Seven Types of Ambiguity*. New York: New Directions.

Foucault, M. (1973/2008). *This Is Not a Pipe*. J. Harkness (Ed. and Trans.). Berkeley: University of California Press.

Frost, R. (1961). The silken tent. In Milton Crane (Ed.), *50 Great Poets*, p. 514. New York: Bantam.

Hillman, J. (1975). *Revisioning Psychology*. New York: Harper & Row.

James, H. (1893/1996). The middle years. In *Henry James: Complete Stories 1892–1898*, pp. 335–355. New York: Library of America.

James, H. (1898). The turn of the screw. In *The Two Magics*. New York: Macmillan.

James, H. (1934). *The Art of the Novel*. New York: Charles Scribner's Sons.

James, H. (1970). *Partial Portraits*. Ann Arbor: University of Michigan Press.

Janowsky, D. S., Leff, M., and Epstein, R. S. (1970). Playing the manic game: Interpersonal maneuvers of the acutely manic patient. *Archives of General Psychiatry*, 22(3), 252–261.

Johnson, S. (1765/2004). Preface to the plays of William Shakespeare. Gutenberg.org.

Jung, C. G. (1968). *Psychology and Alchemy*, Collected Works, Vol. 12, 2nd ed. Princeton: Princeton University Press.

Kael, P. (1963). *I Lost it at the Movies*. Boston: Little, Brown.

Kael, P. (1971a). *The Citizen Kane Book*. New York: Bantam Books.

Kael, P. (1971b). Trash, art, and the movies. In *Going Steady*. New York: Bantam Books.

Kirsch, J. (1966). *Shakespeare's Royal Self*. New York: G. P. Putnam's Sons.

Lewis, R. W. B. (1964). Afterword to Signet Edition of Herman Melville, *The Confidence-man*. New York: New American Library.

Lynn, K. (1959). *Mark Twain and the Southwestern Tradition*. New York: Little, Brown.

Marlon, S. (2005). *The Black Sun: The Alchemy and Art of Darkness*. College Station, TX: Texas A & M University Press.

Melville, H. (1964). *The Confidence-man: His Masquerade*. New York: New American Library.

Meyerowitz, P. (Ed.). (1971). *Gertrude Stein; Writings and Lectures 1900–1945*. Baltimore, MD: Penguin Books.

Radin, P. (1956). *The Trickster: A Study in American Indian Mythology, with Commentaries by Karl Kerenyi and C. G. Jung*. New York: Philosophical Library.

Renker, E. (1998). "A—!" Unreadability in *The Confidence Man*. In R. S. Levine (Ed.), *The Cambridge Companion to Herman Melville*, pp. 114–134. Cambridge: Cambridge University Press.

Sarris, A. (1968). *The American Cinema*. New York: Dutton.

Sarris, A. (1970). Notes on the *Auteur* theory in 1962. *Film Culture Reader*. New York: Praeger.

Sartre, J. P. (1938/2013). *Nausea*. R. Howard (Trans.). New Directions (Kindle edition).

Shakespeare, W. (1998). *The Arden Shakespeare Complete Works*. R. Proudfoot, A. Thompson, and D. Kastan (Eds.). Walton-on-Thames, Surrey: Thomas Nelson and Sons.

Stein, M. (1980). Review of The meaning of Aphrodite by Paul Friedrich. *The San Francisco Jung Institute Library Journal*, 2(1), 18–22.

Tannen, R. S. (2007). *The Female Trickster: The Mask that Reveals*. Hove, UK: Routledge.

Taylor, E. (2011). *William James on Consciousness beyond the Margin*. Princeton: Princeton University Press.

Torczyner, H. (1977). *Magritte: Ideas and Images*. New York: Harry N. Abrams.

Twain, M. (1965). *The Adventures of Huckleberry Finn*. New York: Bantam Books.

Wadlington, W. (1975). *The Confidence Game in American Literature*. Princeton: Princeton University Press.

Weitz, M. (1964). *Hamlet and the Philosophy of Literary Criticism*. Chicago: University of Chicago Press.

West, N. (1962). *Miss Lonelyhearts & the Day of the Locust*. New York: New Directions Publishing.

Wheelwright, J. (1981). *Death of a Woman*. New York: St. Martin's Press.

Willeford, W. (1969). *The Fool and His Scepter: A Study in Clowns and Jesters and their Audience*. Evanston: Northwestern University Press.

Wilson, E. (1934). The ambiguity of Henry James. *Hound and Horn*, April–June, 385–406.

Chapter 2

Astrid Berg

I was born in 1950 to immigrant parents, being the older of two children. My father left Germany before the outbreak of the war in order to pursue his career in South Africa. My mother was a war refugee from Eastern Prussia. My upbringing in Pretoria was within the German cultural and language milieu, with Afrikaans as my second language. I attended Pretoria High School for Girls as it was important for my parents that I would be fluent in English as well. My father died of a stroke when I was 16 years old; not consciously getting to know him left its mark on my psyche.

Successfully matriculating with several distinctions was followed by six years as a medical student at Pretoria University where I graduated with the MB ChB degree in 1968. This multi-language and to an extent multicultural upbringing has made me accustomed to communicate across divides and enabled me to be comfortable in the role of the relative outsider. In a predominantly conservative environment as the University of Pretoria was at the time, I was the German girl with the miniskirt, a "communist" newspaper under her arm, whose closest friends were the left-wing, Jewish students. My move to Cape Town in 1974 with my then fiancé, Heinz Rode, formed the second phase of my life. I was grateful to find myself in the more liberal atmosphere that the city and the University of Cape Town offered.

My interest in paediatrics from my medical school days was reflected in the distinction I received in paediatrics in my final year and subsequent work as a senior "houseman" at the Red Cross War Memorial Children's Hospital. During this time however, I realized that the pursuit of a specialization in paediatrics would not satisfy me intellectually and I became interested in the psychological development of children. This had very much to do with the relative emotional deprivation I had experienced as a young child, born to a mother who was up-rooted and traumatized by a horrific war.

My training as a general psychiatrist was followed by another few years of part time sub-specialisation in child and adolescent psychiatry—I was the first student for the new M Phil degree in child and adolescent psychiatry at the University of Cape Town. My thesis was on the bereaved child, probably unconsciously connecting my research work to my own adolescent bereavement.

DOI: 10.4324/9781003148968-3

Despite family obligations (two children born in 1980 and 1981), I managed to train in Jungian analysis and became a member of the International Association of Analytical Psychology in 1992. The reason for undertaking this extra training was my desire to understand myself better and through this to become a more skilled clinician and psychotherapist. It has always been of central importance to me to be able to establish a connection with the "other," notably my patients, in order to truly gain an understanding of their world view and their experiences. It is this which makes me an able clinician, a sound psychotherapist and a person who is comfortable within culturally diverse settings and who appreciates finding commonalities as well as differences.

I was supervised for many years by Dr Vera Bührmann, who was the driving force behind the establishment of the South African Association of Jungian Analysts (SAAJA). Her interest in and knowledge of the early years of life resonated very much with my inclinations.

In 1995 I was introduced to the area of infant mental health by Mara Sidoli, a Jungian analyst who was visiting Cape Town. My attention was drawn to her presenting us with an infant observation. This was undoubtedly linked to my own experience as a parent of two children, but also linked to my early years with my own mother for whom I had to be the "therapist." This was a natural development from general child psychiatry into a more specific niche within which I could develop new skills. In time I was able to take the lead on a national as well as international level. My election in 2020 to the position of President-Elect of the World Association for Infant Mental Health has provided me with an enormous opportunity to increase global awareness as to the importance of the beginning of life.

My political awareness, my respect for cultural diversity and my concern for "the other," particularly the "other" who cannot speak, that is, the infant, were the driving force behind my engagement in long-standing community work in a township outside of Cape Town. For over 18 years I provided a service to mothers and young children, but at the same time made it into an academic endeavour out of which much of my writing flowed and for which I gained international recognition. This work brought together my passion for those without a voice, my reverence for the delicate beginnings of mental life, and my interest in the way human beings see the world, each in their own way.

I consider my ability to be on the "edge" of different disciplines an important one in the type of work I am engaged in. Child psychiatry, and particularly infant psychiatry, is my chosen field. In order to be an able psychiatrist plus psychotherapist I needed not only a medical training but also an in-depth psychological training which explains my qualification as an analytical psychologist. Living in an ethnically diverse country and working across past political divides has also made me realize that I have to understand the cultures in which the families that consult me are embedded. Analytical psychology has provided me with a framework through which an in-depth understanding of different world views has been possible for me. I have striven to have a thorough knowledge and grasp of these three domains, which come together for me on a daily basis in the consulting room, be this directly with my patients or in supervision and teaching of younger colleagues.

If I were asked "what do you believe in?" my reply would be "in relationships with others." I do not know whether there is a benign creative force out there, I do not know whether my soul will continue to live in another world, but I do know that the relationships I have with those close to me will continue in their minds, even after my body is gone. The notion of ancestor reverence, so present in the African world view, is one that makes more sense to me than any formal religion. My children and grandchildren will know me as their ancestor, and, if I am "on the other side" (as is said in Africa), I will protect them, if that is possible. And perhaps bits of me will remain alive in the work that I have done, which I hope will have contributed to making the world a friendlier place.

Cape Town, April 2020

Psychoanalysis and Primary Health Care

Originally published in the Journal *"Psycho-analytic Psychotherapy in South Africa"* (2014, Vol 22 No 1 p 92–105). Reprinted with permission.

[A]t some time or other the conscience of society will awake and remind it that the poor man should have just as much right to assistance for his mind as he now has to the life-saving help offered by surgery.

(Freud, 1919, p. 167)

Freud spoke these words in 1918 in his address to the Fifth International Psycho-analytic Congress in Budapest. The idea of universal access to psychotherapy was a progressive one which fitted in with the spirit of the time; it was a call for action which Freud and his followers subsequently followed up on. The first polyclinic for psychoanalysis was opened in Berlin in 1920. A list of prominent psychoanalysts agreed to devote a fifth of their working time to the free clinics. However, with the advent of National Socialism in Germany, this had to come to an end. Altman (2006) argues that historical forces subsequent to World War II conspired to bring out the more conservative aspects of psychoanalysis, so that what we have today is a mostly middle-class, Eurocentric discipline offered to persons who can afford to pay for services rendered. In the modern world with its keen awareness of human suffering, this state of affairs is increasingly untenable. If psychoanalysis is about healing the human psyche, it should not be accessible to only an elite few.

Already in 1993 Altman had questioned this conservative state of affairs in a chapter titled "Psychoanalysis and the Urban Poor." Amongst other issues, he challenges the classic notion of insight as the only mechanism for analytic change on the grounds that it places a premium on verbal intelligence which in turn introduces a bias against patients who have not had the kind of upbringing that encourages this ability. He also disputes the rule of strict abstinence observed by the classically orientated psychoanalyst, as it may be seen as culture bound "Calvinist individualism" (p. 33) and may thus not be congruent in a different cultural context where group identification and affiliation are in the foreground. Instead of describing certain patients as "unanalysable" he challenges psychoanalysis to review its practice, especially in public clinics where a psychoanalytic approach is not playing the role it could and should.

Foster (1993), in his response to this chapter by Altman, argues for a postclassical object relationship model of human relatedness that would accommodate a wider spectrum of being. He calls attention to the fact that it is the analyst's task to enter into the patient's world and to learn from it (and not vice versa). If followed through, this way of working would be more inclusive and might ultimately eliminate some of the exclusionary criteria for "analysability" in the classical model.

In a social context such as South Africa's these arguments are not merely theoretical but are crucial to the future of psychoanalysis and its role in mental health practice and advocacy. The call for improved services in public clinics comes from many corners. The policies of the Department of Health aim at addressing the upstream risk factors that impact on health; these can be dealt with within the framework of the primary health care system. Most importantly there is also the ethical, moral imperative, the "ethics of social responsibility" (Gobodo-Madikizela, 2009, p. 83) which we as clinicians have, namely that we need to broaden our mental health services to communities who so desperately need to be seen and heard and about whom Freud's call was made—something which the South African Psychoanalytic Confederation is attempting to address and redress.

On the surface it would appear that traditional, conservative psychoanalysis and primary health care occupy opposite ends of the therapeutic spectrum; from the private consulting room to a public space requires a big jump: office allocation may change from week to week; scheduled appointments which take place within a prearranged time frame give way to unpredictable and unplanned attendances; the intimate one-on-one space is not feasible as language barriers are such that the work needs to take place with a third adult person, an interpreter, in the room. In short, the conditions for the analytic attitude in terms of "the frame" are simply not provided by the outer environment.

Despite these differences it is possible to work psychoanalytically within a primary health care context. While the frame may not be in the outer setting, psychoanalytic theory can provide an inner frame which holds the therapist and enables him or her to approach the patient with the same care and attention that would be provided in the private consulting room.

Many years of working in a parent-infant mental health service ("the Service") in a community near Cape Town have shown that the Service is used, that it works, and that it is appreciated precisely because of the basic analytic attitude that prevails.

A Brief Overview of the Clinical Setting

The Service is part of a general community clinic in a township setting where mothers bring their infants for immunisation. As part of the general screening that is done, the infants' weight is checked at each visit.

Infant-caregiver dyads are seen at the Service upon referral by the clinic staff. Clinical practice has shown the baby's failure to gain adequate weight to be a useful indicator of possible emotional problems; it has become an acceptable entry point into further enquiry into the attachment relationship as well as family circumstances. After basic demographic facts are established, the mother is asked about her problems, while the infant is being observed and interacted with. While direct advice is given where needed and where appropriate, more often than not the mother is simply given the opportunity to unburden herself and to be in conversation with an "other" who is non-judgemental and abstinent from immediate action. Given the severity with which many of the patients in the community are treated by medical staff, this release from being blamed for the child's failure to thrive is profound. Spontaneous comments such as "I feel lighter" or "I can see things differently after coming here" are frequently offered.

In analysing patient demographics and outcomes in a four-year sample, the compliance rate was found to be 75% (Berg, 2012). This means that three-quarters of caregivers returned for follow-up visits and/or followed the recommendations made, such as taking the child for an appointment to the hospital. This is a significant finding, as mothers were not forced to come back and their compliance (or not) with us had no influence on their general clinic visits. We also found an improvement in parent-child relationships and infant functioning (Berg, 2012).

How do we account for this outcome? What are the active ingredients of this infant-parent psychotherapy in this primary health care setting? There are many possibilities for exploring these questions; here, four possibilities are highlighted.

First, the availability of a confidential space with a consistent and reliable clinical team, which allowed for a personal connection to be made, was pivotal. Always present were at least two persons: the clinician plus the community counsellor, in this case Mrs Nosisana Nama, who acted as the clinician's mentor, guide and interpreter, and who was the person the mother most related to. The triangular space that is created in this way will be discussed later.

Second, the sessions were in line with the modality of "unstructured reflective developmental guidance" (Lieberman and Van Horn, 2009). The clinical team responded to the needs of the moment, rather than following a prescribed treatment module; it was reflective because the parent was encouraged to think about her infant and find a different way of viewing her situation and of viewing her child. This way of working is in line with the reflective parenting approach developed by Nancy Suchman and her team at the Yale Child Study Centre and which has been shown to be effective (Suchman et al., 2013).

Third, bestowing personhood onto the infant through talking to the infant made the infant an active partner in the interaction and was an important modelling action for mothers whose sense of competence in their maternal abilities was impaired. Careful observation of the infant's behaviour and gestures enabled the clinician to highlight the moments when the infant was trying to make contact with his mother. The capabilities of young babies are generally not known, and being able to find these as they happen spontaneously often provided even the most troubled mother with a sense of being loved and needed.

Fourth, crisis intervention and case management were indicated particularly in cases of domestic violence. Concrete advice and referrals to appropriate agencies were given.

Psychoanalysis Viewed Through the Community Lens

Psychoanalysis respects and takes into consideration unconscious processes within the patient, within the therapist and in the relationship between them. In order for these processes to become conscious a space is needed in which they can manifest; this space needs to be a containing one as it is only within boundaries that feelings can be expressed and that links can be made.

In the community situation the space and the boundaries are created by the therapeutic team: a regular, predictable and dependable presence on a weekly basis within the same physical space is what matters and what forms a counterpoint to the outside business and often chaotic clinic background.

Besides the challenges of creating space and boundaries, we have an added task in South Africa. We have 11 official languages, and understanding the spoken word of our patients frequently requires us to have a third person in the room who acts as an interpreter. This person, who may initially be simply called in, could in time became a partner to the therapist. This should not be experienced as a hindrance in terms of establishing the therapist-patient relationship, but it should in fact be regarded as an opportunity to learn and widen the interactive space. An interpreter of language is also a translator of meaning: this latter part is often not respected. Without such a person working with us on an equal level we cannot truly bridge difference; if we make the effort of establishing a relationship with this person and accord her respect as the one who knows the lifeworld of the patient, she can come to fulfil the role not only of an interpreter, but also of a "cultural broker" (Dysart-Gale, 2007) or "community navigator" (Henderson and Kendall, 2011). She (or he) is the one who provides the clinician with a fuller and thicker description of the patient's story. If seen in this light, the presence of such a cultural broker becomes a *sine qua non*.

In addition to the obvious advantage of understanding our patients better, two theoretical constructs are helpful in giving us a deeper insight into the benefit which is provided by having an interpreter in the room.

The Concept of the Third

The triangle and the position of the third occupy a central position in psychoana-lytic theorising. In describing the Oedipal constellation in normal child develop-ment, Ronald Britton and colleagues suggested the following:

> The triangular space includes the possibility of being a participant in a rela-tionship, observed by a third person, and of being an observer as a third of a relationship between two other people . . . This provides us a capacity for seeing ourselves in interaction with others and for entertaining another point of view while entertaining our own, indeed, for reflecting upon ourselves while being ourselves.
>
> (Britton et al., 2006, pp. 289–290)

Britton (2004) has also stated that theories and professional training are a "third object" in his mind, one that holds him in the moment of the clinical situation. Thus the third is both manifested concretely in a three-person relationship as well as being an inner psychic position; it could be hypothesised that the three-person relationship starts off as an object constellation in the external world and then moves to the inner world as a triangular psychic space.

In the community setting there are two triangles which alternate in their interac-tion: mother-child-therapist, mother-therapist-interpreter, and various combina-tions thereof. Invariably the conversations are between three of the four persons, mostly seamlessly moving from one triangle to the other. Within these shifting triangles "moments of meeting" (Stern et al., 1998, p. 305) may arise in which something that was implicit is understood more consciously by the participants.

A clinical vignette serves to illustrate this:

> *Twelve-month old Aphiwe was standing between her parents who were in conversation with Nosisana, exploring their marital difficulties. All of this occurred in isiXhosa, thus leaving me out of the exchange. I noted that Aphiwe was offering a key ring which her father had given her to her mother, who absentmindedly took it and then returned it to her. Aphiwe then moved to her father and gave it to him, and so the play continued. When Nosisana and the parents had come to an end of their exploration, I spoke about what Aphiwe had been doing and interpreted her wish to keep both parents con-nected with each other and with her. This was heard and received and the session ended on a positive note.*

Several processes were going on simultaneously during this brief interchange; they could have easily been missed had there not been two therapists in the room. Had Nosisana been in the exclusive role of interpreter she would not have had the freedom to take the initiative to talk with the parents, and I would not have been freed to focus on the child.

The interpreter who fulfils the role of a co-therapist can only add to the richness of the clinical encounter, not just in terms of mediating culture and translating language, but also in opening a psychic space in which links can be made.

In the South African context there is an added dimension of a socio-political nature, namely that of yielding control.

Yielding Control

The medical model focuses on the defect of the patient which is then diagnosed and treated according to an established protocol. The power is clearly in the hands of the doctor who is the one to possess the required knowledge. Psychoanalysis has changed this traditional doctor-patient relationship from one of authority to one of partnership (Rayner, 1991). It is generally accepted that the doctor knows as much or as little as the patient and thus both patient and therapist are involved in an exploration of what is going on for the patient.

While the traditional hierarchical doctor-patient relationship has changed over time in monocultural settings such as in Europe, this cannot be said of settings where there are marked culture, language and economic status differences. Implicit in many of the psychological interventions practised in South Africa is a sense that what is done in the higher-income countries is that which is best and which should be emulated. There is often very little appreciation that not everything coming from Western urban, secular life is superior to that of more traditional ways of viewing the world and that the former could also learn from the latter.

In our attempt to be non-racist we often have a wish to obliterate difference without realising that we are actually continuing to be racist in our assumed (albeit unconscious) superiority that we know what is best. In 1998 Tervalon and Murray-Garcia coined the term "cultural humility" which they describe as coming from a lifelong commitment to self-evaluation and self-critique and of being a self-reflective practitioner (Tervalon and Murray-Garcia, 1998). This means that we not only regard every human being as equal to another, but it also means acknowledging difference, respecting this difference and seeking help in order to bridge the difference. Even with the best intentions, we cannot know it all. Only once mutually respectful interchanges and partnerships have been established will power imbalances be redressed. In South Africa this cultural humility has particular significance, as the built-in superiority of apartheid ideology remains an ongoing, albeit repressed, theme in the collective psyche. Working closely and on an equal basis with an interpreter addresses this traditional asymmetry in a tangible and real way.

Looking at this superiority theme through a psychoanalytic lens, Foster (1993, p. 75) warns of the "dangerous legacy of positivism" that assumes supremacy of the psychoanalytical world view which then "applies the belief system of the Western, European middle class to all patients."

In his plea towards a more relational approach he goes on to state:

> [T]he new view is that relevant meaning and understanding are created in the dialectical discourse between the two members of the dyad—each of whom is embedded and constrained by his or her own inner psychology and view of the world . . . the work must be undertaken as a joint quest for meaning and understanding with the analyst exercising particular caution in rushing to apply his or her assumptions about minds at large.
>
> (Foster, 1993, p. 76)

While Foster speaks within the traditional two-way psychoanalytic relationship, we face the challenge of establishing a relationship between three persons. The triangle that is created between the therapist, patient and interpreter provides us with an opportunity to discover in open and transparent dialogue and trialogue the world view of the patient, thereby enabling the therapist to "affectively . . . enter the patient's world, be impacted by it, be transformed by it, and experience first-hand the host of internalised objects that lie within" (Foster, 1993, p. 74).

In Conclusion

Freud's 1918 address continues:

> [I]nstitutions or out-patient clinics will be started, to which analytically-trained physicians will be appointed . . . such treatments will be free . . . we shall then be faced by the task of adapting our technique to the new conditions . . . we shall need to look for the simplest and most easily intelligible ways of expressing our theoretical doctrines.
>
> (Freud, 1919, p. 167)

The adaptation of psychoanalytic techniques is not only possible but is necessary. One such necessary adaptation is the presence of an interpreter who is also a cultural mediator. This is of particular importance in the South African situation given that power differentials between people continue to exist. As Mamphela Ramphele stated, "apartheid's geography is alive and well" (Cunningham, 2010). Health professionals and patients frequently belong to different language, socio-economic and cultural groups, and bridging this divide requires more than good intentions. Yielding control to a person of the "other" group is vital to breaking traditional asymmetries.

If psychoanalysis is going to be meaningful in the future, we do not have a choice: we have to move forward. We need to revisit many assumptions that were originally made within a middle-class Victorian world view, and we have to ask ourselves whether we can truly afford to remain in our consulting rooms, shielded from realities which may be talked about but not necessarily directly experienced.

Freud's 1918 call for action could only partly be seen through by Freud and his followers and was interrupted by the horrors that were enacted in Europe soon thereafter. In South Africa the situation is different; the "conscience of society" (Freud, 1919, p. 167) has awoken and we do have an opportunity to correct what was wrong. Those of us who have had the privilege of an in-depth training could and should take this challenge on. Similarly psychoanalysis needs to step out of its traditional confines. Only then will it become the progressive social force its forebears intended it to be and only then will it contribute to building bridges between people.

References

Altman, N. (1993). Psychoanalysis and the urban poor. *Psychoanalytic Dialogues*, 3(1), 29–49.

Altman, N. (2006). How psychoanalysis became white in the United States, and how that might change. *Psychoanalytic Perspectives*, 3, 65–72.

Berg, A. (2012). Infant-parent psychotherapy at primary care level: Establishment of a service. *South African Medical Journal*, 102, 582–584.

Britton, R. (2004). Subjectivity, objectivity, and triangular space. *Psychoanalytic Quarterly*, 73, 47–61.

Britton, R., Cused, J., Ellman, S., and Likierman, M. (2006). Panel II: The Oedipus complex. the primal scene, and the superego. *Journal of Infant, Child & Adolescent Psychotherapy*, 5, 282–307.

Cunningham, J. (2010). Rainbow nation: Myth or reality. *South Africa The Good News*. www.sagoodnews.co.za/newsletter_archive/rainbow_nation_myth_or_reality.html

Dysart-Gale, D. (2007). Clinicians and medical interpreters: Negotiating culturally appropriate care for patients with limited English ability. *Family & Community Health*, 30, 237–246.

Foster, R. P. (1993). The social politics of psychoanalysis commentary on Neil Altman's 'Psychoanalysis and the urban poor'. *Psychoanalytic Dialogues*, 3, 69–83.

Freud, S. (1919). Lines of advance in psycho-analytic therapy. In J. Strachey (Ed. and Trans.), *The Standard Edition of the Complete Psychological Works of Sigmund Freud*, Vol. 17, pp. 157–168. London: Hogarth Press.

Gobodo-Madikizela, P. (2009). Exploring the ethical principal of social responsibility and other ethical issues in the context of the mental health professionals' response to xenophobic violence in Cape Town. *Psycho-Analytic Psychotherapy in South Africa*, 17, 79–101.

Henderson, S., and Kendall, E. (2011). 'Community navigators': Making a difference by promoting health in culturally and linguistically diverse (CALD) communities in Logan, Queensland. *Australian Journal of Primary Health*, 17, 347–354.

Lieberman, A. F., and Van Horn, P. (2009). Child-parent psychotherapy: A developmental approach to mental health treatment in infancy and early childhood. In C. H. Zeanah (Ed.), *Handbook of Infant Mental Health,* 3rd ed., pp. 439–449. New York and London: The Guildford Press.

Rayner, E. (1991). *The Independent Mind in British Psychoanalysis*. London: Free Association Books.

Stern, D. N., Bruschweiler-Stern, N., Harrison, A. M., Lyons-Ruth, K., Morgan, A. C., Nahum, J. P., Sander, L., and Tronick, E. Z. (1998). The process of therapeutic change involving implicit knowledge: Some implications of developmental observations for adult psychotherapy. *Infant Mental Health Journal*, 19(3), 300–308.

Suchman, N. E., Decoste, C., Ordway, M. R., and Bers, S. (2013). Mothering from the inside out: A mentalization-based individual therapy for mothers with substance-use disorders. In N. E. Suchman, M. Pajulo, and L. C. Mayes (Eds.), *Parenting and Substance Abuse—Developmental Approaches to Intervention*, 1st ed., pp. 407–433. New York: Oxford University Press.

Tervalon, M., and Murray-Garcia, J. (1998). Cultural humility versus cultural competence: A critical distinction in defining physician training outcomes in multicultural education. *Journal of Health Care for the Poor and Underserved*, 9, 117–125.

Chapter 3

Patricia Berry

I remember when I was very young asking my mother if I had a father. I can't remember what she answered. I do remember a time she told me she was going to "give me back to the Indians." I was surprised and delighted. Could I secretly belong with a tribe of Indians dancing around with feathers and drums? When she realized I had taken her remark seriously, she laughed.

That was in Long Beach, California, where I was born, during the war. We lived in an upstairs apartment next to Seaside Hospital where my mother worked as a nurse. I remember hiding with my mother under a sheet on the bed, with a radio glowing, and my mother warning me to be quiet. An unknown plane, she said, which could be the enemy, was flying overhead. I knew we were in a war. It was a special time, in which my mother got little orange cards so she could buy shoes for me.

Sometimes I went to the hospital with her and rode around in the laundry cart. I went to a community nursery school down the street when it was open. I was proud to look both ways and cross the street all by myself. My mother always insisted I was bigger, stronger, and more able than other children my age. Instead of wasting time on a tricycle, she taught me to ride a small two-wheel bike right away.

Once traveling along a back road pressed against my mother in our Dodge coupe, she swerved and stopped abruptly by the road. A man had fallen out of the back of a pickup truck in front of us. She raced down the hill into the ditch beside the road and bent over the man. He was already dead.

I have never forgotten this event. My mother, the nurse, was without fear of life or death or of anything in between. It seemed. There is something about this, it occurs to me now, that sparked me into a person drawn to danger and depths, albeit for me, it was more legitimately the depths of a psychological and emotional sort.

When I was 4-1/2 we packed the Dodge coupe with our belongings and drove cross country back to the Midwest where my mother had been born and raised and attended high school. There, as we slept on cots in a back room at her brother's house, my mother reconnected with an old boyfriend, married him (I was the flower girl), and then disappeared with him for what seemed forever and ever. I never got over the shock of this abandonment. How could she? I also never called this man who became my stepfather by any name at all. Eventually I would not let him touch me (he was always trying to turn my mother against me) and by

DOI: 10.4324/9781003148968-4

no means would I let him or them speak of adopting me. I told kids my real father had died in the war.

To avoid embarrassment, my mother nevertheless enrolled me in school under my stepfather's surname, which was "Berry." Turns out the name on my birth certificate was Corcoran, Patricia Ann Corcoran. (John Norman Corcoran was a marine with whom my mother fell in love, left her post as a navy nurse, and married. He had been on assignment somewhere when I was born. I do have a picture of him holding me as a baby and his metals, and such, somewhere.

My mother spoke with school officials at each significant advancement point in my schooling and always somehow convinced them my chapters of adoption were just about to arrive. It seems she even managed to get me into college with this ruse. Eventually, when I needed an official U.S. passport to travel to Europe, she did make an appointment with a notary public and we finally managed to get my name legally changed.

Underneath, of course, I always had a sense that I was not legitimate, or not who I pretended to be. Although I had been a good student, active in student activities, had friends, and hung out with my teachers (some of whom kindly mentored me, bless them!), I knew I was different from my family somehow, I also knew I did not belong anywhere really. I graduated from university without bothering to attend my own graduation ceremony. Instead, I left for Zurich. I had just turned 23 and broken up with the boyfriend who had introduced me to Jung. He and I had planned to go to Zurich together, but he still had another semester to go before graduating. So I simply left, took off, more or less fleeing the relationship, the past, and hurtling myself forward towards something new—what, I didn't know.

During what ended up being 12 years in Zurich, I met interesting people, learned a great deal about cultures and lifestyles other than my own, participated in a supervision group with Toni Frey and other activities at the Klinic am Zurichberg. I worked with several different analysts and supervisors. My dreams as well as awarenesses changed during that period. A larger, more sophisticated picture of just about everything began to ripen within me and emerge. I had come to Zurich for analysis because Jung as I read him (bracketing out all the symbolic and cultural stuff) was closer than Freud was to the humanistic, existential psychologies I had experienced in the U.S. Here, however, in Zurich, strange symbols had begun to appear in my dreams. As I learned about these symbols, I realized I was indeed part of a larger interconnected world. I belonged as part of humanity. Such a realization was spiritual without being the result of any particular religion or practice. Something more universal had begun to claim me. I also loved working with others.

As I said earlier, I never forgot the event I had witnessed of my mother racing down into the ditch to help the man who had fallen and died.

Somehow this memory has helped me realize my mother's calling—who she was. Among the many other things she was—such as suffering and injured, limited, sometimes even violent—she also had served her life bravely. I feel as though I carry her inside me and that I have the space and capacity to do so easily. I am indeed stronger than she was. Unlike me, she focused more on physical than on psychological realities. Nonetheless, she was in many ways dependable, and patient in the concrete world in ways I am not. I have a different calling from hers and have had different opportunities and gifts. Nevertheless I feel, as I age, I hold her close and comfort her within me. As I serve my work, the things I love, I feel I also serve a bit of hers. I believe I understand her in ways I never could have when I was younger. I am grateful for that and that I can comfort her. I am glad to have her with me.

Rules of Thumb Toward an Archetypal Psychology Practice

Originally published in *Echo's Subtle Body: Contributions to an Archetypal Psychology* (Thompson, CT: Spring Publications, 2017). Reprinted with permission.

I am sometimes asked if I still consider myself an archetypal psychologist. The question astonishes me. How could I not? I was in at the base level before archetypal psychology was named "archetypal psychology"—first as student adept, later as *soror mystica*, leaning over the edge with those stirring this heady brew. Newts, lizards, our innards were all in the pot. Not only did I feel archetypal psychology was me, I was part it—in it for a toe or two, my whole head and lots of spit.

Yet it is true, in the last years I have not hung out much with the folks talking archetypal psychology. One of the reasons for my absence is that as archetypal discussion has become focused increasingly on ideas, I have become increasingly less so. I certainly honor ideation; theory is important. No school of anything would exist without it. But they are not for all of us—all the time. As I age, I become more often "hands on" about most things. This does not mean I don't think—only that when I do, the thoughts tend to translate into what is being created with the idea, rather than viewing the idea as a thing in itself. This practice of seeing ideas immediately in terms of what they create in a given instance is fun stuff for me. Is that still archetypal psychology? Well, you tell me. Perhaps it is just my archetypal psychology, one of the many archetypal psychologies. Whatever the case, in the following pages I will lay out something of how I have come to think. These are my rules of thumb for practice, as well as I can describe them just now.

Rule of Thumb #1 Any Idea Can Be Used Defensively

Here by "rule of thumb" I mean approximately, or more or less. To my mind, there are no "right" ideas, more or less. The "less" part is that some ideas truly are more useful, rich, interesting, promising, fruitful. But that doesn't mean they are right in any final sense—or wrong either, for that matter.

As a depth psychologist, my focus is on how the psyche works. One of the ways the psyche works, according to depth psychology, is by way of a fragile ego fending off what it perceives to be threats from within or without. To protect itself against these threats, the ego hauls from its arsenal all sorts of defensive weaponry.

Ideas are like the ramparts surrounding a castle. They are designed to keep other ideas from intruding. In times of peace they may give lovers a safe place to meet, wise men a space to converse above the treetops without interruption, a place for women to spin in the fresh air, and wizards to conjure under the stars. But in times of war, ramparts are used to hide behind while arrows fly and boulders are catapulted. So too with ideas. Ideas can nurture life, or they can serve as aggressive and defensive structures.

Rule of Thumb #2 If a Sacred Cow Is Blocking the Path, Shoo It Off

Depth psychology assumes a reality called the unconscious. The "un" part of the unconscious refers to that which is *not*—not conscious, unknown. Making the unconscious conscious, in the Freudian sense, or (in more modern Jungian terms) integrating unconscious contents and dynamics into more workable positions, adding resources, complexity, and richness to the personality—that is certainly a goal of depth psychological work. The means for accomplishing this work requires what Hillman called in his archetypal psychology "seeing through."

The method of depth psychology in general is something of a *via negativa*. By that I mean we more often shoo away what is blocking the path than claim to know what the path ought actually be. Nonetheless, there are some general values, although they may vary in emphasis depending upon the context, particular theory, and from practitioner to practitioner. Some values are the unknown, depth, resonance, complexity, interconnection, integration, richness, mastery. I am sure you can add others.

Values or value-laden concepts can provide orientation, but one must sense and consciously choose when one or another set of values is to be applied. When values are clung to, one tends to get lost in their glow such that one can no longer discern the more subtle, new, or, I would even say, real psychic events. When one or another value-laden feeling is embraced such that the ego hides behind it, then we may need to put aside the value itself, shoo it off the path, even if that value reeks of Truth, Soul, Psyche, Democracy, Identity, America. Whatever the treasured terms of the place or period, its self-righteousness—such values can and will be used to occlude more interesting, challenging, fecund psychological possibilities.

Rule of Thumb #3 Ideas Ought Not Be Applied

The problem with the notion of *praxis* (as in psychological praxis) is that we think of it as an application of theory. When we apply ideas to practical situations, they so easily result in misapplication of one sort or another. In fact, the first few times around, misuse is nearly a given. A new idea is like a new tool or toy one might try out in many places—most of which are not a fit. In my experience, few life situations are such that a single idea does them justice anyway.

My view is that it is best to work from a particular moment, event, context to whatever idea, not the other way round. (1) Begin with the living event, for archetypal psychology the "image," moment, patient, relationship; (2) focus on this image/event, sensing into it; (3) track bits of resonance that begin to form out of the event. Whether these resonances are well-known tropes, mythemes, or simply fragments does not matter. Eventually such bits will begin to create echoes in, through, and around the situation. Remember image is, most importantly, a *way* of seeing, sensing, feeling metaphorically—not simply or only what is perceived on the surface but not without it either.

Rule of Thumb #4 When Possible Think Poetically

For Aristotle, practicality, or praxis, leads to action, whereas making, or poeisis, leads to production. Aside from praxis as in a spiritual practice, which, to my mind, is right on the money, praxis, according to Hannah Arendt, lends itself to political thinking. Marx regarded his dialectical materialism as praxis.

Sometimes, however, one is more about making—simply making—than about anything political. When that is the case, as it almost always is for me, the fantasy of making, creating—just the activity for the sake of itself—is quite appealing. For me, "making" psychological moves, interpretations, interventions, reflections, and moments feels more fitting than any other description for what I am about.

Rule of Thumb #5 Go Connatural

Connatural is a term coined by the Catholic theologian Jacque Maritain. Maritain was interested in the interrelation between artistic processes and the processes of nature. In his view, the task of the artist or craftsman is to align mimetically with "nature's secret workings and inner ways" (Maritain, 1953, 1977). He saw artistic activity, when working properly, as attempting to parallel nature's processes. Human creativity is like nature's creativity. The task is to work *con*-naturally *with* nature—to sense nature's operations, feel them metaphorically, see them, hear them. The attempt to look deeply into natural psychological processes, and attune with and around, is what depth psychological work intends.

Rule of Thumb #6 *Symbols Are Not Symbols of Anything but Symbolic With Many Things*

Islamic scholar Henry Corbin characterized symbols as "symbolizing with" rather than "symbolic to" their referents (Corbin, 1960, 1972). The distinction is important in that no one symbol, image, or level of psychological reality is regarded as *necessarily* prior to or more important than another. The kind of making implied here would develop by way of similarities, reverberations, and improvisations mimetic with, or paralleling, natural movements and processes. In that same spirit, rather like the spirit of Maritain's connaturality, our depth psychological work proceeds with an ear to the ground of nature's reverberations, both natural and symbolic (Berry, 1982, 2008).

Rule of Thumb #7 Stick to the Image

Ok, so this is an old rule. We all know it. I have always attributed it to Rafael Lopez-Pedraza, since he was the guy I heard it from repeatedly (Hillman would then chime in with his descant "save the phenomena"). At this point in my life, my sense may have wandered a bit from Rafael's and Jim's. Today I regard Image as a far more supple notion than I once did. One way to understand its flexibility is to talk about framing.

Rule of Thumb #8 To Know It Is to Frame It

Please, let me be clear. I am not saying things exist only because of their framing. I am saying that frames organize what we see. Organized well, what we see can become fresh, even breathtaking. The way in which a picture is framed becomes part of its effect and meaning. The frame of the window over my desk gives a particular view of the California hills outside. When I frame a picture in my camera viewfinder, I am positioning the view in such a way as to enable something revelatory to come forth. In a moving image, many frames rushing one after another become the film that an editor then cuts and shapes—that is, frames—into the final film. The purpose of framing is to put limits on the view so that what is within those limits can be focused on with greater clarity and freshness.

How we frame a story we tell to a friend or a case presentation to colleagues has to do with what we want to show (and perhaps how we want it and ourselves to be seen). How we frame something also conditions how others approach it, what they get from it, and what activities generate around it. This is not as obvious as it may seem. In a case colloquium, for example, someone presents a situation with a client with whom they are having difficulty. Generally speaking, what astute participants in the group will also hear is not only what the presenter "meant" for them to hear but also what the presenter has not presented and perhaps has not been aware of.

I consider the image here to be both what the presenter presented and what others heard—that is, the unconscious workings behind the presentation and evoked by it. The conscious framing was the framing of the presentation, but that framing also brought other thoughts through the cracks, other insights, and other points of view into the discussion, which widened the intended frame to a larger and different one. As that occurs, the image changes.

If the practitioner had presented the story differently, what the participants perceived would also have been different. Let's say the practitioner had framed the narrative, beginning and end, with a statement about how frustrating this deeply disturbed patient is. The group may then have tended to work on the case noting how the patient's disturbance (diagnosis) had affected the analyst and resulting transference/countertransference dynamics. My point is that situations framed differently become different and ask for different approaches. The comments as well as the dynamics of the group are affected.

Sometimes image situations are framed too small. When too little context is given a situation, working with it tends to get loose, projective, less fitting, and less meaningful. On the other hand, sometimes psychological events get framed so large that it is difficult to work with them using anything but broad, sweeping strokes.

On occasion these large strokes are exactly what you want, as, for example, when working with issues on a cultural or a sociopolitical level. Within these broader, more general contexts, particular and precise image work of an intrapsychic sort becomes sometimes impossible. Overall, what is most important is to be sensitive to *how each framing* is affecting the narrative. Ideally, one wants the depth, latitude, and awareness able to move adroitly among forms. That way one can choose which is most appropriate or helpful at a particular moment.

Rule of Thumb #9 *The Observer and Observed May or May Not Be the Same*

Our perceptual convention is to experience ourselves when we observe—for example, the participants observing a case presentation (as we discussed earlier) as separate from what they are observing. However, we know from contemporary physics, botanical, biological, ecological, and other studies nowadays, how thoroughly we are, in one way or another, implicated in what we observe. However, on a practical level, the positions we assume vis-à-vis "other"—whatever "other" is (dream, client, colleagues, world) varies considerably.

Thus, how we choose perspectives makes a difference. With a client's dream, say, some therapists will work so close to the imaginary aspect of the dream such that they experience its energies in their own bodies. They likely then will give priority to working with the dream using their own experiences, musings, and imaginings as well.

Other analysts prefer to assume a more formal position with the patient and the material, as did Jung and the early Jungians. This can work too—depending on the analyst's skill and ability to connect deeply with the emotional workings of the patient. Again, however, one must be as mindful as possible about the position one is assuming and why. No position is the only true or correct one. So much depends on the secret alchemy between patient and analyst as well as their ability to work effectively with it.

Rule of Thumb #10 Contrast: It's a Setup

Not surprisingly, I find archetypal psychology's notion of multiplicity to be not only a larger, more generous, and more inclusive umbrella, but also a more interesting attitude than, for example, dualism. Yet, at times, one does want to set up strong contrasts. On such occasions one can certainly sound "either/or" dualistic, as to my ear Hillman sometimes does.

But since he explicitly claimed his work to rest on a "poetic basis of mind," let's give him a break. Let's view his more argumentative constructions as ways of making his points stand out most clearly. Imagine a painting with a dark background and white figures in the foreground. The white figures stand out because of the contrasting background. When archetypal psychology sets up oppositions, it is useful to view such oppositions as contrasts rather than literal exclusions. Think of some of archetypal psychology's oppositions: underworld versus day world (Hillman, 1979), imaginal versus heroic ego, world versus consulting room, and (my favorite) psychological versus literal. The good guys are set up at one end of the opposition and the bad guys at the other, good guys foreground, bad guys background.

Aesthetically speaking, these "either/or" exclusions create contrasts to make a point. But let's not forget, these bad guys are merely straw men hauled in to be railed against. In drama, straw men caricatures act as foils for the more complex principal characters. Some dramatists maintain that collective taste requires these figures. Maybe so, but as psychologists we need to remember that it is a setup.

Rule of Thumb #11 Steal Tools When Necessary

Hillman characterized his psychological method as like that of a *bricoleur* (an inventive do-it-yourselfer). I'd say mine is like a thief, though a good thief and for good reasons, I hope. Although archetypal psychology distinguishes itself philosophically from widespread collective psychologies that mix behaviorism, cognitive psychology, counseling psychology, and so on, nonetheless as a practitioner one might on occasion lift a tool or two from their toolboxes.

On occasion those boxes may indeed contain something useful, if not downright essential. The tool may be one that allows us to focus on behavior as such, or to advocate change in behavior before even understanding what the behavior is about. This may sound most unlike depth psychology, but it is sometimes necessary—as in situations of abuse or addiction. Since there are nearly as many explanations for events as there are psychological perspectives for viewing them, sometimes a simple negative reinforcement (such as terminating therapy or not seeing a patient until they are sober) is the way to go.

If we take seriously the Maritain/Corbin image of parallel processes, then perhaps imaginal change can begin with behavioral change as well as the other way round. Sometimes grabbing the stick by the other end is advantageous. It seems to me it is not other psychologies (such as addiction counseling) that are reductive, material, and literal—it is *we who are, whenever we view them with less than a psychological eye.*

If we stand on psychic ground, *in media res*, maintaining our awareness from that position, what we do will be psychologically based. It is a matter of awareness. When we are psychologically aware, our means will be metaphorical and our tools reflective.

Rule of Thumb #12 Don't Take the Literal Literally

Earlier I said that the literal versus the psychological was my favorite opposition. But, you know, one ought not take even the literal so literally. To do so is to become way too literal. That literal voice, insisting on "nothing but," is just one of the many voices in the chorus. Sometimes it is useful for belting out strong, sure tones, but the point is to hear it as one voice—rather than the whole-truth, nothing-but-the-truth it pretends to be.

Rule of Thumb #13 Truth or Daimon

Sometimes I think of truth imagistically, as in a clear, true tone or the "true line" a carpenter might determine, a navigator reckon, or a Zen master draw in the sand. True, as in *authenticity*, is for me a very high value, but I try not to capitalize or even make a substantial noun of the word, such as Truth. In terms of an individual psyche, I think of true as central to the notion of individuation. This old-fashioned Jungian term is vague, subjective, and interior enough to work for me. Some might speak of following one's daimon as guide rather than Jung's notion of individuation, but daimon*es* are by nature flashy. Besides daimon*es* are also demons, and so easy to identify with! So, too, notions like "psyche" or "soul" as personifications don't work for me as they once did. In the beginning of archetypal psychology these words were truly alive, earth-shaking, electrifying, daring as heck. Now they are clichés in the titles of half the books on the self-help shelf. Is the notion (psyche, soul) true? Sure. But it is hard nowadays to inspire in someone like me much feeling of authenticity simply by using those words.

I tend to orient myself with more practical aesthetic notions like "what works." What "works" as a novel, film, painting, or piece of music is determined by the piece itself. Each piece sets up its own criteria. In this way the work is measured against itself and within its own genre—sort of like what individuation implies in personal psychology, where the unique nature of the person is the goal.

Rule of Thumb #14 Layard's Rule

I tend to view dreams through Layard's rule (Berry, 1982, 2008). I may not always share this vision with my client. But I sometimes do, because it is in fact how I see things. John Layard was an English anthropologist and a first-generation Jungian analyst. Hillman admired him greatly and passed along his maxim to me some 50 years ago, crediting it to Layard. This rule of thumb has over the years served me, as well as several generations of my own students. It is my favorite tool, although the hardest to use appropriately.

The rule goes like this: "Everything in the dream is right except perhaps the dream ego." The purpose of this rule of thumb is to shift focus beyond the dream ego. Its use deliteralizes the usual, ego point of view, enabling an ability to look at the dream from the other side.

As with any other rule of thumb, this one applies only loosely and sometimes not at all. Always it is, I think, a helpful perspective for practitioners themselves in deepening their own awareness of other possibilities. It is *not* always the right tool for the therapy. In some cases—for example, when support or stabilization is a priority—moving against the ego perspective is not smart therapeutically. In such situations, Layard's rule is not the right tool. Pick up another. As with any other rule, this one merely one of many in the toolbox.

As an example, let's look at the following dream:

> *I go into my bathroom. My dog, Corky, is lying underwater in the bathtub. I am horrified, knowing he is going to drown. He looks up at me as though nothing were wrong.*

I know nothing about the woman who dreamt this dream—her situation in life, her complexes, where she is in her analytic process—nothing. But that does not mean I cannot get something from the dream.

From a naturalistic perspective (the usual ego perspective), the dog seems as though he is going to drown, and that feels terrible to the dreamer and to us as observers. To apply the Layard rule, however (here, an underwater as well as "underworld" perspective), we bracket out the ego's feeling and look to the dog. Corky acts as though nothing is wrong. Perhaps this is an underwater dog, able to survive under water. Or perhaps he is going to dissolve into the alchemical solution, and that is part of a necessary process here. Psychologically everything is as it should be.

This point of view would seem horrific to an ego or humanistic psychologist. For one thing, the situation is not normal. Dogs are not naturally under water. Thus there is something wrong with this woman's "dog." Her dog instinct is unaware, self-destructive. Another reason the dream would not sit well is that in humanistic psychology, it is the human that is most highly valued. Human perspectives and values are identified with and taken literally.

To flip things such that we are looking from the dog's perspective, trusting the animal over the human viewpoint, can lead us into awarenesses that other, more usual perspectives do not allow. The Layard perspective deepens and enriches our understanding. If everything is right except the dream ego, it is "right" that the dog does whatever it does in the dream. Perhaps the dog is like an old instinct, effective for many years in sniffing out what was what, but no longer needed to sniff in the same way. Perhaps a new dog with fresh senses is in order.

Rule of Thumb #15 Listen to Your Friends. Love Your Teacher

I regularly lead seminars for students in the final stages of depth psychological study. The drill is that each student takes several hours during the weekend to talk about their work with a client.

As the participants interact around the images and processes that arise, I am astonished at how well they have come to understand one another. Of course each arrives at the weekend with particular perspectives and favorite theories. They may not always agree, but eventually they all come to appreciate one another, to understand what is being said and where it is coming from. They listen to one another.

And to me.

Do they know I am an archetypal psychologist? Do they know my background? I don't know. If they do know, it is certainly not in any detail. Yet they are doing what I consider to be archetypal psychology. They are focusing carefully on what appears as image, aware of their framing, the lenses they use. They bracket causal explanations and appreciate mimetic resonances. They have learned to steal. They make inventive use of available resources (the "bricoleur!"). To one degree or another each has an eye for some "true" line. They recite Layard's Rule like a mantra. Is this archetypal psychology? Well, it is certainly one form of it.

In ending I must say, thank you, Jim Hillman. Those years in the mix with you were fundamental to my learning, glorious in reach and spread and lift, beyond inspiration. It was an extraordinary time. I remain deeply and forever grateful to you, my teacher.

References

Berry, Patricia. (2008a). Defense and telos in dreams. In *Echo's Subtle Body: Contributions to an Archetypal Psychology*, p. 83. Dallas: Spring Publications, 1982.

Berry, Patricia. (2008b). An approach to the dream. In *Echo's Subtle Body: Contributions to an Archetypal Psychology,* p. 57f. Dallas: Spring Publications, 1982.

Corbin, Henri. (1960). *Avicenna and the Visionary Recital*, p. 261. Willard R. Trask (Trans.). New York: Pantheon (cf. also p. 31 and "Mundus Imaginalis, of the Imaginary and the Imaginal," trans. Ruth Horine, Spring 1972, p. 9].

Hillman, James. (1979). *The Dream and the Underworld*, p. 127f. New York: Harper & Row.

Maritain, Jacques. (1953). *Creative Intuition in Art and Poetry*. Rpt. Princeton: Princeton University Press, 2008 [1977], p. 127.

Chapter 4

Fanny Brewster

I first came to Jungian psychology through a wish to study dreams and the dreaming life. My dreams had been influential from an early age. When I decided to change my profession from that of a speech-language pathologist to one of psychologist, I wanted the focus to be about dream work as an essential aspect of soul, consciousness and creating change in my life and that of others. I arrived at Pacifica Graduate Institute to study dreams, which I did, and left with a Ph.D. in clinical psychology. My engagement with dreams was equal to my interest in writing—poetry as well as nonfiction. An underpinning of my interest in dreams has been spirituality and seeking to find ways to deepen my understanding for not only human behavior but also the more important unconscious dynamics of being. The path for this was ever changing, grew larger at times, and in some instances seem to just disappear. Those periods of darkness were lit by my dreams. They guided me. On the journey I have studied writing, obtaining an M.F.A. degree in creative nonfiction, studied the enneagram with Helen Palmer and worked in public schools as an educational psychologist. My inner work has led to Zen Buddhist practice as well as the Church of Religious Science. Each of these experiences and more have deepened me as a Jungian analyst. My most recent writings, including *The Racial Complex: A Jungian Perspective on Culture and Race*, have provided me with a psychological lens that hopes to better understand our consciousness regarding race, racism and the deconstruction of ideas that support us in embracing the fullness of ourselves as both human and divine. I'm intrigued by how we do this as individuals and how we can invoke this through our passionate engagement with each other in our collective.

DOI: 10.4324/9781003148968-5

The Racial Complex

Dissociation and the Search for Unification With the Self

An earlier version of this essay first appeared in the *Racial Complex: A Jungian Perspective on Culture and* Race (Routledge, 2019). Reprinted with permission.

A Review of the Complex Theory

In *The Structure and Dynamics of the Psyche*, Jung (1928/1969) wrote the following in his description of the complexes:

> Today we can take it as moderately certain that complexes are in fact "splinter psyches." The aetiology of their origin is frequently a so-called trauma, an emotional shock or some such thing, that splits off a bit of the psyche. Certainly, one of the commonest causes in a moral conflict, which ultimately derives from the apparent impossibility of affirming the whole of one's nature.
>
> (para. 204, p. 98)

We understand from Jung's definition of the complexes as just described that the complexes were originally a part of the psyche as a whole. Due to what Jung labels "so-called" trauma, we develop what eventually become complexes. It is important to note that he says the complexes are most likely caused by a moral conflict that keeps us from having a sense of wholeness. This is similar to what Edward Edinger references in his writing, *The Ego and the Archetype* (1992). I think it brings together our understanding of how complexes—actual traumatized aspects of our psyche—cause a disconnection with the archetype of the Self. It is only through the conscious affirmative working of an alienated ego, burdened with psychological complex issues, that the archetypal aspect of psyche can appear seeking balance. I would call this, as Jung did, the archetype of the Self.

We have a better understanding of complexes, as depth psychologists have studied these for more than 100 years since first Pierre Janet, then Freud and later Jung helped us look into the Unconscious. Our attempts to understand our human nature and the Unconscious, I believe, lead us into that place Jung called Shadow.

Today, as our understanding of Jungian psychology has grown, we also have a greater understanding of the Shadow as archetype functioning within us on an individual as well as a collective level. I believe that our complexes hide behind Shadow until they choose to no longer remain hidden. Jung (1928) himself says, "The complex can usually be suppressed with an effort of will, but not argued out of existence, and at the first suitable opportunity it reappears in all its original strength (v. 8, para. 201, p. 96)."

Jung (1928) says that the complexes play "impish tricks." These are some of the examples he provides in this chapter on the complexes in paragraph 202:

> They slip just the wrong word into one's mouth, they make one forget the name of the person one is about to introduce, they cause a tickle in the throat just when the softest passage is being played on the piano at a concert, they make the tiptoeing latecomer trip over a chair with a resounding crash. They bid us congratulate the mourners at a burial instead of condoling with them, they are the instigators of all those maddening things.
>
> (v. 8, para. 202, p. 98)

Jung (1928) states, "unconsciousness helps the complex to assimilate even the ego," resulting in "a momentary and unconscious alteration of personality known as identification with the complex (v. 8, para. 204, p. 98)." He later says that this identification was spoken of as possession during the Middle Ages—being driven mad by the devil or "hag-ridden."

I was drawn to Jung's very limited mention of what I have termed racial complexes through his comment in the *Collected Works*, v. 10, paragraph 963, in which he said the following:

> Just as the coloured man lives in your cities and even within your houses, so also he lives under your skin, subconsciously. Naturally it works both ways. Just as every Jew has a Christ complex, so every Negro has a white complex and every American (white) a Negro complex.

At the time of these words Jung had begun writing about America's ethnic situation—the differences between whites and blacks. Though he did not say very much, he emphasized the negative results from the influence of the "primitive" on white American society. His focus was mostly on skin color differences, intellectual functioning and levels of consciousness. I think that our American Jungian society has been uncomfortable with Jung's words from the 1930s; these words with their negative racial commentaries generally about the African diaspora and specifically about Africans. As a result, I believe that we African Americans have developed, like the larger Collective, a racial complex. In discussing how Freud became the discoverer of the unconscious, Jung (1928) addresses the issue of complexes. He says:

> The via regia to the unconscious, however is not the dream, as he thought, but the complex which is the architect of dreams and of symptoms. Nor is this via so very "royal", either, since the way pointed out by the complex is more like a rough and uncommonly devious footpath that often loses itself in the undergrowth and generally leads not into the heart of the unconscious but past it.
>
> (v. 8, para. 210, p. 101)

I like this idea and image of the complex as a devious footpath because it suits very well my idea regarding a racial complex. I would like to return to Shadow for a moment—the place where we hide in the "undergrowth" all the things we cannot tolerate seeing—and say that I think our racial complexes also can live in that dark place of shadow. African Americans, I believe, have known more consciously regarding this fact because of being at the negative symptomatic end of the racial complex. The very convoluted racial relations in America have been well documented, while there is still so much more to tell. Within the last 150 years, we have intensely begun to open up Pandora's Box regarding ethnic issues and racism in America.

Actually, today I believe we have more of a dialogue than ever before. But if we are to believe Jung, these conversations will not eliminate our racial complexes, and I agree with Jung. One important circumstance is that as psychic material from the unconscious, complexes develop and have a free will of their own. I think the only control we can exercise on these autonomous split-off parts of psyche is first learning about them and unveiling them further through Shadow work and ego strengthening. Jung believed that it was through the analytical relationship and the transference that complexes could be addressed. My immediate question was: what happens when one is not engaged in a therapeutic relationship? How are complexes then remediated? We can perhaps speak more of this in terms of promoting healing of racial complexes later in our discussion.

Trauma and Dissociative Cultural Trauma

What exactly are our racial complexes? As an African American, I have a white American complex—or so Jung believed. How does it haunt me? When I was a child, my grandmother used to talk about haunts riding people and the things one needed to do in order to *not* incur the wrath of haunts or spirits. She also used to speak about the healing remedy for getting rid of haunts. Let's say my racial complex, with its white complex haunting me, lives in my unconscious self. How might I be uncomfortable in my own skin, certainly with my black-skinned identity? How does my ethnicity cause me a repetitive experience of the psychological trauma of identity tied to race as an individual, as well as tied to my American group identity?

Growing up African American means that there are racial lessons to be learned at a very early age. The lesson of skin color differences brings with it the sociological and psychological wounds and trauma of racism. This is a fact of living in America. It is a personal experience as well as a known part of our American history.

The hiding of racial complexes has contributed to the wounding of the American psyche in terms of how physical and psychological pain has been inflicted, because of a constructed idea, regarding differences due to ethnic lineage.

Collective cultural trauma shows itself as having a cultural racial complex that has been formed and nurtured by slavery and survived through decades because of the racist aspects of American life. Jung's idea of the theory of Opposites has done much, in probably an unintended way, to promote American racism. Sam Kimble, author of *Phantom Narratives* (2014), has spoken eloquently regarding the racial issues inherent in groups that have their own cultural rituals and rites of passage.

One landmark critical event in early America was the passage of Africans to the Americas as slaves. This event, I believe, remains a very uncomfortable topic for many Americans, even though we have not even begun to fully bear witness to the psychological trauma still being experienced by the descendants of those slaves. Slavery was a holocaust event that lasted for centuries. Unfortunately, we continue to live out this event via our fears through racial complexes expressed many times through unconscious racist actions. Jung (1928) says, "Complexes are something so unpleasant that nobody in his right senses can be persuaded that the motive forces which maintain them could betoken *anything* good (v. 8, para. 211, p. 101)." There is no wonder we have avoided within our own area of Jungian psychology a deep discussion of racial complexes.

Archetype of the Self

In his autobiography, *Memories, Dreams, Reflections* (1961/1993), Jung wrote the following from Chapter 6, entitled "Confrontation with the Unconscious."

> During those years, between 1918 and 1920, I began to understand that the goal of psychic development is the self. There is no linear evolution, there is only a circumambulation of the self. Uniform development exists, at most, only at the beginning; later, everything points toward the center. This insight gave me stability, and gradually my inner peace returned. I knew that in finding the mandala as an expression of the self I had attained what was for me the ultimate. Perhaps someone else knows more, but not I.

Jung concludes this chapter with a dream that came to him years later in 1927. I think of it as his *Liverpool Dream* because the location of the dream is Liverpool. He describes the city as dark and "sooty." However, in the distance, Jung sees a small island on which grows one magnolia tree in a "shower of reddish blossoms." He recognized this image as an expression of the symbol of his own life's work. He understood, by this dream, that he had achieved the goal of his deepest yearnings of self-exploration and the search of his life's meaning.

Jung speaks further of the dream, referencing his breakup with Freud that began a period of dissociation, psychic experiences and numinous encounters that later developed into the Red Book. In *Memories, Dreams, Reflections* (1961/1993), we hear of how Jung conceived of this dream of the Self as an "act of grace." Jung believed that the Self archetype provides the direction we require to make order out of what oftentimes can be total emotional chaos. Jung says, "After this dream I gave up drawing or painting mandalas. The dream depicted the climax of the whole process of development of consciousness."

"It satisfied me completely . . . the clarification brought about by the dream made it possible for me to take an objective view of the things that filled my being" (*MDR*, p. 199). The development of the Self within each of us begins before life and carries us through a lifetime. There is no bias or prejudice in how elements of the life are chosen—the Self does not discriminate on the side of good or bad. Choices are made almost as if with the toss of a coin—that is until we awaken and choose consciousness, to be awake to the demands of the ego and the necessary mediation of Shadow in relationship to the ego. The Self pushes towards individuation, and in this push can gain support from both ego and the unconscious.

When we are in a disjointed relationship with the Self, we are generally in a place of disease and *dis-ease* with ourselves. We can also call this a dissociated state. This is not the disease of pathology but rather the uncomfortable egoic life of the Self moving, pulling us towards a mandala psychic center and therefore psychological balance. The event that brings us into therapy and analysis is not generally because we are feeling happy, so great that we want to visit a therapist. We show up in distress, thrown into suffering by an intensification of neurosis, complexes or an archetypal possession. The autonomous nature of the elements of our psyche can drive us to distraction. It does feel like a possession—something our ego cannot control and as Jung states most often want to forget, to repress.

Though Jung at different periods refused to allow for the religiosity of the Self archetype, Edward Edinger in *Ego and Archetype* (1992) develops the idea of the significance of the spiritual nature of the Self. His text focuses on the relationship between the psychological role of the ego and the divine role of the archetype. Through detailed descriptions, Edinger provides words and images of this necessary relationship and how crucial it is for human inner peace, recognition of emotional struggles and for creating a path—individuation—in the lifetime. Edinger has given us a way to envision our lives because of an engagement with the Self archetype. He writes that without this conscious engagement we fall into alienation from ourselves—dissociation, or an inflation of ego that does not allow for an integrative human context for truly living. Edinger's writing expands our understanding of the importance and vitality of that something—that Self within us that Jung first spoke of and how its acknowledgment is required in order to deepen consciousness.

Dissociation in the s/Self Relationship

Identity is crucial to our psychological health and well-being. We understand that from the very beginning of our biological and I would say psychic lives, including the DNA of the archetypes, we need recognition in the form of identity. Due to the issue of racial relations in America, we are taught early on about ethnic differences. Jung pointed to something that was present in our shadowed Collective unconscious that was and continues to be acted out through negative racial acts. I believe that when we cannot recognize or see ourselves because of a complex taking over ego consciousness, then we are limited in developing a healthy connection between our ego selves and the archetypal Self.

The constellation of the complex creates a psychic disturbance that touches ego functioning. An internal repetitive traumatic moment repeats itself—repetition compulsion—and eventually shows itself in our behaviors. This dissociation in the s/Self relationship, in the situation I am referencing, belongs originally to the traumatic holocaust event of slavery and all that has followed in terms of racial identity problems—individually on a psychological level and within the American Collective. We have seen the struggle to find the "right" identity for African Americans, first called African, then colored. Nigger emerged and has re-emerged, then black—the negative one and the one of beauty of the 1960s. Finally we have arrived at African American. Our cultural collective has struggled with finding its identity in terms of how we will and must be treated because of skin color differences and all that goes along with the cultural meaning of such a circumstance.

The psychological trauma of being Other has its impact on people of color. We can be Other, but a part of our consciousness makes the Other—the white person also Other. One of the aspects of white privilege is that it perceives itself as the only one that can confer qualities. In the case of African Americans these qualities, both consciously and unconsciously, in the Shadow would have us be primitive and not rational minded or reasonable human beings. We would be unintelligent and slow to learn. I believe that these beliefs come from our racial complexes that have lived minimally explored, within Shadow, for many centuries since the arrival of slaves in the 1600s.

The cultural collective that is African American has been bound not just by the act of physically being bound for centuries, but also the psychological suffering of being individuals held within a racist societal structure. This structure has controlled and promoted through conscious habits the educational, financial and emotional deprivation of this cultural collective. Ironically enough, the projection onto this cultural collective is that we have created our own deprivation through a lack of something—be it intelligence or a higher level of consciousness. I believe that this external imposition of a negative racial construct has supported the development of a negative racial complex within individuals and in group psychic consciousness. I think that lynching and development of groups such as the KKK are examples of this type of a negative group consciousness—a cultural complex that erupts into American society.

Jung has stated that complexes are split-off parts of psychic material originally caused by trauma. I have considered a specific complex, that of the racial complex partly because it has not been discussed in any manner within Jungian psychology with the exception of Jung's reference to it in 1930. I would not look to Freudians or other American psychology groups to open up a dialogue on one of Jung's theories, and I feel that it is left to us as Jungians to begin these conversations. Secondarily, I have considered a discussion of the racial complex because I believe we are caught in this complex, in a constant struggle attempting to forget about its existence. The pain of such a complex has left us no peace.

The very real suffering of racial discrimination and even physical death due to one's identity can cause severe emotional trauma on an individual and a cultural level. It can feel like the never-ending wave of a tsunami because thus far it has not come to an end. The days of mass lynching of African Americans have passed. However, the words: alt-right, states' rights, voter suppression and white nationalists in the White House all date back to a time when physical trauma was a very real event.

I believe that each African American has not only the Collective fear of such events held in psyche but also the individual anxiety at the not unrealistic possibility of being harmed due to skin color.

As I stated earlier, I think there has been a reluctance to discuss a racial complex in our Jungian collective. Jung himself predicts that this could happen due to the very "devilish" nature of complexes—they appear to be adequately suppressed by the ego only to come back stronger. Jung identified the Germanic cultural complex that could be seen in the rise of Nazism leading to the Second World War. This rise of a group of people who participated in the murder of millions showed a distinct manner in which complexes can take hold of us. Individuals made up the armies, medical staff and military administrators that formed Hitler's Nazi Party. The trauma victims of this persecution were also individuals. Sometimes, I think we can lose sight of the importance of the individual—not just in terms of a process of individuation, which the Self promotes, but also when dealing with complexes—concerning the suffering that can occur. The numbers of those who have been tortured or murdered are so great that it is difficult to comprehend and stay within our own ego's place of comfort. Denial seems very necessary.

When we are haunted by complexes we lack not only comfort but also peace of mind. The trauma of racism and its effects does not disappear but accompanies one on a daily basis. I propose that any racial complex of African Americans will be closely "identified" with this type of trauma-racism. How can we create less pain originally caused by an initial traumatic event such as slavery?

I believe that we must first open ourselves to conversations about historical Collective trauma and intergenerational psychic pain lived out in everyday contemporary life and experienced as complexes. The reoccurring trauma experienced as a racial complex moves in relationship with the Self. I propose that this relationship creates anxiety and a fear specific to the trauma that initially caused such a complex to develop.

The tension and anticipatory anxiety caused by issues of racial identity, discrimination and fear of physical harm could only intensify psychic pain and a separation or dissonance with the Self.

Healing Racial Complexes/Connecting With the Self

Complexes do not go away. We bring them into consciousness out of the Shadow. We make the unconscious conscious. This is our healing work. In the comprehension of Jungian theories, it is incumbent upon us to explore, discuss and examine those things that continue to haunt us. This is our healing. To me this is the true work of being Jungian. I believe myself and others like me follow in

Jung's footsteps when we pick up the slender threads of his beautifully woven tapestry and begin to create a different textile with a familiar pattern. I think about the development of ideas regarding racial complexes as being in alignment with this proposition. How do we begin to think about healing these places of psychic pain—of long-standing psychological suffering? I think the beauty of analytical psychology is that it usually provides the answer to our suffering. The remedy is in the poison!

The path will usually be in the form of a labyrinth—it will of course not be easy. The acceptance of this fact and both the painful realization of the complex and the divinity of the Self continue to offer hope.

References

Brewster, F. (2019). *The Racial Complex: A Jungian Perspective on Culture and Race*. New York and London: Routledge.

Edinger, E. (1992). *Ego and Archetype* (C.G. Jung Foundation Book Series). Boston: Shambhala.

Jung, C. G. (1928/1969). The structure and dynamics of the psyche. In *Collected Works*, 2nd ed., vol. 8. Princeton, NJ: Princeton University Press.

Jung, C. G. (1930/1968). Civilization in transition. In *Collected Works*, vol. 10. Princeton, NJ: Princeton University Press.

Jung, C. G. (1961/1993). *Memories, Dreams, Reflections*, 13th ed. New York: Random House.

Kimbles, S. (2014). *Phantom Narratives: The Unseen Contributions of Culture to Psyche*. Lanham, MD: Rowman & Littlefield Publishers.

Chapter 5

Joseph Cambray

In a reflective glance over my life's course, a set of interweaving threads suggest a set of inflection points marked by relocations at key times; in short, a becoming that remains in flux. Practically from birth, I've lived in a series of punctuated equilibria: settling into what initially seemed permanent locations, which subsequently proved to be more ephemeral as larger forces propelled me onto the next destination. My family moved four times before I had gone to school, then we built a house and lived there until we outgrew it by the time I began high school. These early, formative experiences hold the seeds of symbolic life and underscore the seeking of a sense of home and self.

During a period in middle childhood I had an illness that required decreased overt activity. While frustrating for a boy, it created a slowing down that served as the entrance into the world of myth through reading and introversion. Chief among the narratives I discovered was the tale of Odysseus—that wanderer in a post-war world, seeking a passage home and undergoing numerous adventures and trials in the attempt to arrive there. The illness spontaneously remitted, curiously after I completed a tour of books on world myths—retrospectively it seems my first orientation in the preparation for becoming an analyst, through this intersection of psyche, soma, pathology and myth.

After emerging from this initiatory period, I moved towards science and the world of "knowing." My natural inclinations led me to chemistry with its secrets on the behaviour of matter, especially how transformations between substances occur. Refining this knowledge throughout my undergraduate career led me towards theories seeking root causes. However, in addition the human sciences, especially anthropology and psychology, increasing drew my attention, so that I graduated with a major in chemistry and a minor in psychology, along with a brief opportunity to undergo a bit of psychoanalysis.

Graduate school took me across the US and deepened my burgeoning interests, in particular quantum theory as applied to small organometallic systems. This occurred at a time when computer graphics were beginning and so I spent much time generating and puzzling over electron density maps. Visualizing fields of force and energy became a fascination and a basis for future endeavours in analytic theory and practice. During this period, I also intensified my reading of the

DOI: 10.4324/9781003148968-6

history of science, including early chemistry, and explored its roots in alchemy. By this time, I had read *Memories, Dreams, and Reflections* and saw the film *The Wisdom of the Dream*, so my interest in Jung began to add a historical reflection onto my areas of interest and touched into my personal psychology.

As a post-doctoral fellow these parallel tracks deepened with applications of chemical model of complex biochemical catalysts containing metals ion at the active site. Simultaneously I read Jung's *Psychology and Alchemy*. Intuiting that I was reaching another inflection point, I took a position as a visiting faculty at a Japanese university where I continued research on biochemically transformative metal ion–containing catalysts, while also exploring Zen meditation. The practice of Zen was quite psychoactive and a wealth of dreams emerged, sending me after several years back to the US.

In transition, I both taught science at several universities and pursued personal Jungian analysis. Ever the itinerary seeker, I travelled the US on analytic adventures and ultimately decided to retrain in psychology with an emphasis on becoming a psychotherapist. This quickly led to the further step of Jungian analytic training. Perhaps not surprisingly, this entailed several relocations and developing a new set of rewarding relationships.

As I settled into analytic practice, national and international opportunities arose. I thoroughly enjoyed the widening community of like-minded souls. While the scholarly side of my life had been more in the background through clinically focused training and establishing a practice, it now resurfaced. Soon this brought involvement with the *Journal of Analytical Psychology*, and I enthusiastically took on editorial tasks and responsibility. Holding conferences in my role as US editor opened new doors and brought further enriching friendships; it felt as if I were much closer to my psychological home now. Hence, my involvement with the IAAP flowed from these roots, and the administrative part of my psyche strengthened in unanticipated ways as it resonated with history and mission of the organization.

Nevertheless, during these years I was struggling with constructing a bridge between my careers. Fortunately, as I reengaged in scholarly life, the field of complexity science had recently been developed. There were some key writings that linked it to depth psychology, and I turned to them when I had a cluster of severely traumatized clients whose analyses were marked by curious anomalous events, what Jung would have referred to as synchronicities. By careful reading of Jung's primary essays on the topic, I was able to envision a contemporary way to express the insights offered by his concept, now amplified through the lens of complexity. This has proven personally rich and rewarding and has kept me in dialogue with many dear friends and colleagues. I also sought ways to apply the concepts to systems of management of organizations, starting with the leadership of the IAAP. Complexity allowed a vision of cultivation of collective wisdom, that is, how knowledgeable, skilful colleagues when working in concert could as a group manifest levels of understanding and wisdom beyond the capacity of any one individual. Helping facilitate such group activities has fulfilled many hopes and wishes.

Upon completion of my tenure as IAAP President, opportunities to relocate and resume a full-time academic life arose. Again, relocating across the US, I with my wife Linda Carter made our way to Santa Barbara, CA, where I became Provost and then President/CEO of Pacifica Graduate Institute. Complexities abound, but the richness of the experience has proven most rewarding. Hence I continue on this Odyssean pathway, which has brought me psychologically and spiritually more fully into the 21st century. The journey continues. . .

Moments of Complexity and Enigmatic Action

A Jungian View of the Therapeutic Field

Originally published in the *Journal of Analytical Psychology*, 2011, 56(3), 296–309. Reprinted with permission.

Jung's Intersubjective Model

Throughout his writings, Jung's discussions of clinical matters contain an intersubjective thread that readily lends itself to contemporary considerations across schools of analysis. From the 1930s on, Jung increasingly attended to the interactive field engendered between therapeutic partners. His theories of therapeutic action drew on multiple sources, as diverse as cultural anthropology, the history of symbolism, especially of alchemy, as well as modern physics, through his friendships, especially with Einstein and Pauli. Thus, for example, in a supervisory letter to James Kirsch, who was asking advice about an explicit transference dream of one of his patients, Jung commented:

> With regard to your patient, it is quite correct that her dreams are occasioned by you . . . In the deepest sense we all dream not out of ourselves but out of what lies between us and the other.
>
> (Jung, 1973, p. 172; 29 September 1934)

This was more fully developed in his abstract, symbolically dense monograph *The Psychology of the Transference*, first published in 1946. The dyadic relationship with multiple channels of communication, including the intrapsychic, was given form together with detailed discussion of the archetypal basis for this model. The therapeutic couple is seen to become joined in entanglements that can lead to the emergence of a new element, the analytic third, often appearing in symbolic form, such as in a linking dream. Attending to the personal and the archetypal aspects of this third as it plays through the therapeutic field can lead to transformative encounters, not only between the individuals in the dyad but also within each partner. As I've discussed elsewhere (Cambray & Carter, 2004), the methodology Jung used to explore the analytic third can be formulated in general systems theory as the means to detect and engage emergent properties of complex adaptive systems, especially when the interactive field is undergoing a phase transition or significant shift of states, as during a psychic reorganization arising in the therapeutic encounter. The appearance of a dynamic third then is often indicative of increasing interactional complexity, itself a signal of developmental possibilities seeking expression.

One indicator of such a field being activated, especially in long term analytic work which I've noticed over the years, has been the way essential features of a dream often enter the therapeutic process even before the dream has been explicitly told to the therapist. Not infrequently a patient will be discussing a dilemma with considerable affective charge, which activates a reverie process in me and leads to an exploratory comment. This in turn brings us, the therapeutic dyad, into the orbit of the unarticulated dream and often serves as its point of entry into the process, at times with a comment from the patient such as "that reminds me of a dream I recently had." The clinical use of the therapist's reverie can be a valuable intuitive tool for exploring what is emerging in the interactive field as some Jungians have been discussing since the 1960s in terms of the technique of "active imagination"; more recently, some psychoanalysts, in particular Thomas Odgen, have been extending the use of the therapist's seemingly mundane reveries as a guide to insight on the state of the field.

Field Theory

Before proceeding to an updated version of this model, I would like to provide a thumbnail historical background to Jung's use of field theory. He was most likely introduced to the importance of modern field theory by Albert Einstein, who was a houseguest of Jung's several times in the years between his publication of the special and the general theories of relativity. Jung commented on this in a 1953 letter: "It was Einstein who first started me off thinking about a possible relativity of time as well as space, and their psychic conditionality" (Jung, 1975, p. 109). Einstein was of course the greatest field theorist of the 20th century, if not of all time. His theories of relativistic fields were themselves developments of classical field theories of science first articulated in the 19th century in attempts to study and then link electric and magnetic properties of matter and light. These began in 1820 with serendipitous observations by Hans Christian Orsted on how an electric current could deflect a nearby magnetic compass. Michael Faraday greatly expanded these observations experimentally and proposed the first field theory in 1845 to explain electrical and magnetic phenomena more generally. In the process he rejected Newton's idea of space as wholly empty; instead he saw how lines of force described a field which could carry light and extended this to an account of gravitation, thereby overcoming Newton's mysterious and troublesome "action at a distance" view of gravity. Faraday subsequently began a correspondence with a young James Clerk Maxwell who from 1862 to 1865 worked out a complete, rigorous mathematical expression for the electromagnetic field, not only providing the equations that unify electric and magnetic phenomena but also verified that light was a form of electromagnetic radiation with a spectral range extending far beyond visible light in both directions (which Jung was to borrow in metaphoric descriptions of archetypes, having both infrared, i.e., somatic, and ultraviolet, i.e., spiritual, aspects). Einstein then radically revised Maxwell's classical field equations into the relativistic field theory of 20th-century physics. (For more details of this history see chapter two of my book on synchronicity [Cambray, 2009].)

The initial pathway for the importation of these ideas into psychology comes via Williams James. By 1875 James was known to have been carefully reading the latest in physics, which probably included Maxwell's 1873 *Treatise on Electricity and Magnetism* (Richardson, 2006). He went on to speak of "the field of consciousness" and in *The Varieties of Religious Experience*, from his Gifford Lectures of 1901–1902, he writes:

> The expression 'field of consciousness' has but recently come into vogue in the psychology books. Until quite lately the unit of mental life which figured most was the single 'idea', supposed to be a definitely outlined thing. But at present psychologists are tending, first, to admit that the actual unit is more probably the total mental state, the entire wave of consciousness or field of objects present to thought at any time; and, second, to see that it is impossible to outline this wave, this field, with any definiteness . . . The important fact which this 'field' formula commemorates is the indetermination of the margin. Inattentively realized as is the matter which the margin contains, it is nevertheless there, and helps both to guide our behavior and to determine the next movement of our attention. It lies around us like a 'magnetic field', inside of which our center of energy turns like a compass-needle, as the present phase of consciousness alters into its successor.
>
> (1961, pp. 190–191)

Thus James is articulating a holistic field theory of the mind with operations outside consciousness, though it lacks a detailed articulation of dynamic unconscious processes. Jung is known to have been influenced by James, including having spent time with him when he was a guest along with Freud at Clark University's 20th anniversary celebration in 1909. In fact Jung quotes from this same material in his essay "On the Nature of the Psyche" (see 1954, para. 382, n. 47). Thus, James is clearly a major source for Jung's formulation of a field model.

A Contemporary Model of Therapeutic Action in Analytical Psychology

Descriptions of the therapeutic process occurring in an interactive or intersubjective field have received much interest in recent decades. Psychoanalysts from various camps have debated the merits and difficulties with relational, interpersonal and intersubjectivist points of view. Some parallels with Jung's views can readily be found in these discussions, though are rarely made explicit. While the recent discussions draw upon more fully elaborated theories and are exemplified with greater clinical details, they are generally missing the broader, collective dimensions of Jung's theory. Thus, Thomas Ogden's idea of a co-constructed analytic third emerging in the therapeutic process (Ogden, 1997), while having many resonances to Jung's field model, does not include reflections on the dyad's embeddedness within cultural or social milieus beyond the overt contents of the sessions, nor an acknowledgement of potential archetypal patterns. Alternatively we could say that recent research on how individuals are influenced by larger social networks has not yet been integrated into most field models. Similarly, some contemporary Kleinian and Bionian analysts have also taken up a field model with enthusiasm as in the edited collection *The Analytic Field: A Clinical Concept*, by Antonio Ferro and Roberto Basile (2009). The clinical use to which they and their authors put the bipersonal field model is impressive, though theoretically they only trace the field concept back to Madeleine and Willy Baranger, psychoanalysts from Latin America, without reference to the origins of the idea in 19th-century science and thereby miss the opportunity to locate the model within the larger multidisciplinary discussions that have been emerging in the last decade.

Of particular relevance for my topic have been the contributions from the Boston Change Process Study Group, with their descriptions of the implicit domain of relational knowledge. In their views developed from microanalysis of therapeutic encounters, progressing from "present moments," of being present to the lived subjective experience of a moment, to affectively charged "now moments," which when taken up therapeutically can lead to a unique, transformative "moment of meeting" (Stern, 2004). The latter is marked by a sudden qualitative change in the way the therapy partners experience one another in the implicit relational domain. Now moments tend to occur "when the traditional therapeutic frame risks being, or is, or should be, broken" and passes through "an unknown and unexpected intersubjective space" which as noted can lead to a "moment of meeting" (Stern et al., 1998, p. 912). Additionally a now moment is understood by the group as being "a potential emergent property of a complex dynamic system" (Stern et. al, 1998) which they related to the Greek concept of *kairos* (Stern et al., 1998, p. 911), a seizing of the right moment, ideas I shall return to shortly. Thus therapeutic action pivots on the responses to such charged moments, which when skilfully handled can foster increasing psychological complexity and richness in the dyad. The Boston group's attention focuses on the experience of the therapeutic partners, acknowledging the asymmetries involved in the mutual process of transformation occurring within the intersubjective matrix.

Recently George B. Hogenson has written a series foundational chapters (2005, 2007, 2009) in which he has been considering the notion of symbolic density in relation to psychological transformation and has applied this idea to synchronicity constructing a potential bridge to clinical studies involving moments of meeting. I would like to expand on this cluster of ideas and shift focus onto transformations of and within the field itself; that is, I will take the field as an analytic object for exploration as this can, I believe, provide a unique perspective on the more enigmatic aspects of the therapeutic process.

While the recent interest in the study of emergent properties of complex adaptive systems has been a product of scientific research in the later portion of the 20th century, most notably from the Santa Fe Institute, there had been an early wave of publications on emergent phenomena at the end of the 19th and into the first several decades of the 20th century. These chapters, however, were speculative as the computational power needed to study such systems was more than 60 years in the future. Thus, the American developmentalist James Mark Baldwin wrote a series of chapters in the 1890s on the interactions between culture, or learned behaviour, and evolutionary processes. These have been rediscovered with much acclaim in the last two decades, with chapters and books now written on the "Baldwin effect." His descriptions of these interactions indicate a key role for emergent properties, those that arise out of the interactions between components in a system but cannot be reduced to these, such as the way the experience of mind arises out of our neurophysiology. These ideas were elaborated on by Baldwin's friend and colleague, the British scientist-psychologist Conway Lloyd Morgan. In fact, Morgan's (1927) Gifford lectures in 1921–22 were entitled *Emergent Evolution*. C. G. Jung was familiar with Morgan's writings, incorporating the example of the leaf-cutting ant from Morgan's *Habit and Instinct* to demonstrate how an instinct "[a]lways . . . fulfils an image and the image has fixed qualities. . . [s]uch an image is an *a priori* type" (1954, para. 398, and n. 112). He continued on to note "the image represents the meaning of the instinct" (1954) and thus building this biological concept into his archetypal theory thereby providing it surreptitiously with an emergentist core as detailed by Hogenson in 2001.

Extending such revisions by employing complexity theory, especially as developed at the Santa Fe Institute, a number of contemporary Jungians have been drawing out modern emergentist elements implicit in Jung's theories. Among the benefits of this approach has been the opportunity to evaluate and revise these theories in the light of contemporary neuroscience, biology and attachment research, to good effect. Archetypes are themselves seen as emergent properties in the field of body-mind, environment (natural and cultural) and narrative; they are also being reconsidered as "epigenetic rules" which would operate at the core of multilayered, nested complex systems.

My own work has involved a re-examination of Jung's synchronicity hypothesis with these tools. By reassessing the basis for his theory in terms of complexity and emergence, much of the anomalous phenomena that Jung was trying to comprehend through this hypothesis can be better described as emergent phenomena in systems undergoing self-organization. However, this is not meant to identify synchronicity with emergent phenomena completely. It would no longer be wholly surprising to find that there are actually a wide variety of phenomena classified as synchronicities; the notion might be productively analysed into various categories, some emergent, while others remain acausal even from a contemporary perspective (exactly what constitutes acausality may be a shifting horizon). Further, some of these phenomena can also be formulated as transformations of the interactive field involving enigmatic communications. Similarly a re-examination of empathic communication in therapy in terms of interactive fields suggests significant self-organizing properties are operative in which mirror neurons may serve as field resonators.

The intensity of transformations of the field can be quite variable: from sudden reorganization with high intensity, as in phase transitions associated with moments of meetings, to slow changes that build over extended periods of time through series of micro-shifts, as from disruptions and repairs that have a cumulative, mutative impact. However, from the perspective of where a treatment begins there will be a feeling of enigma whenever the engagement leads to a thorough-going transformation with emergent properties; emergence is inexplicable from the viewpoint of contributors/agents but only makes sense in terms of the whole, which can be most easily described in field terms—in therapy this need not just be dyadic, it can also be intrapsychic, as when parts of the personality are reorganized into a more integrated whole. Emergence in complex systems is known to most readily occur at the edge of order and chaos; too much order leads to rigidity, while too much chaos is dissolutive. Therapeutic action designed to foster emergence would then of course be best oriented toward this edge, not as a fixed goal but as a rudder to guide the therapeutic couple. More generally, I would like to suggest the use of the phrase "the moment of complexity," to capture the orienting possibilities of the field itself. The term is borrowed from the philosopher of religions and cultural critic, Mark C. Taylor, who has a (2001) book so titled.

Taylor was looking at the emergence of network culture, noting the increasing rate of change, that is, acceleration of transformations being engendered by the expansion of connections between things (people, information, disciplines, etc.). Several of his definitions of the moment of complexity may help clarify this: it is " 'the tipping point' where *more is different*" (p. 5); "[it] is the point at which self-organizing systems emerge to create new patterns of coherence and structures of relation" (p. 24). These moments are intimately linked with moments of decision when "some possibilities are realized and others are cut off" (p. 149). As we make choices in these key moments, for example in therapeutic work, whether to intervene overtly or not, and if so, how, *at just this moment* (i.e., with awareness of *kairos* as the psychological quality of the moment), we alter the flow of the field. Each potential choice will lead to alternative pathways, some holding greater richness, others truncating the evolving complexity. While we cannot know with certainty which paths are optimum for any given moment in therapy, attending to intuitions about the quality and flow of complexity can provide some guidance. Moments of complexity are moments in which linear time is resisted; instead as systems self-organize a multiplex of temporal possibilities can be encountered. Such moments often occur at the onset of a transference/countertransference enactment in therapy; or when something new is about to emerge beyond the transference/countertransference field; similarly they occur often in the supervisory encounter when a "parallel process" is at play. Let's now turn to a clinical example.

The Case of "Melanie"

On a spring day while having lunch with a psychiatrist colleague, we were interrupted by a call from the police. They were trying to help locate a patient of my colleague who had disappeared and, as I discovered, was feared to be in the midst of a psychotic episode. Thus I was unexpectedly given some details of the case of a young woman who had suddenly vanished and so I tried to help my colleague reflect on the dynamics operating in this upsetting situation. Later that year, in the autumn, I received a call from this colleague explaining that the patient had eventually returned to the area but after several months decided to terminate treatment (medications and psychotherapy) because she felt her medications had not been adequately monitored and so had been a major factor in her psychotic break. I was then asked if I would be willing to take the patient for psychotherapy. Since both parties had agreed that termination was appropriate I agreed to an evaluation interview, if the patient would contact me. The patient was not told of my prior knowledge of her case.

Initially Melanie presented as an attractive, petite woman, groggy from a host of psychotropic medications, and anxious about her chances of recovery. The break had occurred over the Easter weekend and she had spent several months in a distant hospital, with what today would be termed a Bipolar I diagnosis. In her late 30s at the time, she was single and without children. As a university professor Melanie was worried about her ability to continue doing research given her decreased capacities for attention and concentration; she was struggling desperately to regain her higher cognitive functions. For the time being she had restricted her professional activities to teaching which felt manageable despite occasional intrusions of delusional thoughts and quick flashes of hallucinatory activity.

As a prerequisite for working with Melanie psychiatric care was essential. In fact, she had already procured another psychiatrist who worked at a local hospital with admitting privileges. She was to see him on a biweekly basis. I requested permission to contact him as needed, especially should I have any concerns about her mental status. She expressed relief with my conditions, and in fact, her self-monitoring was so scrupulous that when she did begin to decompensate, she was able to quickly report this to me as well as seeking out her psychiatrist. She was understandably terrified of having another psychotic episode, while I felt a parallel concern about treating someone in her condition in a private practice setting.

Silently, I wondered about the connections between us that appeared to have been operating at the time of her break. Retrospectively, I could now see the lunch as having held a moment of complexity, in which my future patient and I were being brought into relationship through a lapse (in therapeutic oversight) and a disappearance; hence, our initial contact was made through negation rather than meeting. Nevertheless, a powerful psychological field had been constellated between us prior to any direct encounter. This field was to become affectively charged at key moments both during the therapy and, as I have discovered, long after it formally ended. Experiences of this sort have led me to subsume the notion of a moment of meeting into the broader category of a moment of complexity which has an irreducible element of serendipity associated with it, often coming with the feeling of an enigma, something not emphasized in most discussions of moments of meeting. In the present case this also helped me to contain my own countertransferential anxieties about working with Melanie.

In the initial phase of our work together we explored Melanie's family history; the therapeutic focus was on establishing basic trust: she asked to tape record the sessions ostensibly to capture the details but also scanning for potential abandonments—I agreed to her request and the taping persisted for about three months until we could shift from a recitation of historical facts to more direct engagement. Melanie's early life was marked by trauma and loss. Her father died when she was three years old; sadly, she discovered the body. She then had a nanny for about a year after this, which fortunately provided her with some much needed care and affection. This woman was black, whereas Melanie was white; the significance of this will become clearer when we hear her dreams. Later she endured sexual abuse while in the care of a neighbour and had to contend with erratic, at times psychotic, behaviours in her mother. A keen intellect was one of her saving graces as it brought her academic acclaim and positive attention, though in a limited arena. Gradually she revealed that she had had a previous psychotic episode about eight years earlier; both that break and the more recent one were precipitated by the loss of a love relationship with a man. Thus the slow, cautious approach we pursued was allowing her to move into more current feeling states with me; nevertheless the interactive field was constrained and subdued during this phase.

As trust built between us through establishing constancy of psychological contact and metabolizing her shame reactions especially with regards to her psychotic episodes, Melanie risked discussing some of the details of her delusions during these episodes. The quality of the field changed markedly, becoming charged and somewhat erratic, though her overt behaviours remained subdued. Soon she brought in dreams spontaneously and the intensity of psychological work accelerated. A figure she called "the beautiful woman dressed in black" appeared in several dreams. Manifesting in various guises this figure was to become a potent entity in the analysis—a composite of memory traces of the black nanny who cared for her in her childhood despair, mingled with black moods of grief and depression, clothed in the garb of mourning, yet holding the potential for transformation. Although this figure included manic defences against grief, she also offered genuine hope of establishing a more secure sense of self.

Through acknowledging this beautiful feminine figure within her, we moved into a "now moment" where Melanie asked me, in what felt to be a more authentic voice than I previously had heard from her, if I could genuinely see this figure in her. Although a complex and delicate question, laden with transferential significance, I felt the most important thing was to validate what was occurring and not to offer an interpretation. I suggested the dream figure seemed to be both a true aspect of herself, what could come out of the work on her suffering, and a way for us to value that potential in our interactions, that such a possibility was indeed a thing of beauty. With my affirmation Melanie proceeded to give the first detailed account of the hallucinations she experienced during her recent psychotic episode—they were truly terrifying, filled with devouring demons of madness and failed attempts at salvation. The woman in black then emerged as an image symbolizing a holding and transformative presence for what was to unfold; she embodied this moment of meeting between us.

Together we noted parallels between the cyclical extremes of her bipolar swings and seasonally based archetypal events. Springtime with Easter festivals was resonant with death and rebirth myths, most directly available to her through the Christ story. The wish to redeem others, and herself, had led her to an inflationary identification with a saviour; the influx of numinous psychic energy unleashed in her then crescendoed into an unsustainable manic crisis. This was followed by the collapse of her ability to contain the affect. No longer able to function in the mundane world, Melanie had plunged into a psychotic depression. Contra Jung at this point, the encounter with the numinous was disintegrative not therapeutic[1]—I would say that there was not yet sufficient psychological complexity available to employ this energy in the service of enhancing self-organization.

On one occasion Melanie spoke of the demons as being like bugs, or cockroaches, and surely these contents and associated affects did drive her "bugs." However, they were not to be read as wholly destructive, for on the Easter morning exactly one year after the onset of her second break she had the following dream:

> I was in the beautiful woman's home. She had wooden (plank) floors. We were lying on the floor talking when I noticed a brown centipede circling us.
>
> I asked her if I should kill it and she said, 'No, it's our friend'. We went on talking until I noticed that it was quite close to me and it had something . . . She said, 'This is wonderful, he's starting to trust you'.
>
> He had turned darker and uglier. Then he came between us and crawled on my arm. The beautiful woman said I was really lucky, 'because look at what he can do'. With that he clicked open an ornate box. He held it open for us to

look. Inside the box were incredibly beautiful jewels, bright shiny colours. I saw a red jewel, a huge ruby. The beautiful woman said to me, 'Whenever I can't find something I go to him'. She loved him.

In her associations she noted that the beautiful woman's appearance now was rather similar to her own, and that the wooden floors were reminiscent of those in my office. The drama of revealing and engaging the madness was truly entering the analytic space. Processing the dream was worrisome and deeply troubling as this dream was a harbinger of an impending psychotic break. While the analysis seemed to offer solid ground and a space where terrifying internal experiences could be explored and understood, it remained to be seen whether the jewels would become a psychological reality for her. Some solace could be found in the beautiful woman serving as a companion and guide helping us see that there was also something of value and meaning in the frightening experiences. However, Melanie did suffer a third psychotic episode about a month after this dream, but this time it was much less debilitating and destructive than the previous two.

In my struggles with how to proceed during this difficult time, I came to realize that there had been another moment of complexity captured in the dream imagery. Following my curiosity in exploring the enigmatic figure of the insect, and employing Jung's method of amplification, applying relevant cultural and historical analogies to unconscious imagery, I did some research which included the following finding:

> In Tahiti the two indigenous centipedes are regarded as shadows of the medicine gods, and are never disturbed or killed. If one can be induced to crawl over a sick person, that person will surely recover.
>
> (Leach, 1972, p. 206)

This might seem just a fortuitous coincidence of questionable relevance; however, what strengthened my resolve to continue with the course we were on was the fact, wholly unknown to the patient, that my first wife's family was Tahitian (I kept this to myself until long after the treatment was over—by 20 years; I have written elsewhere about the issue of enactments in the use of amplification [Cambray, 2001]). Again, Melanie and I were profoundly linked through a relational field in a moment of complexity involving a third person and outside awareness for either of us at the time of its occurrence. The enigma of that moment, however, held the key to therapeutic action in Jung's sense that there was now a way of being in relation to the numinous that could foster transformation. Unfortunately, I don't have time to explore the rest of the work we did on the dream but want to conclude the case with two brief dreams that speak to the transformation itself.

As she rapidly recovered from the last break, Melanie reported that at the onset of each of her last two psychotic episodes she had had dreams that were close to being repetitive. At the time of the break that eventually brought her into treatment with me she had dreamt:

> A black fiery woman came up out of the earth; she watched me then walked on past me, over to a hill to where people and children followed her. She was like a teacher.

Whereas this last time the dream was:

> A black fiery woman comes up out of the molten ground. She walks behind me, as if she is my shadow. I'm walking in stride with her.

In struggling to respond to the eruption of the psychotic process, to take it "in stride," Melanie was no longer a passive victim but able to mobilize herself (she actually took herself to the hospital, collapsing as soon as she stepped on the grounds). She employed her new sense of agency to get into a more viable relationship with the numinous energy of the emergent self. While the effort required to accomplish this was enormous, Melanie's active response, positioning herself more favourably for what she was about to endure, bears witness to the increased complexity of her psychological processing. I believe this to be an outgrowth of the gradual integration of a series of moments of complexity of varying intensity, even if not always consciously articulated. Such moments, which often could not be readily accounted for by causal mechanisms, manifested in her pressing need to be joined with a loving other, to the point of unconscious fusion, or what I prefer to see as massive compensatory attunements. There were a series of "now moments" which led to moments of meetings embedded in moments of complexity, which generally were not made explicit but remained in the implicit domain between us, though certainly riveting my attention. By my orienting towards and privileging the interactive field in its enigmatic aspects, Melanie was able to use the therapy to learn to get into a transformative relationship with what was emerging in the field and in herself. To date, this has been the last psychotic break she has suffered in more than 20 years. We were able to go past subsequent Easters without incident.

The latest development in this story came when I was first asked to give this presentation. As I began to consider how I might address the topic of therapeutic action, I found myself thinking back to Melanie's case but as I had not asked for permission to present her material, I felt I could not use it. Then about six weeks later, I got a telephone call, seemingly out of the blue. Melanie was planning a trip back east and wanted to see me for a single session—it had been more than 15 years since we had last spoken. We did in fact meet and discuss her current situation, but what she was really interested in hearing was how I had managed to stay with her and keep her in treatment when she had the break during the course of our work. I explained what I had learned about the dream with the beautiful woman and the centipede and how that had impacted me. She said she was grateful that I had not shared this at the time for it could easily have been taken into her delusional system then, but that now it was helpful to recognize that the deepest resource for her came from within her own psyche. It seems that the field between us has not dissipated but continues to manifest moments of complexity in unexpected ways.

Final Reflection

To end I would like to briefly reflect on moments of complexity and analytic boundaries. In my experience as an analyst, supervisor and teacher, I've found that such moments are not uncommon in cases where unconscious dynamics have been significantly activated or constellated. These often occur at the margins of or outside our usual clinical boundaries as in the presented case. The transgressive nature of unconscious processes to our normal, egoic sense of time and causality can be made evident in moments of complexity. While such breaches of our ordinary ways of experiencing the world challenge boundaries and seemingly disrupt our attempts at neutrality, they are generally not based in behavioural violations, nor are they reducible to enactments (albeit, as noted earlier, enactments often have a core of complexity), but can be viewed as challenges to expand our notion of boundaries so as not to rule out the impact of unconscious processes. Moments of complexity therefore have the potential to enlarge our view of analysis, helping to broaden but not degrade boundaries while bringing us experientially into an encounter with the radical otherness of the therapeutic field in which each of the partners may find themselves in their own unique ways. Seeking to integrate these moments into our clinical understanding of the way meaning is made and discovered may also encourage us to incorporate their significance into our analytic attitude.

Note

1 This theoretical discussion has been considerably expanded for publication. The commentaries therefore refer mainly to the case presentation of 'Melanie'. Jung's source for the concept of the numinous was Rudolf Otto (1958). For clarity, numinosity is enigmatic for ordinary consciousness. Jung went so far, in certain moments, as to equate this with therapeutic action: 'the fact is that the approach to the numinous is the real therapy and inasmuch as you attain to the numinous experiences you are released from the curse of pathology. Even the very disease takes on a numinous character' (Jung, 1973, *Letters* Vol. 1, p. 377; to P. W. Martin on 20 August 1945). This view is at the heart of a classical Jungian approach and accords with much current interest regarding the role of spirituality in psychodynamic therapy. However, it is important to also look at the date of this letter; it is highly significant, as it was written within a fortnight of the dropping of the atomic bombs on Hiroshima and Nagasaki, darkly numinous events for many, raising the spectre of annihilation for a world already exhausted by war. Jung has clearly been impacted, perhaps traumatized by these momentous events (in the 1957 interview by Richard Evans in the midst of the Cold War, he comments, 'The world hangs on a thin thread, and that thread is the psyche of Man . . . There is no such thing in nature as an H-bomb—that is all man's doing. We are the great danger. The psyche is the great danger' (Jung, 1977, pp. 303–304).

References

Cambray, J. (2001). Enactments and amplification. *Journal of Analytical Psychology*, 46(2), 275–303. (*JOAP.046.0275A*)

Cambray, J. (2009). *Synchronicity: Nature & Psyche in an Interconnected Universe*. College Station: Texas A & M University Press.

Cambray, J., and Carter, L. (2004). *Analytical Psychology: Contemporary Perspectives in Jungian Analysis*. Hove and New York: Brunner-Routledge. (*JOAP.047.0001A*)

Ferro, A., and Basile, R. (2009). *The Analytic Field: A Clinical Concept*. London: Karnac Books.

Hogenson, G. B. (2001). The Baldwin effect: A neglected influence on C. G. Jung's evolutionary thinking. *Journal of Analytical Psychology*, 46(4), 591–611. (*JOAP.046.0591A*)

Hogenson, G. B. (2005). The self, the symbolic and synchronicity: Virtual realities in the emergence of the psyche. *Journal of Analytical Psychology*, 50(3), 271–284. (*JOAP.050.0271A*)

Hogenson, G. B. (2007). From moments of meeting to archetypal consciousness: Emergence and the fractal structure of analytic practice. In A. Casement (Ed.), *Who Owns Jung?* pp. 293–314. London: Karnac Books.

Hogenson, G. B. (2009). Synchronicity and moments of meeting. *Journal of Analytical Psychology*, 54(2), 183–197. (*JOAP.054.0183A*)

James, W. (1961). *The Varieties of Religious Experience*. New York: Collier Books.

Jung, C. G. (1946). The psychology of the transference. *CW* 16.

Jung, C. G. (1954). On the nature of the psyche. *CW* 8.

Jung, C. G. (1973). *Letters. Vol. 1: 1960–1950*. Gerhard Adler and Aniela Jaffé (Eds.). Princeton: Princeton University Press.

Jung, C. G. (1975). *Letters. Vol. 11: 1951–1961*. Gerhard Adler and Aniela Jaffé (Eds.). Princeton: Princeton University Press.

Jung, C. G. (1977). *C. G. Jung Speaking: Interviews and Encounters*. William McGuire and R. F. C. Hull (Eds.). Princeton: Princeton University Press.

Leach, M. (Ed.). (1972). *Funk & Wagnalls Standard Dictionary of Folklore, Mythology, and Legend*. New York: Funk & Wagnalls.

Morgan, C. Lloyd. (1927). *Emergent Evolution*, 2nd ed. London: Williams and Norgate.

Ogden, T. (1997). *Reverie and Interpretation*. Northvale, NJ: Jason Aronson. (*PAQ.066.0567A*)

Otto, R. (1958). *The Idea of the Holy*, 2nd ed. Oxford: Oxford University Press.

Richardson, R. (2006). *William James: In the Maelstrom of American Modernism*. Boston and New York: Houghton Mifflin.

Stern, D. N. (2004). *The Present Moment in Psychotherapy and Everyday Life*. New York and London: W. W. Norton.

Stern, D. N., Sander, L. W., Nahum, J. P., Harrison, A. M., Lyons-Ruth, K., Morgan, A. C., Bruschweilerstern, N., and Tronick, E. Z. (1998). Non-interpretive mechanisms in psychoanalytic therapy: The 'something more' than interpretation. *International Journal of Psycho-Analysis*, 79, 903–921. (*IJP.079.0903A*)

Taylor, M. C. (2001). *The Moment of Complexity: Emerging Network Culture*. Chicago: University of Chicago Press.

Chapter 6

Joan Chodorow

Approaching my mid-eighties now: I begin by going back to the age of seven, when I asked my father to build me a swing. I had in mind an ordinary swing. But when I used the word "swing," my father had vivid memories of the trapeze artists in the Russian Jewish circus that he remembered from peaceful times in his childhood (between the First World War and the Russian Civil War). When I came home after school that day, I found the great gift of a trapeze in the backyard. From then on, I spent many happy hours swinging back and forth, often upside down. To this day I have vivid memories of the rhythmic swinging, fluctuating between sensations of density and strength in descent, toward the breathtaking sensations of weightlessness and flying at the top. Rhythmic fluctuations between earth and sky led to my first conscious awareness of an ongoing flow of inner fantasies. I played with images as they floated up, and they seemed to play with me. Some were visual. Some were auditory (fragments of voices or songs). Sometimes a whole orchestra or chorus seemed to come from sounds of the air rushing by. And always there was the delicious and challenging world of rhythmic movement and felt bodily sensations. Fantasy inspired and shaped the way I moved. At the same time, moment evoked a continuing flow of fantasy.

I had good witnesses, actual and imaginal. As the only child of my parents and the only child in my small extended family of recent and first-generation Jewish immigrants from Eastern Europe, I had a dim sense that my play on the trapeze carried for people I loved something about freedom and hope for a better future. Father, mother, grandmother, two aunts, best friend next door, and other neighbors liked to watch. They also stood by to keep me from falling when I tried out new ways to move. The family atmosphere was infused with a complex mixture of love, creativity, and zest for life, together with dread about the spread of fascism, loss of my beautiful young uncle who fought and died in Spain, and the devastating Second World War. In the midst of play on the trapeze, my wishful fantasies brought into the safety of our backyard children and grownups from cities and villages in Nazi-occupied Europe. Some were relatives and family friends I knew from faded photos and stories but had never met. Around the same time I also discovered the imaginal presence of teachers and classmates I admired — and some I did not like — as well as animals, both beloved pets and wild ones. All these and many more were my witnesses.

DOI: 10.4324/9781003148968-7

Continuing to play on the trapeze, I was also drawn to study ballet with a teacher who understood the importance of both technique and improvisation. Similar to the trapeze, ballet required careful attention to balance, coordination, flexibility, and strength, while at the same time moving — and being moved by — the ongoing flow of inner feelings and fantasies. From early on, the experience of listening to the body to discover the shape changing flow of multisensory images while at the same time expressing imagination through movement led me to understand that meaning and physical shape changing could be two aspects of the same thing.

Another early influence on my understanding of the union of expressive action and meaning was the atmosphere of the family, infused with emotion and its many creative transformations. A swirl of languages flew around the table, mainly English, punctuated with phrases and songs in Russian and Yiddish, also some from Ukraine, Poland, France, China, and other parts of the world. In addition to the alphabet we use for English, someone was always reading or writing in the Cyrillic or Hebrew alphabet. The multilingual sounds and sights were familiar and comforting, but my curiosity was not drawn to follow the exact meaning of the words; I was instead drawn to the way people expressed what they were feeling. Over the years, I learned increasingly to appreciate the way people's faces, bodies, and tone of voice were able to express what they were feeling, with or without words.

I first heard about the psychology of C. G. Jung from Carmelita Maracci when I was sixteen. One of the great ballet teachers of her time, she dedicated each class to teaching technique as an essential tool. Yet of equal value and at the heart of her work, she invited her students to reflect on and be moved by the beauty of the music, art, poetry, the horrors of war, and humanity's painful and slow development toward social justice. Containing it all was the relationship between motion and emotion. For Carmelita, dance is not limited to entertainment. For Carmelita, dance is a way to open to the inner landscape, to experience and express the passions and mysteries of the human soul. She shared a long friendship with Martha Graham, who was in town, and the two of them had a conversation about Jung. As Carmelita put it: Martha had always been interested in the idea of psychoanalysis but over the years had noticed a pattern that concerned her. Several artist friends in psychoanalysis told her that as they retrieved previously repressed contents and reflected on it from a rational point of view, certain neurotic symptoms subsided—and so did their creative drive. However, a psychoanalyst in Switzerland named C. G. Jung understood something artists have always known, that is, the unconscious is a creative resource. In Jung's view, the unconscious includes a top layer of personal repressed material, and then as you go deeper there is so much more in the personal, cultural, and collective unconscious; it will never end. With Jung, you don't have to worry about losing your creativity.

I remember being impressed with Carmelita's story and was drawn to Jung's view of the unconscious. Although it did not occur to me back then to become a Jungian analyst/psychoanalyst, in the years that followed something seemed to move me through dance to dance therapy. Life itself led to analysis and continuing development that led eventually to analytic training and practice, together with invitations to teach in many parts of the world and writing books and chapters along the way.

The Body as Symbol
Dance/Movement in Analysis

Originally published in in N. Schwartz-Salant and Murray Stein (Eds),
The Body in Analysis. Ashville: Chiron Publications. Reprinted with
permission.

> *The dance is the mother of the arts. Music and poetry exist in time; painting
> and architecture in space. But the dance lives at once in time and space. The
> creator and the thing created . . . are still one and the same thing.*
> (Sachs, 1937, p. 3)

This chapter will discuss the use of dance/movement as a form of active imagination in analysis. The history of this work emerges out of two traditions: depth
psychology and dance therapy. The roots of both can be traced to earliest human
history, when disease was seen as a loss of soul and dance was an intrinsic part of
the healing ritual.

The importance of bodily experience in depth psychology has not been fully
recognized, despite Jung's interest in and experience of the body and his understanding of its relationship to the creative process. I will take up some of this
material; look at the early development of dance movement therapy, with attention to Mary Starks Whitehouse and her contribution to the development of active
imagination through movement; and explore the process of using dance/move-
ment in analysis. This will lead to discussion of dance/movement as a bridge to
early, preverbal stages of development.

Depth Psychology

Throughout his life, C.G. Jung seemed to listen to the experience of his own
body: "I hated gymnastics. I could not endure having others tell me how to move"
(1961, p. 29). "My heart suddenly began to pound. I had to stand up and draw a
deep breath" (ibid., p. 108). "I had a curious sensation. It was as if my diaphragm
were made of iron and were becoming red-hot-a glowing vault" (ibid., p. 155).
His visions, too, were clearly experienced in his body:

> Suddenly it was as though the ground literally gave way beneath my feet, and
> I plunged down into dark depths. I could not fend off a feeling of panic. But
> then, abruptly, at not too great a depth, I landed on my feet in a soft sticky
> mass. I felt great relief.
> (Ibid., p. 179)

From his boyhood realization that he had two "personalities," Jung was interested in questions about the relationship of body and psyche. His earliest psychological study included observations of unconscious motor phenomena (1902, par. 82). His work with some of the severely regressed patients at Burghölzli led him to question and eventually discover the meaning of their peculiar, perseverative, symptomatic actions (1907, par. 358). His word association studies involved measurement of physiological changes that occur when a psychological complex is touched. His later speculations about the existence of a psychoid level and his alchemical studies continued to explore the relationship between instinct and archetype, matter and spirit. In an evocative chapter entitled "Giving the Body Its Due," Anita Greene (1984) writes, "For Jung, matter and spirit, body and psyche, the intangible and the concrete were not split or disconnected but always remained interfused with each other" (p. 12).

Adela Wharton, an English physician, told Joseph Henderson that during one of her analytic hours, Jung "encouraged her to dance her mandala-like designs for him when she could not draw them satisfactorily." The room was not large, but a small clear space was sufficient (Henderson, 1985a, p. 9, 1985b). We know very little about the details of her dance, or what it stirred in each of them, or how they came together afterwards. But in his "Commentary on 'The Secret of the Golden Flower,'" Jung wrote:

> Among my patients I have come across cases of women who did not draw mandalas but danced them instead. In India there is a special name for this: *mandala nrithya*, the mandala dance. The dance figures express the same meanings as the drawings. My patients can say very little about the meaning of the symbols but are fascinated by them and find that they somehow express and have an effect on their subjective psychic state.
>
> (1–29, par. 32)

Jung touched on this theme again in his 1929 seminar on dreams:

> A patient once brought me a drawing of a mandala, telling me that it was a sketch for certain movements along lines in space. She danced it for me, but most of us are too self conscious and not brave enough to do it. It was a conjuration or incantation to the sacred pool or flame in the middle, the final goal, to be approached not directly but by the stations of the cardinal points.
>
> (1938, p. 304)

As early as 1916, Jung suggested that expressive body movement is one of numerous ways to give form to the unconscious (1916, par. 171). In a description of active imagination, he wrote that it could be done in any number of ways: "according to individual taste and talent . . . dramatic, dialectic, visual, acoustic, or in the form of dancing, painting, drawing, or modelling" (1946, par. 400). As with so many aspects of his work, he was far ahead of his time. The idea of using the arts as part of a psychotherapeutic process must have been startling in 1916. The original chapter was circulated privately among some of Jung's students and remained unpublished until 1957. Still more time had to pass before the creative art therapies could emerge and be recognized by the mental health community.

Dance Movement Therapy

Dance therapy became a profession in 1966, with the formation of the American Dance Therapy Association. The pioneer dance therapists were all women: dancers, choreographers, and teachers of dance, they shared a common passion and deep respect for the therapeutic value of their art. At first, they were without any kind of clinical training, and they lacked a theoretical framework. But each of them knew the transformative power of dance from personal experience. Although isolated from each other, they taught in private studios and made their way into psychiatric hospitals and other clinical settings throughout the 1940s and '50s. Some of them started as volunteers; part-time or full-time jobs were created for them after they established themselves. Dancers, psychotherapists, and others came to study and apprentice with the early practitioners, who began to develop theories to support their keen observations. The need to develop a theoretical framework led most of them to psychological and other related studies (Chaiklin and Gantt, 1979).

Mary Starks Whitehouse was one of the early movement therapy pioneers. She received her diploma from the Wigman School in Germany and also was a student of Martha Graham. Her personal analysis with Hilde Kirsch in Los Angeles and studies at the Jung Institute in Zurich resulted in the development of an approach that is sometimes called authentic movement or movement-in-depth. In a chapter entitled "Reflections on a Metamorphosis" (1968), she told the story of this transition:

> It was an important day when I recognized that I did not teach Dance, I taught People . . . It indicated a possibility that my primary interest might have to do with process, not results, that it might not be art I was after but another kind of human development.
>
> (p. 273)

Her work has many aspects. She was the first to describe movement from different sources in the psyche:

> "I move" is the clear knowledge that I, personally, am moving. The opposite of this is the sudden and astonishing moment when "I am moved." It is a moment when the ego gives up control, stops choosing, stops exerting demands, allowing the Self to take over moving the physical body as it will. It is a moment of unpremeditated surrender that cannot be explained, repeated exactly, sought for, or tried out.
>
> (1979, p. 57)

The core of the movement experience is the sensation of moving and being moved. Ideally, both are present in the same instant. It is a moment of total awareness, the coming together of what I am doing and what is happening to me.

(1958)

As she developed her approach to movement, she taught her students to become aware of a specific inner impulse that has the quality of a bodily felt sensation:

Following the inner sensation, allowing the impulse to take the form of physical action, is active imagination in movement, just as following the visual image is active imagination in fantasy. It is here that the most dramatic psychophysical connections are made available to consciousness.

(1963, p. 3)

She was also interested in visual images that come out of the movement experience, as well as images from memories, dreams, and fantasies. Whether the images were Godlike, human, animal, vegetable, or mineral, she encouraged her students to remain in their own bodies and interact with the interior landscapes and personified beings that appeared. There were times when the images themselves seemed to want to be embodied, as if the image could make itself better known by entering the body of the mover. Then her students would experience not only *dancing with*, but they would allow themselves at times to *be danced by a compelling inner image*.

She developed much of her work through an extremely simple structure. It involves two people: a mover and a witness. Whitehouse was primarily concerned with exploring and understanding the inner experience of the mover. Some of her students, other dance therapists, and analysts have been developing the work further, toward a deeper understanding of the inner experience of the witness and the relationship between mover and witness. When this work is brought into the analytic temenos, many questions arise about how the dance/movement process weaves into the larger context of a Jungian analysis.

Dance/Movement in Analysis

The use of dance movement in analysis is similar in many ways to use of sandplay. Both are a nonverbal, symbolic process that usually takes place within the analytic hour. The analyst serves as participant/witness. It is the quality of the analyst's attentive presence that can create the "free and sheltered space" that has been so beautifully described by Dora Kalff.

As with other forms of active imagination, the use of dance/movement relies on a sense of inner timing—inner readiness. Sometimes the timing is wrong. For example, when tension or discomfort is building in the verbal work, the idea of moving may be an unconscious form of avoidance. But most people are able to sense when it's time to imagine an inner dialogue, when to move, when to build a sandworld, or use art materials, or write, or bring in a guitar to sing their own song of lamentation or celebration.

The various forms affect each other. For example, when sandplay and move-ment are both part of the analytic process, analysands may sometimes experience themselves moving as if they were inside one of their own sandworlds, interacting with some of the tiny figures. When this happens, it tends to evoke in the mover an Alice-in-Wonderland quality, as she or he meets the imaginal world with inten-sified interest and curiosity. Whether the mover has grown smaller, or the sand-world larger, things are getting "Curiouser and Curiouser." The mover usually meets such a novel situation by becoming even more alert and attentive, learning all she or he can about this strange, yet familiar, landscape and its inhabitants.

Alice may be a particularly useful model of a strong, young feminine ego who is learning how to follow her curiosity (down the rabbit hole, or through the look-ing glass) into an unknown realm—the unconscious. She is wide awake, ques-tioning everyone and everything. The story offers a helpful image for any form of active imagination, that of the ongoing, interwoven relationship between Alice (curiosity) and Wonderland (imagination).

Another similarity between dance/movement and sandplay is that specific themes emerge that seem to follow stages of development in early childhood. More about this later.

Analysts and analysands find individual ways to introduce dance/movement into the analysis. When initiated by the analysand, it may be as spontaneous as the mandala dance described above. Or, there may be much previous discussion and exploration of feelings and fantasies about moving.

When initiated by the analyst, movement may be as spontaneous as a moment of playful, nonverbal interaction. Or it may be as subtle as the mirroring and synchronous breathing that naturally occurs when we open ourselves to a state of "participation mystique." An analyst may invite the analysand to enact a specific dream image (Whitmont, 1972, pp. 13–14) or psychosomatic symptom (Mindell, 1982, pp. 175–197, 1985). Analytic work on a body level may be grounded in a specific approach that includes the use of gentle touch techniques (Greene, 1984). Or, dance and movement may be introduced through a series of workshops and continued in the individual analytic hours that follow (Woodman, 1982, 1983).

When the analyst is familiar with and interested in dance/movement as active imagination, his or her analysands are likely to want to move at some point in their work. But there are also analysands who are fully committed to work with the unconscious, yet never or rarely feel the need to leave their chairs. Some people move every hour, some a few times a year. Some get involved with a particular body level theme and work on it intensely for weeks or months, and then continue on a verbal level.

The movement itself may take no more than ten minutes, or it can go on for an hour or more. Sometimes it is helpful to decide in advance on a time period, per-haps twenty minutes, and have the analyst serve as timekeeper, letting the mover know when to (gradually) bring the movement process to an end.

Physical safety issues need to be discussed. The mover closes his or her eyes in order to listen for the inner sensations and images. But if he or she begins any kind of large swinging, spinning, leaping movements, any kind of momentum that could lead to a collision with windows, furniture, or what have you, it is essential that the eyes be open. Even when the quality of movement is smaller and slower, movers have to learn to open their eyes from time to time to keep an orientation to the room. It is difficult to do this without losing the inner-directed focus. But if the work involves a true meeting of conscious and unconscious, maintaining a sense of where one is in a room becomes part of the conscious standpoint. This is easy to say, but often extremely difficult to do. When one is moving in this way, the eyes usually want to stay closed. To open the eyes (even a tiny slit) takes a major effort. At times, one's eyes feel as if they are glued shut.

A photograph of a Siberian shaman depicts him in a garment that has ropes hanging from his waist. Heavy metal weights are tied to the end of each rope. The shaman enters an ecstatic state as he begins to dance, whirling around. The ropes with their heavy weights fly out around him; a person could be badly injured, if hit by even one of them. The shaman is in a trance, but at the same time, remains conscious and restricts his dancing to an area that is safe. No one gets hurt (Henderson, 1985b).

This aspect of the shamanic tradition is similar to the process of active imagination. The essence of both processes requires the capacity to bear the tension of the opposites, that is, to open fully to the unconscious, while at the same time maintaining a strong conscious standpoint.

The Mover and the Witness

Dance/movement usually needs a brief warm-up period. A time to stretch, relax, and attend to the depth and rhythm of one's breathing helps to prepare the physical body for inner-directed movement. It may also serve as a rite d'entree into the experience—a time when both mover and witness may become more fully present. After the warm-up, the mover/analysand closes his or her eyes, attends inwardly, and waits for an impulse to move, while the witness/analyst finds a corner in the studio where she or he can sit and watch. Movers are encouraged to give themselves over to whatever the body wants to do, to let themselves be moved by the stream of unconscious impulses and images. At the beginning, the witness/analyst carries a larger responsibility for consciousness while the mover/analysand is simply invited to immerse in his or her own fluctuating rhythms of movement and stillness. In time, the mover will begin to internalize the reflective function of the witness, and develop the capacity to allow the body to yield to the unconscious stream of impulses and images, while at the same time bringing the experience into conscious awareness.

In movement, the unconscious seems to manifest in two recognizable ways: in images and in bodily felt sensations. Some movers experience the unconscious predominantly through a stream of inner visual images. Others may experience it primarily through the body. The initial preference seems related to typology. But the movement process tends to develop an increasingly balanced relationship to both realms. As we learn to listen and respond, our attention usually fluctuates back and forth. Each realm may constellate and enrich the other. A woman describes a movement experience that has the quality of such a dialectic:

> My left hand became hard fisted. It was like a phallus. I moved through all levels with this strong, hard, left forearm and fist. Then, the fist opened. It opened so slowly that it was like a reversal from numbness. As my hand relaxed slowly into openness, a large diamond appeared in my palm. It was heavy. I began to move my left arm in slow spirals around myself. I was aware of feeling the sequential, overlapping rotations of shoulder, elbow, wrist, and even fingers. Both arms came to stillness together, joined behind my back. The left hand continued to hold the diamond. Then, the image of the diamond came in front of my eyes. It grew larger, until I could see through it with both eyes. It showed me a vision of everything broken up by its facets. The diamond grew larger, until I was inside it looking out. The light was bright—almost golden. I bathed in it and felt that it was a healing kind of light. Now, my body shape took on the diamond's many facets. I was myself, my own shape, but each part of me had many cut surfaces. It was as if I could "see" through the myriad facets of all of me. There was a sense of wonder and suspension and peacefulness.

This mover describes a fluctuation and constant interchange between two sources of movement, the world of the body and the world of the imagination.

The experience of the analyst/witness ranges along a continuum that has at its poles two modes of consciousness. They are sometimes described as Logos or directed consciousness, and Eros or fantasy consciousness (Jung, 1912; Stewart, 1986, pp. 190–194). They are known by many names. The alchemists spoke of a mysterious marriage between Sol and Luna.

Let us take a moment and imagine how the same landscape might be affected by sunlight and by moonlight. Sunlight, or a solar attitude, offers us clarity. It enables us to divide what we see into its separate parts. But when it gets too bright, everything becomes harsh, glaring, dry. When the sun is at its peak, we live in a world without shadow. The moon, on the other hand, reflects a mild light. It reveals a moist, shimmering landscape. Everything merges. In the darkness we find an unsuspected unity (Jung, 1963, par. 223).

What does this have to do with witnessing movement? The witness fluctuates between a solar, differentiated, objective, definitive way of seeing to a lunar, merging, subjective, imaginative way of seeing. The same movement event may be seen and described in many ways:

> As I watch, I see the mover crouch low with her face hidden. Only her arms reach forward, with wide-spread hands pressing flat on the ground. With an increasingly deep cycle of breathing, she slowly drops forward onto her knees and elbows, and finally slides flat onto her stomach, stretched full length on the ground. Her arms draw together in a long narrow shape, slipping between her body and the floor. She rests, breathing deeply.

As I watch, I let myself imagine and remember what it is like to go deeply inside. I know that this woman was largely ignored during the early years of her life, due to a series of illnesses in her family. As I watch, I feel an ache in my throat and my heart goes out to her. I now see her as if she were a very young infant. I imagine holding her close to my body, we rock back and forth with merging rhythms. As I imagine holding and rocking her, I slowly become aware that I am actually rocking slightly. Later on, I realize that our breathing has become synchronous.

As she presses her hands into the ground, I experience mounting tension and for a moment, I'm fearful that she'll press harder and harder and suddenly explode. But instead, she slides forward and lies on her stomach. She has now withdrawn so much that there is very little movement. My mind wanders. I pick at a hangnail. I feel irritated with her, then guilty and irritated with myself. I imagine she is sitting on a volcano. In any case, it feels as if I am: my shoulder muscles are contracted, my jaw is tight, I'm not breathing very much. My mind dimly wonders whether I might be picking up something about her father's cycle of violent outbursts and subsequent remorse. Or is her withdrawal too close to my own way of avoiding anger?

As she kneels low, the shape of her body reminds me of the Moslem prayer ritual. Another image comes: one of the paintings Jung did for his Red Book shows a little figure that bows low, while covering its face. An enormous fire spout is erupting out of the earth in front of the little person. It fills the upper half of the painting with intricately formed red, orange, and yellow flames.

We know from ancient tradition that the Feminine Mysteries are not to be spoken. Yet consciousness demands that we reflect on and at some point name our experience. When and how do we speak about the experience of dance/movement? How do we understand the meaning of the symbolic action? Do we interpret it from the perspective of transference and countertransference? When and how do we allow the symbolic process to speak for itself? When and how do we respond to it in its own language?

Dancers know instinctively that there is danger in "talking away" an experience that is not ready to be put into words. Isadora Duncan was asked to explain the meaning of a particular dance. Her reply: "if I could tell you what it meant, there would be no point in dancing it."

Analysis offers a different perspective, but analysts, too, know the danger of making premature interpretations that would analyze feelings away (Greene, 1984, pp. 14, 20–21; Machtiger, 1984, p. 136; Ulanov, 1982, p. 78).

There are three aspects of dance/movement in analysis that we gradually learn to remember: (1) What was the body doing? (2) What was the associated image? (3) What was the associated affect or emotional tone? There are heightened moments when all three are clearly known and remembered by both mover and witness. When we're aware of both physical action and inner image, we are likely to be conscious of the emotion as well. But there are times, just as with dreams, that we remember very little. When the mover is conscious of his or her experience, it can be told. Telling it to the analyst is not unlike telling a dream. But a dream is different from active imagination. Active imagination is closer to consciousness. Also, in dance/movement as active imagination, the analyst is literally present and able to witness the experience as it unfolds. The analyst/witness may be unaware of what the motivating images are until after the movement, when the two participants sit together and talk. Or, the analyst/witness may be so familiar with the mover's previous dream and fantasy images that he or she can sense and imagine the nature of the images while watching. Sometimes, the movement comes from such depths that mover and witness experience a state of participation mystique.

When an untransformed primal affect is touched, the mover may "space out," or feel dazed, or stuck, or in some other way become numb to it. Or, if the mover goes with it—if she or he merges with the affect/archetypal image—she or he is likely to be taken over by a primal affect, or by resistance to it, or a logjam of both. At such a moment, the emotional core of the complex is experienced as toxic, even life threatening. At one time, it may well have been that.

Sylvia Perera (1981) writes so beautifully, as she tells the story of our descent to a realm that has been unimaginable and unspeakable:

> Work on this level in therapy involves the deepest affects and is inevitably connected to preverbal, "infantile" processes. The therapist must be willing to participate where needed, often working on the body-mind level where there is as yet no image in the other's awareness and where instinct and affect and sensory perception begin to coalesce first in a body sensation, which can he intensified to bring forth memory or image. Silence, affirmative mirroring attention, touch, holding, sounding and singing, gesture, breathing, nonverbal actions like drawing, sandplay, building with clay or blocks, dancing—all have their time and place.
>
> (p. 57)

Because much that goes on in the analytic relationship at this level is preverbal, we will turn to some of our earliest experiences as they appear in dance/movement and relate them to certain stages of normal development in infancy.

Sources of Movement

An earlier chapter (Chodorow, 1984) discussed the origins of movement from different aspects of the psyche. Four sources were suggested and illustrated: movement from the personal unconscious, the cultural unconscious, the primordial unconscious, and the ego-Self axis. Although every complex has elements that are personal, cultural, and primordial, themes that emerge through the body are so immediate that it seems possible and helpful to sense from which level or source it is constellated.

Dance/movement is one of the most direct ways to reach back to our earliest experiences. Movers frequently lie on or move close to the ground. By attending to the world of bodily felt sensations, the mover recreates a situation that is in many ways similar to that of an infant who swims in a sensory-motor world. The presence of the analyst/witness enables reenactment and reintegration of the earliest preverbal relationship(s). It is here that images of the transference and the countertransference may be most clearly recognized.

This chapter will introduce five symbolic events that appear and reappear in the movement process of many individuals. They seem to represent certain stages of developing consciousness through the preverbal, presymbolic developmental period of infancy, that is, from birth to approximately sixteen months. The symbolic actions and interactions are (1) patterns of uroboric self-holding; (2) seeking the face of the witness and, when found, a smile of recognition; (3) the laughter of self-recognition; (4) disappearance and reappearance; and (5) full engagement in the symbolic process via free imaginative use of mime.

Two sources have been essential to my recognition and understanding of these events. Louis H. Stewart (1981, 1984, 1986) has been updating Jung's model of the psyche from the perspective of child development and recent studies of the affects and their expression. Charles T. Stewart, a child psychiatrist, has been developing a theory of play and games as universal processes in ego development (1981). Working individually and in collaboration (C. T. Stewart and L. H. Stewart, 1981; L. H. Stewart and C. T. Stewart, 1979), they have gathered a wealth of material from Jung, Neumann, Piaget's observations, Tomkins's study of the affects, and anthropological research into play and games. From these and other sources, they have brought together certain phases of ego development described by Neumann, with fully embodied observations of real babies.

Infant and child development is most often studied from the perspective of patriarchal values. For example, Piaget wanted to understand the development of the intellect, so even though his observations demonstrate a development of both imagination and intellect, his theory shows a one-sided emphasis on logos functions. Louis H. Stewart and Charles T. Stewart give us a way to understand the development of the imagination. Together, both perspectives form a whole, an ongoing dialectic between the twin streams of life instinct. One stream is Eros as imagination, divine relatedness; the other is Logos as intellect, divine curiosity (L. H. Stewart, 1986, pp. 190–194).

In the following pages, we will discuss each theme as it appears in dance/movement and explore it from the perspective of infant development. The ego-Self axis is constellated at the threshold of each stage. The experiential core of each passage in the development of consciousness is a startling, even numinous moment of synthesis and reorientation.

Uroboric: Patterns of Self-Holding

Movers tend to explore a very wide range of uroboric self-holding. We see all kinds of patterns: one hand holding the other; thumb holding; arm(s) wrapping around the torso to hold rib(s), elbow(s), hip(s), knee(s), foot, or feet. All of these seem reminiscent of those earliest body experiences when we at first unintentionally find, then lose, and find again and gradually discover what it is to hold ourselves. In infancy, the first primal recognition of self may well be that powerful and comforting moment when thumb and mouth find each other:

> We may see that the infant, while sucking its fingers or its toes, incarnates the image of the mythical Uroborus that, according to Neumann, represents the "wholeness" of that undifferentiated state of self-other consciousness that is characteristic of this developmental state. We can also see in this early behavior the earliest evidence of that aspect of the autonomous process of individuation that Neumann, following Jung, has called centroversion. In this light we may understand the infant's behavior in the discovery of sucking its thumb as representing the first synthesis of the psyche following upon the rude disruption of life within the womb, which had more impressively represented a paradisiacal absorption in the purely unconscious processes of life itself.
>
> (L. H. Stewart, 1986, p. 191)

When the mover is immersed in self-holding, his or her eyes are closed or have an inward focus. There is usually rocking, swaying, or some other kind of rhythmic pulsation. The quality is usually complete self-containment. If the analyst/witness opens himself or herself to a state of participation mystique, he or she may join the mover in a timeless state and experience a similar kind of rhythmic self-containment. Shared rhythms of holding, touching, lulling, and lullabies are the psychic nourishment of this earliest phase.

If the analyst/witness does not enter into a state of participation mystique with the mover, he or she may feel excluded, irritated, uneasy. Alternatively, or even concurrently, he or she may feel shy, embarrassed to watch an experience of such intimate union with self. As with any other analytic work, witnessing requires opening to the unconscious, and at the same time maintaining a conscious analytic standpoint to reflect on the meaning of the symbolic action and the associated countertransference response.

At times, the experience has a different, perhaps more conscious quality. There is a sense of wonderment as the mover's hands discover and explore the shape of his or her own body. As the mover's hands shape themselves to the bulges and the hollows, the hard bones and the soft flesh, there is a profound sense of self-recognition—as if meeting oneself for the first time. Both mover and witness often feel as if they are participants in an ancient ritual form. After many years of witnessing women and men spontaneously discovering the shape of their own bodies with their hands, I learned of a myth that demonstrates so clearly such a return to our uroboric origins. The myth of Changing Woman, who presses and molds her own body as she comes of age, is still reenacted throughout the American Southwest in the form of an initiation ceremony.

First Smile: Recognition of Other (Approx. Second Month)

The movement process frequently evokes a special smile that is reminiscent of the infant's earliest recognition of the "other." When the movement comes to an end, it is almost always followed by continued inner attentiveness—a period of natural self-containment similar to the uroboric quality. Then, as the mover makes the transition to everyday consciousness, it is as if she or he is gradually waking up. When the mover's eyes open, she or he usually begins to search the room for the analyst. When the analyst's face is found, there is a mutual sense of reconnection and, most often, the smile(s) of recognition. The mover may have just experienced painful emotions; his or her face may still be wet with tears. But as he or she gradually comes back to the dayworld and scans the room for the analyst's face, there is a meeting and a clear-eyed smile. Even when the quality of the therapeutic relationship is primarily that of two adults, any fully spontaneous smile has at its core the infant's smile when she or he first consciously recognizes the now famil-iar face of the mother or other primary nurturing adult.

Louis H. Stewart (1984) reflects on the infant's first smile:

> What are the first signs of love in the infant and child? Our Western image of childbirth has been that the mother must suffer and the child come crying into the world. All this has more recently been questioned and there are those who talk about infants entering the world with smiles on their faces and wide awake mothers ready to smile back immediately upon birth. We are far from knowing then what may be the possible potential of the development of love in the child. However, what is observable today is that the mutual smile of recognition between mother and infant does not occur for several weeks after birth. Before that the child smiles under certain conditions of satiety, half awake, half asleep, but in a dazed, glassy-eyed manner. Then there comes a moment, as early as the end of the first month sometimes, when the infant, awake and clear eyed, smiles in what is unmistakably a pleased recognition of the familiar sounds and face of the mother. Soon, within days or weeks, the infant's first joyful laugh occurs.
>
> (p. 1)

First Laugh: Recognition of Self (Approx. Third Month)

From time to time, usually in the midst of movement, the mover laughs. There are many kinds of laughter. This one expresses joy in the sheer exuberance of bodily motion, and/or a particular image appears and there is the laughter of self-recognition (Stewart and Stewart, 1981). Piaget describes such a laugh:

> It will be remembered that Laurent, at 0;2(21), adopted the habit of throwing his head back to look at familiar things from this new position. At 0;2(23 or

24) he seemed to repeat this movement with ever-increasing enjoyment and ever-decreasing interest in the external result: he brought his head back to the upright position and then threw it back again time after time, laughing loudly.

(Piaget, 1962, p. 91)

Charles T. Stewart draws an analogy between the infant's first laugh and a similar moment in the analysis of an adult, reported by D. W. Winnicott. Winnicott's patient was described as a schizoid-depressive man who could carry on a serious conversation but lacked any kind of spontaneity. He rarely, if ever, laughed. In the midst of one of his analytic hours, the patient imagined himself doing a backward somersault, similar to the movement made by Laurent when he threw his head back and laughed. Winnicott (1954) writes of his patient:

> On important but rare occasions he becomes withdrawn; during these moments of withdrawal unexpected things happen which he is sometimes able to report . . . The first of these happenings (the fantasy of which he was only just able to capture and to report) was that in a momentary withdrawn state on the couch, he had *curled up and rolled over the back of the couch.* This was the first direct evidence in the analysis of a spontaneous self.
>
> (p. 256, emphasis added)

Joan Blackmer writes of a dream in which two small, agile tumblers, trained acrobats, turn somersaults. Among her amplifications, she describes their trickster quality: "They certainly are transformers . . . The somersault, in itself a moving circle, is a mandala, a symbol of the Self, which causes change *through human motion.* Psychologically, this represents a change in attitude" (1982, p. 8, emphasis added).

The laughter of self-recognition always turns our world around.

Disappearance and Reappearance: Object Constancy (Approx. Ninth Month)

There are so many ways that the mover/analysand hides from the witness/analyst—and reappears. The dance/movement structure itself is a game of disappearance and reappearance (as the mover's eyes close and open again). But within the movement, even with eyes closed, the mover may turn away and do some small, intricate gestures that the witness cannot see. If the witness follows his or her curiosity and moves to where the gestures can be seen, the mover may turn away again, and the cycle can repeat itself. Often, if the witness stays put, the mover turns around again to where she or he may be seen. Sometimes peek-a-boo and other hiding games and activities emerge as overt, central, conscious themes in dance/movement enactment.

Separation anxiety develops in the third quarter of the baby's first year. At the same time that the infant begins to struggle with the pain of separating from beloved persons, she or he immerses herself or himself in games of peek-a-boo, and intensely investigates problems of disappearance and reappearance.

At 0;8 (14): Jacqueline is lying on my bed beside me. I cover my head and cry "coucou"; I emerge and do it again. She bursts into peals of laughter, then pulls the covers away to find me again. Attitude of expectation and lively interest.

(Piaget, 1952, p. 50)

0;9(05): Jacqueline wails or cries when she sees the person seated next to her get up or move away a little (giving the impression of leaving).

(Piaget, 1952, p. 249)

0;9(20): Jacqueline is lying down and holds her quilt with both hands. She raises it, brings it before her face, looks under it, then ends by raising and lowering it alternately while looking over the top of it: Thus she studies the transformations of the image of the room as a function of the screen formed by the quilt.

(Piaget, 1954, p. 193)

As the first smile is the beginning of mother-child differentiation, peek-a-boo, and later games of hide-and-go-seek, continue an ongoing process that leads toward the development of object constancy.

Pretend Play: Separation of the World Parents (Approx. Sixteenth Month)

Jung describes this major passage of consciousness as:

the first morning of the world, the first sunrise after the primal darkness, when that inchoately conscious complex, the ego, the son of the darkness, knowingly sundered subject and object, and thus precipitated the world and itself into definite existence . . . Genesis 1:1–7 is a projection of this process.

(1963, par. 129)

A number of passages in the infant's first year create the base upon which a clear separation of dayworld and dreamworld can occur. Neumann (1954, 1973) refers to this differentiation of conscious and unconscious as "separation of the world parents." In the infant's life, this passage comes not through the word but rather through the discovery of nonverbal, symbolic play—that is, the baby discovers that she or he can pretend. It is this first, independent discovery of symbolic action that coincides with the beginning of real curiosity about language.

Around sixteen to eighteen months of age, the child becomes aware of the semiotic function through the experience of pretense, for example in the miming of an already adaptive behavior pattern like the ritual behavior adopted to ease the transition into sleep (e.g., thumb-sucking and fingering the satiny edge of a blanket). The child laughs with joy at this new recognition of Self; and this is pretend play (Piaget, 1962). But let us reflect for a moment on the sleep ritual. This is not a neutral pattern of behavior. It represents one of the landmarks in the child's development. If the transition to sleep and waking is not easily accomplished, the child may be forever prone to sleep disturbances, to excessive fear of the dark, needing a night light, etc. And why is going to sleep difficult? Because it brings together the child's most feared and distressing fantasies, that of being deprived of the presence and comfort of those most dear, and of being left alone in the dark which is peopled by who knows what ghostly phantoms. Thus we consider it no accident that the child discovers pretense in the recognition of the sleep ritual; pretend play begins with the miming of a behavior pattern which has assisted the child in warding off fear of the unknown and soothing the anguish of separation. Subsequent pretend play will be seen to reenact all the emotionally charged experiences of the child's life.

(Stewart and Stewart, 1979, p. 47)

Similar to the infant's first discovery of pretend play, the dance/movement process in analysis often begins with the miming of a familiar behavior pattern that has served to ward off emotional pain. Also similar to children's play, imaginative mime can lead the mover toward and eventually through the emotional trauma that lies at the heart of a complex.

The following descriptions are of three women, each in the early stages of analytic work.

A woman begins to move by expressing a happy-go-lucky attitude, "moving on." Then she pauses and her chest seems to collapse. With a feeling of increasing heaviness, she lowers herself to her knees and becomes overwhelmed by a deeply familiar sense of despair.

A professional dancer puts on a show that would dazzle Broadway. She then sinks to the ground, becomes very quiet and begins to move slowly. The slow movement is halting and looks increasingly painful. Her body convulses and she seems to be in a trance.

A busy, active executive enacts her over scheduled life. For a moment, she pauses, looks down to the ground and realizes how tired she is. She struggles briefly with her yearning to lie down, and overcomes it by returning to the portrayal of her active life.

Each woman in her own way struggles with the tension between an overly bright, adaptive persona and its shadow. As in any analytic process, a pair of opposites will be constellated. Out of the experience of that twofold tension, a third reconciling symbol will eventually be born: a new inner attitude that contains yet also goes beyond both perspectives.

Carolyn Grant Fay describes the emergence of such a moving symbol. The mover is a woman who has had many years of analytic work. She does not begin with avoidance of pain, nor does she seek it. She begins by listening deeply:

> I lay for what seemed like a long time, listening inwardly to myself. My throat brought itself to my attention. It hurt and felt constricted and tense, so I let my throat lead me into movement. It led me up to kneeling, then forward, and then slowly across the floor in a sort of crouching position. In my imagination I became aware as I concentrated on the throat that it was red with blood. The heart area was also aching and bloody. Finally my throat brought me up to standing and propelled me farther along. It stopped me suddenly, and I just stood there. At this point, I collapsed onto the floor and lay there motionless. There was no movement . . . not an image . . . nothing.
>
> After a while I became aware that the color red from the blood was there at my throat and breast. Little by little it became many shades of red from light pink to deep crimson. A rose began to take shape, rising out of the throat and heart through movements of my arms up, out, and around. The rest of my body down from that area seemed, in the fantasy, to be forming the stem and leaves of the flower. All sorts of superlatives come to me now as I try to express how I felt at that moment: warm, happy, fulfilled, in order, at one with myself.
>
> (Fay, 1977, pp. 26–27)

Closure

More important than whether we use dance as a form of active imagination is the question of how we can fully engage the imagination. Jung suggests giving free rein to fantasy, according to the individual's taste and talent. Some people have what he called "motor imagination" (1938, p. 474). It is the nature of such an individual to experience life in terms of spontaneous movement activity and to imagine with and about the body. Thus a dialogue is initiated between interest and imagination as twin streams of libido: interest in the body the way it &, and fantasies of what the body might be about (Stewart, 1986, pp. 190–194).

As the process of individuation leads us to become who we are, certain analysts and analysands are inevitably led to use dance/movement as part of their analytic work. For those with a motor imagination, dance/movement is simply the most immediate, natural way to give form to the unconscious. Some find dance/movement essential because they feel alienated from the body, or because they only know how to direct the body and now sense deeply that they must learn to listen to it. Some turn to dance/movement because it is a direct way to work with certain complexes that were constellated in infancy. It seems that complexes of a preverbal, presymbolic nature are less often touched by the verbal aspects of analysis.

Eliade (1963) wrote, "Life cannot be repaired, it can only be recreated" (p. 30). In analysis, active imagination is that re-creative process; dance movement is one of its forms.[1,2]

Notes

1 Personality Number One was grounded in the concrete reality of everyday life, the facts of the world the way it is, Personality Number Two lived in eternal time, the world of the ancestors and spirits, a mythic realm. Jung wrote, "The play and counter play between personalities No. 1 and No. 2, which has run through my whole life, has nothing to do with a I split' or dissociation in the ordinary medical sense. On the contrary, it is played out in every individual" (1961, p. 45).

2 The initiation cerement is called the Kinaalda by the Navaho. The Apache call it the Sunrise Dance (Quintero, 1986). It is an elaborate ritual-a time of rejoicing to mark a girl's onset of menstruation. Her passage to womanhood is announced to the whole community in a dramatic four-night ceremony.

   Changing Woman had a miraculous birth and grew to maturity in four days. At this time, she had her first menstrual period. The Holy People were living on the earth then, and they came to her ceremony and sang songs for her. She originated her own Kinaalda. One of the most important parts of the ceremony was molding her body. Some say that at the first Kinaalda, Changing Woman molded her own body. The pressing or molding was done to honor the Sun and the Moon. Changing Woman was molded into a perfect form.

   When the first-born human girl became Kinaalda, Changing Woman did the same things for her. She pressed and molded the younger woman's body, thus gifting her with beauty, wisdom, honor, and self-respect. The Kinaalda is part of the Blessing Way Ceremony. It is done today as it was done in the beginning (Frisbie, 1967; Henderson, 1985b; Sandner, 1979, pp. 122–132; Quintero, 1980).

References

Adler, J. (1973). Integrity of body and psyche: Some notes on work in process. In B. Govine and J. Chodorow (Eds.), *What is Dance Therapy, Really?* pp. 42–53. Columbia, MD: American Dance Therapy Association.

Adler, J. (1985). Who is the witness? A description of authentic movement. Paper presented at movement therapy seminars in Los Angeles and San Francisco, January 1985.

Bernstein, P. L. (1984). *Theoretical Approaches in Dance-movement Therapy*, Vol. 11. Dubuque: Kendall/Hunt.

Bernstein, P. L., and Singer, D. L. (1982). *The Choreography of Object Relations*. Keene: Antioch New England Graduate School.

Blackmer, J. D. (1982). *The Training and Experience of a Modern Dancer: Exploration into the Meaning and Value of Physical Consciousness*. Diploma thesis, C. G. Jung Institute, Zurich.

Chaiklin, S., and Gantt, L. (1979). *Conference on Creative Arts Therapies*, pp. 8–10, 30–32. Washington, DC: American Psychiatric Association, 1980.

Chodorow, J. (1974). Philosophy and methods of individual work. In K. Mason (Ed.), *Dance Therapy: Focus on Dance V11*, pp. 24–26. Washington, DC: American Association for Health, Physical Education and Recreation.

Chodorow, J. (1978). Dance therapy and the transcendent function. *American Journal of Dance Therapy*, 2(1), 16–23.

Chodorow, J. (1982). Dance/movement and body experience in analysis. In M. Stein (Ed.), *Jungian Analysis*, pp. 192–203. La Salle, III and London: Open Court.

Chodorow, J. (1984). To move and be moved. *Quadrant*, 17(2), 39–48.

Eliade, M. (1963). *Myth and Reality* New York: Harper and Row, 1975.

Fay, C. G. (1977). *Movement and Fantasy: A Dance Therapy Model Based on the Psychology of C. G. Jung*. Master's thesis, Goddard College, Vermont.

Frisbie, C. J. (1967). *Kinaalda: A Study of the Navaho Girl's Puberty Ceremony*. Wesleyan University Press.

Greene, A. (1984). Giving the body its due. *Quadrant,* 17(2), 9–24.

Hall, J. (1977). *Clinical Uses of Dreams: Jungian Interpretations and Enactments*. New York: Grune & Stratton.

Henderson, J. L. (1985a). The origins of a theory of cultural attitudes. In *Proceedings of the 1985 California Spring Conference*, pp. 5–13. San Francisco: C. G. Jung Institute.

Henderson, J. L. (1985b). Private conversation.

Jung, C. G. (1902). On the psychology and pathology of so-called occult phenomena. *Collected Works* 1:1–88. Princeton: Princeton University Press, 1975.

Jung, C. G. (1907). The psychology of dementia praecox. *Collected Works* 3:1–151. Princeton: Princeton University Press, 1972

Jung, C. G. (1912). Two kinds of thinking. *Collected Works* 5:7–33 Princeton: Princeton University Press, 1967.

Jung, C. G. (1916). The transcendent function. *Collected Works* 8:67–91. Princeton: Princeton University Press, 1969.

Jung, C. G. (1927). The structure of the psyche. *Collected Works* 8:139–158. Princeton: Princeton University Press, 1969.

Jung, C. G. (1929). Commentary on "The secret of the golden flower". *Collected Works* 13:1–56. Princeton: Princeton University Press, 1976.

Jung, C. G. (1935). The Tavistock lectures: On the theory and practice of analytical psychology. *Collected Works* 18:5–182. Princeton: Princeton University Press, 19–6.

Jung, C. G. (1938). *Dream Analysis*. W. McGuire (Ed.). Princeton: Princeton University Press, 1984.

Jung, C. G. (1940). The psychology of the child archetype. *Collected Works* 9/1:151–181. Princeton: Princeton University Press, 1977.

Jung, C. G. (1946). On the nature of the psyche. *Collected Works* 8:159–234. Princeton: Princeton University Press, 1969.

Jung, C. G. (1961). *Memories, Dreams, Reflections*. New York: Random House, 1965.

Jung, C. G. (1963). *Mysterium Coniunctionis*. Princeton: Princeton University Press, 1974.

Kalff, D. (1980). *Sandplay*. Santa Monica: Sigo Press.

Machtiger, H. G. (1984). Reflections on the transference/countertransference process with borderline patients. *Chiron: A Review, of Jungian Analysis*, 119–145.

Mindell, A. (1982). *Dreambody*. Los Angeles: Sigo Press.

Mindell, A. (1985). *Working with the Dreambody*. Boston: Routledge & Kegan Paul.

Neumann, E. (1954). The separation of the world parents: The principle of opposites. In *Origins and History of Consciousness*, pp. 102–127. Princeton: Princeton University Press, 1973.

Neumann, E. (1973). *The Child*. New York: G. P. Putnam & Sons.

Perera, S. B. (1981). *Descent to the Goddess: A Way of Initiation for Women*. Toronto: Inner City Books.

Piaget, J. (1952). *The Origins of Intelligence in Children*. New York: W. W. Norton & Co., Inc., 1963.

Piaget, J. (1954). *The Construction of Reality in the Child*. New York: Basic Books, Inc., 1971.

Piaget, J. (1962). *Play, Dreams and Imitation in Childhood*. New York: W. W. Norton & Co., Inc.

Quintero, N. (1980). Coming of age. *National Geographic*, 157(2), 262–271.

Sachs, C. (1937). *World History of the Dance*. New York: Norton & Co.

Sandner, D. (1979). *Navaho Symbols of Healing*. New York: Harcourt, Brace, Jovanovich, Inc.

Schoop, T. (1974). *Won't You Join the Dance?* Palo Alto: National Press Books'.

Schwartz-Salant, N. (1982). *Narcissism and Character Transformation*. Toronto: Inner City Books.

Stein, M. (1984). Power, shamanism, and maieutics in the countertransference. *Chiron: A Review of Jungian Analysis*, 67–87.

Stewart, C. T. (1981). The developmental psychology of sandplay. In G. Hill (Ed.), *Sandplay Studies*, pp. 39–92. San Francisco: C. G. Jung Institute of San Francisco.

Stewart, C. T., and Stewart, L. H. (1981). Play, games and stages of development: A contribution toward a comprehensive theory of play. Presented at the 7th annual conference of The Association for the Anthropological Study of Play (TAASP). Fort Worth, April 1981.

Stewart, L. H. (1981). The play-dream continuum and the categories of the imagination. Presented at the 7th annual conference of The Association for the Anthropological Study of Play (TAASP). Fort Worth, April 1981.

Stewart, L. H. (1984). Play-eros. In *Affects and Archetypes II*. Paper presented at active imagination seminar in Geneva, Switzerland in August 1984.

Stewart, L. H. (1986). Work in Progress: Affect and archetype: A contribution to a comprehensive theory of the structure of the psyche. *Chiron: A Review of Jungian Analysis*, 183–203.

Stewart, L. H., and Stewart, C. T. (1979). Play, games and affects: A contribution toward a comprehensive theory of play. In A. T. Cheska (Ed.), *Play as Context*, pp. 42–52. Proceedings of The Association for the Anthropological Study of Play (TAASP). West Point, NY: Leisure Press, 1981.

Tomkins, S. (1962). *Affect Imagery Consciousness, Volume I*. New York: Springer Publishing Company, Inc.

Tomkins, S. (1963). *Affect Imagery Consciousness, Volume II*. New York: Springer Publishing Company, Inc.

Ulanov, A. (1982). Transference/countertransference. In M. Stein (Ed.), *Jungian Analysis*, p. 6885. La Salle, IL and London: Open Court.

Whitehouse, M. (1958). The Tao of the body. Paper presented at the Analytical Psychology Club of Los Angeles.

Whitehouse, M. (1963). Physical movement and personality. Paper presented at the Analytical Psychology Club. Los Angeles, 1963.

Whitehouse, M. (1968). Reflections on a metamorphosis. In R. Head et al. (Eds.), *A Well of Living Waters-Festschiffit for Hilde Kirsch*, pp. 272–277. Los Angeles: C. G. Jung Institute, 1977.

Whitehouse, M. (1979). C. G. Jung and dance therapy. In P. L. Bernstein (Ed.), *Eight Theoretical Approaches in Dance-movement Therapy*, pp. 51–70. Dubuque: Kendall/Hunt.

Whitmont, E. (1972). Body experience and psychological awareness. *Quadrant*, 12, 5–16.

Winnicott, D. W. (1954). Withdrawal and regression. In *D. W Winnicott: Collected Papers*.

Woodman, M. (1980). *The Owl was a Baker's Daughter: Obesity, Anorexia Nervosa, and the Repressed Feminine*. Toronto: Inner City Books.

Woodman, M. (1982). *Addiction to Perfection: The Still Unravished Bride*. Toronto: Inner City Books.

Woodman, M. (1983). Psyche/soma awareness. *Quadrant*, 17(2), 25–37.

Chapter 7

Warren Colman

So where did it all begin? All my grandparents were Jewish immigrants from Russia and Romania who escaped poverty, pogroms and enforced conscription and came to London's East End in the early years of the 20th century. Beyond the mid-19th century, my personal ancestry dissolves into the collective history of the Jewish people, a history of persecution, migration and a rich spiritual, intellectual and emotional heritage bequeathed to me by my parents and grandparents.

After the war (WWII), my parents moved out to the suburbs where growing up as a Jewish boy in a non-Jewish neighbourhood heightened a sense of being an outsider that has stayed with me all my life. Yet nor could I completely identify with my Jewish heritage either. Even in the world of psychoanalysis (the "Jewish science"), I found myself in the outsider group of the Jungians—an outsider amongst the outsiders, neither quite one thing nor the other. Not being a "proper analyst" chimed in perfectly with my doubts and conflicts about not being a "proper Jew." But to live in the spaces between is fertile ground for an analyst, so despite the pain, it's served me well.

I feel incredibly lucky to have grown up in the 1960s when rock music was bursting forth with unparalleled creative energy. As I was growing up, so was rock'n'roll—from Buddy Holly to the Beatles, from the Rolling Stones to Chuck Berry, Eric Clapton and the blues. My parents bought me my first guitar for my 14th birthday and it's been a lifelong passion ever since, even though eclipsed by my passion for psychoanalysis for many years.

Until my mid-twenties, I hoped to be a professional musician, but I was eventually forced to recognise that the Self was pointing me in another direction when I applied for a job in a day centre for drug addicts. Somehow I knew this was where my real future lay even though it was painful to accept that my hopes and dreams of being one of the great rock guitarists was just that—a dream. Later on, I was able to re-channel my creativity, ambition and love of performing into writing—almost everything I've written has first been given as a spoken presentation. Recently, though, after decades writing about the psyche, my creative interest ("libido") has returned to music again, my first love. During the past year, I've written more songs than I have since the 1970s. I live

DOI: 10.4324/9781003148968-8

in hope for the end of the current pandemic when I can go out and perform them live.

I was 26 when I saw the path to becoming a psychotherapist open up before me and knew that, unlike being a musician, this was a mountain I could successfully climb. I trained carefully and thoroughly—first as a counsellor and social worker and then as a couples psychotherapist and finally as a Jungian analyst. Those fifteen years of training for my life's calling brought me into the orbit of a whole other set of ancestors—from Sigmund and C. G. through D. W. Winnicott and my conflictual relationship with Big Mamma Klein to those I knew personally, who nurtured and taught me, almost all of whom are now deceased. A couple of years ago, I had a dream about them all:

I'm in an old part of the SAP building that hasn't been used for a long time. On the wall is a Scythian carpet that I recognise from a recent British Museum exhibition as the oldest carpet in the world. The main room reminds me both of my school hall and of the ballroom from my university. I get chatting to a rather ramshackle looking old man, asking him what's going on. It seems it's some kind of pantomime that's put on every year over the Christmas holidays. Then an elderly lady appears who is organising the pantomime. I recognise her from when I first joined the SAP, someone rather tall and imposing who was known as an old-fashioned stickler for correct analytic practice. I have a very good feeling about having stumbled upon this quaint, long forgotten but enjoyable and good value event.

I think this dream has to do with my own "initiation" into the world of elders and ancestors. It has that quality of Hermann Hesse's *Journey to the East* of an esoteric group who pursue their spiritual path unknown to the quotidian world of everyday life or, as in *Steppenwolf*, of a doorway marked "entrance not for everyone."

The various references to my own past (school, university etc.) gave me a strange feeling of both grief and joy that "my whole life is here." And there's something in it about the shadow-like aspect of the ramshackle old man and the pantomime that has to do with "playing the game." For me this has to do with letting go of the drive for achievement that has fuelled so much of my professional life for so many years. At a certain stage in life we begin to retire from the deadly seriousness of it all, and also begin to take ourselves less seriously. We carry on playing the game, not only for the sake of those who come afterwards, but also out of our genuine love and affection for all that it has meant to us. Yet, if all goes well, we will be ready to leave it behind when the time comes.

As one of my recent songs puts it:

Do the things you like to do
And they will grow inside of you
Before you know it, you'll look back and that's your life

All those tangled bits of memory
Become the stuff of history
You'll find you're walking on the path of all those who came before

Reflections on Knowledge and Experience

Originally published in *Journal of Analytical Psychology*, 2013, 58(2), 200–218. Reprinted with permission.

Introduction: Becoming an Analyst

For many years, I struggled with a nagging doubt that I was not really a "proper analyst" since, in various ways, my practice did not seem to conform to recognisable descriptions of what analysts do. Ironically, only as I have become more accepting of the kind of analyst I really am have I realised the ubiquity of my doubts. For example, Joseph Sandler refers to "the conscious or unconscious conviction of many analysts that they do not do 'proper' analysis." He argues,

> The conviction that what is actually done in the analytic consulting room is not 'kosher', that colleagues would criticize it if they knew about it, comes from the reality that any analyst worth his salt will adapt to specific patients on the basis of his interaction with those patients.
>
> (Sandler, 1983, p. 38)

Similar remarks were made by Bion in his clinical seminars posthumously published in 1987:

> It is only after you have qualified [as an analyst] that you have a chance of becoming an analyst. The analyst you become is you and you alone; you have to respect the uniqueness of your own personality—that is what you use, not all these interpretations (these theories that you use to combat the feeling that you are not really an analyst and do not know how to become one).
>
> (Bion, 1987, p. 15; quoted in Gabbard and Ogden, 2009, p. 311)

The irony implicit in Bion's remarks is that only someone who has given up trying to be an analyst can actually become one. The emphasis on the analyst's own personality is also redolent of Jung's much earlier remark:

> The personalities of the doctor and the patient are often infinitely more important for the outcome of the treatment than what the doctor says or thinks.
>
> (Jung, 1929, para 163)

Nevertheless, relying on one's own personality is a potentially risky option, not least because it exposes us to the vagaries of our own limitations and blind spots.

Where is the dividing line between "adapting to specific patients" and departing from the boundaries of good analytic practice if neither psychoanalytic theory nor established practice are reliable guides to fall back on? This question immediately confronts us with the ethical dimension of analytic work: in this regard, reliance on being a "proper" analyst may be a defence against the effort to discern what constitutes being a good analyst, in the philosophical sense of the quest of "the good." This is inevitably a stressful activity. On the one hand, we need to maintain a flexibility and openness to the unknown that avoids having too definite an idea of the task in order to allow for the more unpredictable and inexplicable aspects of psychic life. On the other hand, analytic work demands an attitude of continual questioning in which nothing can be taken at face value and the analyst is continually engaged in an intensive effort to discover what is "really" going on. Furthermore, the recognition of the complex interplay between transference and countertransference extends this exploration to rigorous self-scrutiny, requiring analysts to be ruthlessly honest with themselves regarding their fallibility, countertransference illusions, limitations, blind spots and so on. The dangers of falling into error, complacency or rote behaviour or acting out one's own complexes are rife—hence the need for consultation with colleagues, although the uniqueness of each analyst/patient relationship and the difficulty of conveying its complexity, detail and implicit dimensions to others means that the guidance offered by colleagues is inevitably limited. This can sometimes make being an analyst a very lonely business.

As a result of these pressures, analysts live with high levels of anxiety and uncertainty. In a previous chapter (Colman, 2006) I suggested that this is one of the main reasons for the pervasiveness of an analytic super-ego that generates further levels of persecutory anxiety about who is and who is not a "proper analyst." In the conclusion of that chapter, I suggested that the functioning of a more benign super-ego might be considered as being "akin to a council of elders consulted by a ruler" (ibid., p. 113). This idea of "eldership" implies that the internalisation of an external set of "rules" may be gradually transformed into something that is based on the kind of knowledge that comes from long experience. Although such knowledge is rooted in analytic theories and traditions, it is oriented more towards "learning from experience," in Bion's phrase. This quality is akin to Aristotle's concept of *phronesis*, translated as "prudence" or "practical wisdom." The role of long experience in *phronesis* is made plain by Aristotle's remark:

> a young man of practical wisdom cannot be found. The cause is that such wisdom is concerned not only with universals but with particulars, which become familiar from experience, but a young man has no experience, for it is the length of time that gives experience.
>
> (*Nicomachean Ethics*, bk. 6, ch. 8)

In other words, there is a transformation of the generalities with which all theories are concerned ("universals") into becoming familiar with the particulars out of which such theories are made. The more one becomes able to recognise theory in practice, the less relevant the theory seems to become since the universal generalities are replaced by a long series of unique particulars, albeit these are organised in terms of a range of increasingly preconscious schemas. This also enables the analyst to apply old theoretical principles in new and unexpected situations they could not have foreseen. The result is similar to that described by Michael Parsons (2000) as "the refinding of theory." But it is also a question of making the theory one's own—the same point that Sandler was making in his 1983 chapter.

Phronesis may also be regarded as the outcome of a super-ego function that has been made one's own. Aristotle refers to the "phronimos," as "the normal, ideally good agent; the man whose goodness is intelligent" and says of him that "the rules which the phronimos finds and applies for himself are based upon his own intelligent moral experience." This may echo the distinction Jung made between the collective conscience embodied in Freud's super-ego and the personal conscience which is a function of the individuated self (Jung, 1940, para 390).

In this chapter I aim to outline the development of *phronesis* in my own practice and explore some of the implications and dilemmas of working in this more personally oriented way. While this confers a greater freedom, openness and authenticity, its shadow aspect appears when freedom slides into laziness and licence. So it is important to remember that *phronesis* is an *ethical* attitude concerned with "intelligent goodness," a theme to which I return at the end of the chapter with a brief consideration of the values underlying analytic practice.

The Surprise and Discomforts of Being Oneself

Inevitably, many of the most important changes in life happen outside conscious awareness. Often this is because they occur very gradually and only become noticeable in retrospect. As John Lennon put it shortly before he was murdered, "Life is what happens while you're busy making other plans"[1] (Lennon, 1980).

Over the past few years, I have noticed a change in the way I practise that seems to have occurred between ten and fifteen years after qualification. Having become much less internally persecuted by the need to justify myself to my analytic super-ego, what went on in my consulting room now seemed to be getting further and further away from what might be recognisable as "analysis."

Despite the discomfort I continue to feel about this from time to time, I have come to feel that the overall sense of being more at ease in the work and the apparent decoupling from explicit theoretical formulation is mainly a sign of the integration that occurs through long years of experience. It also reminds me of an intangible quality I had noticed in the senior training analysts I consulted in the course of seeking election to more senior levels of membership of my analytic society, a process that provided opportunities to take stock of my own level of professional development. These "elders" did not seem to *know* more in the sense of theoretical knowledge but they still had a great deal to teach me. I realised that what they possessed was a kind of clinical wisdom apparent not so much in *what* they said about my work as in the pertinence of it and the way it deepened my own understanding. This intangible quality was probably what Hanna Segal was getting at when she described one of the qualities needed in a psychoanalyst as "intuition but also a kind of knack" (Segal et. al. 2012). An indication of what Segal might have meant is given in a conversation reported by one of my supervisors, Hugh Gee, about Kenneth Lambert, one of the first analysts to train at the society of analytical psychology (SAP) in the late 1940s. One of Lambert's previous patients remarked to a colleague that Kenneth hadn't made any transference interpretations throughout his analysis. The colleague replied, "Ah, but Kenneth was a very subtle man." I took this to mean that Lambert's way of interpreting the transference was so integrated into his overall discourse that it could no longer be differentiated by the label "transference interpretation."

Recently, I have begun to notice this intangible, even ineffable quality in some of my own work, particularly as a supervisor, and this has led me to feel that perhaps I too have become "a senior training analyst," by which I mean nothing to do with status but rather a quality of deep integration that comes from long experience and generates a kind of clinical wisdom. One of these experiences was quite dramatic.

The House Is Having an Orgasm

> The supervisee had made very detailed notes, most of which consisted of a long dream in which the patient being presented found herself in a wooden house in the forest. Her powerful female boss was holding court there with several male figures and after a series of incidents, they all had to leave the house because it was shaking violently as if about to fall down, perhaps due to some kind of earthquake. Throughout this lengthy presentation I found myself entirely bereft of thought and eventually the supervisee expressed her concern that she had overwhelmed me, like in the dream where the male figures were weak and fragmented. The session was nearly over and I had still not come up with anything when I had what felt like a mad thought. I suggested to my supervisee that the shaking house was not falling down but that *the house is having an orgasm*. The supervisee understood this immediately and was able to link it with her patient's feeling that her sexuality is a (destructive) witch. Only now does it also occur to me that the dream was also being re-enacted in the supervision when the supervisor, apparently overwhelmed by the supervisee's excited presentation, suddenly bursts into life and makes an orgasmic interpretation. Even this, though, barely conveys the emotional experience in the room with my supervisee which I can perhaps best convey by comparing it to that sense of shocked amazement that occurs with the more remarkable examples of synchronicity. I suggested to my supervisee that we must have been working together in the deep unconscious—hence the 'mad' thought that arose as if from nowhere into my conscious mind.

Although there may be various ways in which an experience like this may be "explained"—for example by reference to "implicit relational knowing" (Stern et al., 1998; Lyons-Ruth, 1999), "moments of complexity" (Cambray, 2011) or "symbolic density" (Hogenson, 2009)—my emphasis here is on the phenomenology of the experience in which I had *no idea* where my thought had come from. The experiential impact of this is hard to describe. I could see that my "mad thought" had in some way arisen out of a well-practised use of metaphorical interpretation, especially the sexual metaphors that are so prominent in psychoanalytic thought (Colman, 2005). But at the same time, I had a strange feeling as if this knowledge had nothing to do with me and I was as surprised as anyone else by where it had come from. There was an odd sense of being both strange and familiar to myself in seeing that the person who could do this was "me." Although pleased that I could do it, I felt as if I could not take any particular credit for it. To put it in Jungian terms, such insights appear to come out of the Self and have a distinctly non-ego character.

By this I do not mean to imply any kind of *a priori* Self that thinks and acts independently of the ego. Rather I am thinking of a dynamic, fluid and contextualised self that is responsive to the environment but in a way that exceeds conscious knowledge and control. This may be thought of in terms of Fordham's model of a self that learns from experience via the ongoing sequence of deintegration and reintegration. Another perspective may be found in developmental theories concerning the implicit dimensions of cognitive development. According to Lyons-Ruth (1999), cognitive-developmental research shows that "thinking progresses to highly complex, formal modes through the development of enactive procedures that are not easily, and never completely, translated into a verbal, explicitly retrievable medium." This is most apparent in non-verbal domains such as artistic or athletic skills but also occurs in scientific work and in clinical practice where "implicit clinical knowing . . . proceeds to high levels of complexity outside the medium of words" (p. 599). So the Self out of which such spontaneous, non-rational insights and interventions arise is a highly trained and skilled self—something which can only develop through many long hours of practice.

This process requires a kind of radical "unknowing" and an inner trust that "something will turn up." I was initially perplexed when I began to notice this in myself while supervising groups of trainee psychodynamic counsellors. The other members of the group would have lots of ideas and find much more to say about their colleagues presentations than I could, even though I was supposed to be the "one who knows." Quite appropriately, they were all keen to try out their newfound knowledge, whereas I was casting around in the smoke rings of my mind (in the foggy ruins of time) for something that seemed relevant and useful. It would seem that in this process there is a lot going on that has become subliminal so that it may be that many possibilities are rejected out of awareness before something gets selected as worth saying—and even then, that which I feel most certain of may need to be treated as a hypothesis to be tested against further knowledge and experience, and discarded if need be. To this extent, analysis is a scientific discipline, although very similar processes go on in artistic work as well.[2]

Not Knowing Beforehand

Thinking about this has led me to wonder whether I am finally beginning to understand what Bion may have meant by working without memory, desire or understanding. In my experience, this is something that *happens* rather than being *intended* and can only be understood once it has already occurred. If I can feel confident and relaxed enough to settle into a reverie of knowing nothing, something might occur that catches my interest and attention and seems worth pursuing, even if I don't know why. Examples of such "selected facts," as Bion calls them, might include an incongruous image in a dream, an odd choice of words or non-sequitur in what the patient is saying. It takes time to be able to trust that the "selected facts" which interest us are also likely to be analytically relevant, regardless of whether they seem like "mad" thoughts or an irrelevant enquiry into aspects of the patient's external life.

This underscores the futility of attempting to make Bion's eschewal of memory, desire and understanding into a deliberate "instruction" of how to work, a difficulty that is apparent in one of Michael Fordham's last chapters on "Not Knowing Beforehand" (1993). He certainly seems to be addressing the kind of experiences I have described when he writes (regarding the process of "digesting" projective identifications):

> At this point it is desirable to trust one's unconscious and wait further developments, rather than fall back on technical, i.e. conscious knowledge. It is out of that emergent experience that a communication by the analyst, relevant to the patient, can develop, because it relates immediately to the patient's emotional experience.
>
> (Fordham, 1993, p. 130)

Yet he also describes his "investigation" of mutual projective identifications in terms of a conscious "trying to perceive the patient as if he had never seen him before and had no knowledge of him" (ibid.) and recommends this to trainees, saying that they should imagine that they have a "mental filing cabinet" which should remain locked during the time they are with the patient. He acknowledges that it is rare for trainees to achieve this and adds that it is an ideal to be approximated (ibid., p. 131). However, I have come to feel that this is an impossible recommendation that can only increase the trainee's "severe bewilderment that the not-knowing behaviour . . . can evoke" (ibid.). The more the trainee tries, the more they will fail since something which can only arise through a natural process of development becomes instead yet another super-ego injunction, especially when issued by as august a figure as Michael Fordham. I sometimes need to reassure supervisees that they need to accept where they are rather than struggle to be where I am. Rather than trying to perceive the patient in a particular way, the key thing is to allow oneself to recognise the way one *is* perceiving the patient even if that includes recognising one's own self-critical judgements. It's a question of accepting what is. Gradually it becomes possible to recognise what is happening in the room through *not* trying to perceive or do anything in particular. This usually leads to a much greater freedom in the way we relate with patients, the sorts of things we say and, more broadly, how we are with them. This is the meaning of having the freedom to "be oneself" with the patient.

Analytic Freedom and Its Limits

This is not without its difficulties, since it carries the ever-present danger of "wild analysis" when the analyst abandons the analytic attitude and unconsciously acts out with the patient either out of the countertransference pressures induced by the patient's transference or out of the analyst's own needs, especially their own narcissism. Of course, it may be hard to distinguish between the two since it is where one's own vulnerabilities are touched that one is most likely to act out the countertransference pressures evoked by the patient.

It is now generally recognised that minor incidents of this kind, known as enactments, occur frequently and that they can provide useful information about the current state of the transference/countertransference. However, enactments are still usually considered as "errors" of some kind that are only useful as a way of informing the analyst's subsequent understanding expressed either through interpretation or a re-adjustment of the analyst's stance.[3] It is less often recognised that enactments can advance the therapeutic process as a direct expression of the analyst's mainly unconscious response to the patient's needs. Jean Knox (2009) has discussed this in terms of patients who need to establish a sense of self-agency through being able to have an impact on another person. Such patients cannot grasp the analyst's intentions towards them except through their actions, so they cannot feel they have an impact on anyone unless they can "coerce" the other into responding.

Enactments may also be valuable with patients who are not necessarily functioning at this early stage of development since they are an expression of an implicit relational communication that is often more powerful in effecting change than verbal interpretations. This opens up much wider possibilities for the ways in which we are able to help our patients while remaining within the overall discipline of psychoanalytic work. This latter point is an essential caveat because, without it, there would be no boundary between an analytic relationship and the umpteen other ways in which the patient's needs might be met. Nor would there be any distinction between helpful enactment and unhelpful acting out. So it is vital that analysts have a well-functioning schema of what analytic work looks like, especially when they begin to depart from it. This is sometimes expressed in the phrase "you have to learn the rules before you can break them." This may be true, but one of my abiding concerns is that the rules should be taught in a way that opens up the novice therapist to learning from their own experience rather than closing down these opportunities through super-ego-induced guilt and anxiety. In my experience as a teacher and supervisor it is much more common to find therapists who are too inhibited with their patients than those who are too uninhibited and throw caution to the wind.

Nevertheless, those occasions when analysts depart too far from standard analytic boundaries and commit ethical boundary violations offer salutary warnings to us all. Nor is it surprising to learn that it is senior male analysts who are most at risk of transgressing in this way since the additional freedom and confidence that comes with experience can easily tip into the omnipotent belief of those who believe the rules do not apply to them (Gabbard and Hobday, 2012).

Here the distinction between boundary crossing and boundary violation is most helpful (Gutheil and Gabbard, 1998). Analytic boundaries are not like the defined boundaries of a football pitch, and it is sometimes difficult to know precisely where they are; sometimes there may be good reason for behaving differently. For example, there is a wonderful account of working at the implicit level of relational knowing in Beebe and Lachmann's book on *Infant Research and Adult Treatment* (2002). Lachmann describes his work with a suicidal borderline patient who made him so anxious that he phoned her a couple of hours before every session to remind her to come (p. 59). Perhaps even more telling is a similar account by the Kleinian analyst, John Steiner (1993, pp. 18–23), who phoned a patient who had stopped coming to sessions for a few days. From the highly boundaried perspective of Kleinian analysis, this must have been rather more unorthodox than it would have been for Lachmann, and Steiner includes his "uneasy sense of doing something improper" (ibid., p. 23) in his clinical report while nevertheless concluding it was what the patient needed at the time.

Clinical Example: "Don't Let the Bastards Grind You Down"

I would now like to give an example from my own practice of a more or less deliberate enactment that I felt was beneficial to the patient. Although I became aware of the transference implications during the session, I chose to enact the countertransference rather than interpret it. In doing so, I was allowing something to unfold that had a deep relational significance despite the "outer world" content of the discussion.

> The patient is a young man with whom there has been a strong father/son transference/countertransference relationship from the start. Even before I met him, I imagined him as a younger version of myself merely on the basis of his initial phone call. His own father is a rather narcissistic man who tends to be self-preoccupied and unreliable. This is already hinted at in the countertransference fantasy of the patient being 'a younger version of myself'. So I have had to pay attention to this in order to differentiate the patient from my own expectations of him. This necessary work on my own countertransference also has the effect of providing an experience of a father who can allow him to develop in his own way.

In this session, the patient talks about the stresses of his job in the public welfare services, many of which are due to cuts in funding and wider political pressures bearing down on his area of work. He regrets not speaking out at a meeting, feeling that he should have mounted a challenge to political views he abhors and which will adversely affect the client group he works with. He feels that his values are being gradually chipped away in the current climate. I comment that this is a case of 'don't let the bastards grind you down' and that he needs to be clear about what's really important in this situation—for example, maybe it's better to keep a low profile than make an open challenge and risk being shot down. (I felt this might be a rather adolescent and ineffective kind of protest.)

He wonders if he's being naïve—perhaps this is just the way of the world? That's how it is in business (his father's world), and he's been shielded from it by working in the welfare services. I now make a statement that expresses a more personal understanding rooted in my own experience and values. 'That's just the problem' I say. 'In business, the ultimate aim is to make a profit and it doesn't really matter what the product is, whereas in the public services, the product is the end and not the means'. He picks this up and asks if I've seen this kind of thing before?

I refer to the social changes brought about by Thatcherism in the 1980s, and his response makes it apparent that he knows virtually nothing about this fairly recent history that took place when he was a child and I was the age he is now. At this point I feel a strong prompting to fill in this important gap in his knowledge with particular reference to the changes I had experienced myself in social work. In doing so, I am alerted to the fact that an enactment is taking place since I am speaking much more personally than usual and in a way that reveals my own emotional investment. I tell him about the way Thatcher attacked the social welfare ethos of the previous era, replacing it with the law of the market, how she didn't believe in society and about her attack on professional autonomy. I contrast the autonomy and responsibility I had as a newly qualified social worker in the 1980s with the situation now in which social workers are drowned in bureaucratic control and unable to exercise their own judgement. He concurs, telling me of a social work department he's heard about where the staff have to account for every minute of their day and if they fail to reach a certain target, are called to supervision—so supervision has become policing rather than facilitation.

In this discussion which took up the remainder of the session, I knew that I was answering him just as I would answer a son of my own. In doing so I was expressing my own values and beliefs which are implicitly in opposition to his father's values but, perhaps of greater significance, his own father had never taken the time and trouble to talk to him in this way and there were a number of areas in which his father had invaluable knowledge and experience to pass on to him and had not done so. So I was enacting a particular aspect of the father, concerned with passing on the fruits of knowledge and experience in a context of personal values. In so doing, I was implicitly affirming his need for a paternal relationship of mutual identification at this point in his therapy and his life.

It seemed to me that to have stepped back from the enactment towards a more neutral, disengaged stance that merely *interpreted* this need would have missed the opportunity for a "moment of meeting" and would have been experienced as withholding and repetitive of his original deprivation. It may well have elicited the negative father transference but I would be concerned that this might be an iatrogenic artefact of abstinent analytic behaviour. As for the value-laden aspect of my comments, it is, in any event, well known that analysts cannot help but reveal their own values. An amusing example of this is the patient of Ralph Greenson's who knew his analyst was a Democrat because whenever he said anything critical towards the Democrats Greenson interpreted it, but whenever he said anything positive about them he accepted it without comment (Greenson, 1967, p. 273; cited in Orange and Stolorow, 1998). There is also an oft-quoted comment of Karl Menninger that "what the psycho-analyst believes, what he lives for, what he loves, what he considers to be good and what he considers to be evil, become known to the patient and influence him enormously" (Menninger, 1958, p. 91).

One aspect of the enactment of which I wasn't aware at the time was the implicit reference to the earlier discussion about whether to speak out. Although I had counselled caution, my own behaviour represented an endorsement of speaking out and laying claim to the things you believe in. I was giving him an experience of a way of being and relating that was influenced consciously and unconsciously by a sense of something for which he seemed desperately hungry. The elements of personal disclosure were simply a medium for the experience of a particular kind of relating that was taking place in the session. This does not diminish the importance of remaining aware of the transference/countertransference aspects and the fact that there is an enactment going on. This awareness does two things—firstly, it acts as a measure of my behaviour and enables me to keep a sort of running tally as to where we are in the therapy and, secondly, it provides food for later thought: the interpretation of the father/son transference could be made at a later date, referring back to this session as an example.

One concern about this way of proceeding might be the risk of colluding in the patient's wish for an idealised benevolent relationship that would confirm his view that his father was to blame for his difficulties. Subsequent developments in the analysis and in the patient's life do not bear this out. In fact, it seems more likely that the enactment in the analysis was indicative of the early emergence of a different kind of relationship that was later replicated elsewhere. For, despite ongoing difficulties, the patient was able to reach a better understanding with his father as well as being able to recognise some of the disliked aspects of the father in himself. I might also have been more wary of enacting this kind of identificatory relationship if it was a consistent feature of the transference. However, at other times, I had been experienced in very different ways (e.g. rigid and unreasonable) and had felt very differently towards the patient (e.g. irritated and impatient).

Subsequently, the patient became more dependent and regressed for a while, and it is possible that the implicit support provided by my identificatory response facilitated this development. Out of this he was able to have the insight that his earlier tendency to try and pick fights with me had maintained him in a position of always having a father to blame, enabling him to avoid having to grow up and accept responsibility for his own difficulties. Having some of his father hunger provided for in his therapy seemed to have helped him give up his grievance with his father, whereas a more abstinent stance may have entrenched a negative transference in which he continued to feel "justified" in blaming the father-analyst for his difficulties.

The transference is thus always operating in a fluid and multifaceted relational context: it can be understood to some extent but there is always more going on than we know. Enactments and open expressions of emotion may sometimes be a vital part of this. The development of a clinical *phronesis* facilitates this since the growth in the analyst's capacity to think about and metabolise emotion enables him or her to move more freely between the intellectual and affective elements in "thinking feelingly," where the emotion *is* the meaning (Fisher, 2002).

Practical Wisdom ("Phronesis")

I do wish to emphasise that far from giving permission for the abrogation of analytic boundaries, this way of proceeding *requires* good boundaries as the frame within which any effective analytic work takes place. Analytic freedom is quite different from analytic licence. This is one reason why I retain my respect for the analytic tradition of theory and practice in which I was trained and continually refer back to it. This constitutes a form of internal dialogue which every analyst needs to practice as a form of ongoing internal supervision (Casement, 1985). It was this that enabled me to recognise firstly that I was attempting to justify myself to an ideologically rigid analytic super-ego and, secondly, that I had done good work despite practising in a much more open, non-interpretative and self-disclosing way than I used to believe was necessary. I have also realised that the competencies I have developed are those which are best suited to my character (Wiener, 2007) and that trying to work in some other way would only succeed in making me *less* than the analyst I could be. This "continuation of one's own analysis by other means"[4] has gradually had the effect, not of "getting rid" of the analytic super-ego, but of transforming it from a stern judge to a wise counsellor. Increasingly, too, the wisdom of the super-ego counsellor is derived from my own knowledge and experience and is therefore better adapted to my own way of working.

This brings me back to the relation between *phronesis* and personal knowledge, rooted in long experience. This does not come about through knowledge or experience alone but through what is *done* with knowledge and experience, a process of thought informed by a fundamentally ethical intention, the pursuit of the good *of* analysis and the good *in* analysis. Joachim's commentary on Aristotle's

Nichomachean Ethics (Book VI, paras 1138–1139) notes that the possession of phronesis also requires a principle—*logos*—whose rightness is determined by its having the right aim—*scopos* (Rees, 1951, pp. 88–89). I regard the analytic attitude as the best embodiment of this aim through its implicit commitment to a consistent disciplined process of thinking about the patient, one's relationship to the patient and the work as a whole in a way that is informed by past knowledge (theory) and experience (technique) but is radically open to question and ulti- mately concerned with what is right, not in the technical sense of "correct" but in the ethical sense of "good."

For this reason, I consider the analytic attitude to be fundamental, sacrosanct and non-negotiable in my work as an analyst.

Conclusion: Analysis as a Wisdom Tradition

The idea that analysis is defined more by the analyst's attitude than their theory or technique is borne out by research evidence that shows good outcomes for psychotherapy to be independent of theoretical perspective. The evidence for this has been summarised by Jean Knox, who refers to the finding of randomized controlled trials that no one type of psychotherapy can be shown to be better than another, known as the Dodo effect: "Everybody has won and all must have prizes" (Knox, 2011, p. 184). Knox also quotes Jonathan Shedler's (2010) review of the empirical evidence that demonstrates the crucial significance of the qualities and style of the individual therapist with the individual patient and the unique patterns of interaction that develop between them. Furthermore, rigid adherence to specific theories is correlated with poorer outcomes due to "implementation of the cogni- tive treatment model in dogmatic, rigidly insensitive ways" (Knox, 2011, p. 187). Knox uses this evidence to argue persuasively in favour of a relational approach to therapy that is supported by a wealth of observational studies of parent-infant relating and the long-term consequences of adverse relational experience in early life (ibid., p. 190).

Nevertheless, theories and techniques of some kind are clearly indispensable. One cannot practice psychotherapy based on relational support alone any more than one could play a violin concerto based on a love of music. Analytic technique (*techne*) does not constitute wisdom (*phronesis*) any more than perfectly played scales con- stitute musicality, yet the one is vital to the other. Perhaps the closest analogy to the consistent disciplined practice of an analytic attitude is the practice of meditation.

In this respect I would suggest that psychoanalysis belongs to a philosophi- cal wisdom tradition that is fundamentally concerned with how to live. However much we may need to be informed by current scientific research, our day-to-day work goes beyond research towards the development of "*phronesis*"—a prudent, practical wisdom rooted in an ethical consciousness in which feeling and values are ineluctably at the heart of thought and practice (Whan, 1987).

Primarily, the kind of wisdom that analysts develop is clinical wisdom, that is, a deepened understanding of the kind of situations that arise in analysis and how best to think about and respond to them. But it is important to acknowledge too that our therapeutic practice is not isolated from the rest of our lives and that, if analysis has taught us anything, it will also be facilitating the development of greater wisdom in the practice of our own lives as well as understanding the lives of others. So "practical wisdom" is not just the wisdom of analytic experience but also the wisdom that develops through one's own life experience. Being an analyst offers unique, privileged opportunities to learn about this with and through the experience of others; in helping them make sense of their lives, we learn about ourselves and our own life and *vice versa*, the lessons we learn in our own lives feed back into our work with patients.

Psychoanalysis is therefore far more than a technical procedure—it is a way of living informed by values about what constitutes a good life.

In a chapter published over 40 years ago on "The Promise of Psychoanalysis," Harry Guntrip (1971) addressed very similar issues in a context that seems prescient of the crisis facing psychoanalysis today. He begins by asking "what is life about?" thus placing psychoanalysis squarely in the context of the search for meaning and purpose in life. He goes on to outline pessimistic anxieties about the demise of psychoanalysis that were current even then but contrasts this pessimism with his own point of view:

> a psychoanalysis which is closely related to the realities of everyday living, that penetrates to the depths of suffering human beings, has nothing to fear for the future and will flourish . . . However, psychoanalysis will hold the attention of the public only insofar as it speaks truly to the human condition, and insofar as people realize that the psychoanalyst should not be just a professional man with a theory—a psychotechnician—but a human being with a developing experience of understanding, able to help others with their struggles to be real persons living meaningful lives with their fellowmen.
>
> (Guntrip, 1971, p. 45)

And in a message that echoes directly down the decades to our current concerns he concludes: "Psychoanalysis will decline only if it becomes a closed society of the initiated defending an older, undeveloping theory as dogma" (ibid., p. 55). That is a warning that is, if anything, even more relevant to the challenges facing the psychoanalytic profession today than it was then. Ancestors may be revered but they should never be merely imitated.

Notes

1 Tragically, in his case, the same was true of his death.
2 For example, David Lean is said to have discarded the best scenes of *Doctor Zhivago* because they did not fit in with the whole; the ceramic artist, Edmund de Waal, regularly enjoys breaking up pots that are not good enough (*Desert Island Discs*, BBC Radio 4, 25/11/2012).

3 This view can be found even amongst relational analysts who generally have a more neutral view of enactments. See Benjamin, 2009.
4 I believe it was Winnicott who first coined this adaptation of the phrase 'politics is the continuation of war by other means', but I have been unable to find the reference.

References

Beebe, B., and Lachmann, F. (2002). *Infant Research and Adult Treatment. Co-constructing Interactions*. Hillsdale, NJ: Analytic Press.

Benjamin, J. (2009). A relational psychoanalysis perspective on the necessity of acknowledging failure in order to restore the facilitating and containing features of the intersubjective relationship (the shared third). *International Journal of Psychoanalysis, 90*(3), 441–450.

Bion, W. (1987). Clinical seminars. In *Clinical Seminars and Other Works*. London: Karnac.

Cambray, J. (2011). Moments of complexity and enigmatic action: A Jungian view of the therapeutic field. *Journal of Analytical Psychology, 56*(3), 296–309.

Casement, P. (1985). *On Learning From the Patient*. London: Routledge.

Colman, W. (2005). Sexual metaphor and the language of unconscious phantasy. *Journal of Analytical Psychology, 50*(5), 641–660.

Colman, W. (2006). The analytic super-ego. *Journal of the British Association of Psychotherapists, 44*(2), 1–16.

Fisher, J. V. (2002). Poetry and psychoanalysis: Twin sciences of the emotions. *Journal of the British Association of Psychotherapists, 40*(2), 101–114.

Fordham, M. (1993). On not knowing beforehand. *Journal of Analytical Psychology, 38*(2), 127–136.

Gabbard, G. O., and Hobday, G. S. (2012). A psychoanalytic perspective on ethics, self-deception and the corrupt physician. *British Journal of Psychotherapy, 28*(2), 235–248.

Gabbard, G. O., and Ogden, T. (2009). On becoming a psychoanalyst. *International Journal of Psychoanalysis, 90,* 320–327.

Gerhardt, S. (2005). *Why Love Matters*. London: Brunner-Routledge.

Gray, J., and Williams, R. (2012). Cathedral conversation—belief and belonging. Episode 5 in *The People's Passion,* produced by Peter Everett. BBC Radio 4, 6th April. www.bbc.co.uk/programmes/b01f6bf8.

Greenson, R. (1967). *The Technique and Practice of Psychoanalysis*. New York: International Universities Press.

Guntrip, H. (1971). The promise of psychoanalysis. In B. Landis and E. S. Tauber (Eds.), *In the Name of Life. Essays in Honor of Erich Fromm,* pp. 44–56. New York: Holt, Rinehart and Winston. www.erich-fromm.de/biophil/joomla/images/stories/pdf-Dateien/Festschrift/Festschrift05.pdf

Gutheil, T. G., and Gabbard, G. O. (1998). Misuses and misunderstandings of boundary theory in clinical and regulatory settings. *American Journal of Psychiatry, 155,* 409–414.

Hogenson, G. B. (2009). Synchronicity and moments of meeting. *Journal of Analytical Psychology, 54*(2), 183–197.

Jung, C. G. (1929). Problems of modern psychotherapy. In *Collected Works,* Vol. 16, pp. 53–75. London: Routledge & Kegan Paul, 1966.

Jung, C. G. (1940). Transformation symbolism in the mass. *CW* 11.

Knox, J. (2009). When words do not mean what they say. Self-agency and the coercive use of language. *Journal of Analytical Psychology,* 54(1), 25–41.

Knox, J. (2011). *Self-Agency in Psychotherapy. Attachment, Autonomy and Intimacy.* New York and London: W.W. Norton.

Lambert, K. (1981). Individuation and the personality of the analyst. In *Analysis, Repair and Individuation.* London and New York: Academic Press.

Lennon, J. (1980). Beautiful boy (darling boy). From *Double Fantasy.* Parlophone Records.

Lyons-Ruth, K. (1999). The two-person unconscious: Intersubjective dialogue, enactive relational representation, and the emergence of new forms of relational organization. *Psychoanalytic Inquiry,* 19, 576–617

Menninger, K. (1958). *The Theory of Psychoanalytic Technique.* New York: Basic Books.

Oord, T. J. (2005). The love racket: Defining love and *agape* for the love-and-science research program. *Zygon,* 40, 919–938. www.calvin.edu/~jks4/city/Oord~Defining%20 Love.pdf

Orange, D. M., and Stolorow, R. D. (1998). Self-disclosure from the perspective of inter-subjectivity theory. *Psychoanalytic Inquiry,* 18, 530–537.

Parsons, M. (2000). Refinding theory in clinical practice. In *The Dove That Returns, the Dove That Vanishes: Paradox and Creativity in Psychoanalysis.* London and Philadelphia: Routledge.

Rees, D. A. (Ed.). (1951). *Aristotle: The Nichomachean Ethics. A Commentary by the Late H. H. Joachim.* Oxford: Clarendon Press.

Sandler, J. (1983). Reflections on some relations between psychoanalytic concepts and psychoanalytic practice. *International Journal of Psychoanalysis,* 64, 35–45.

Segal, H. et. al. (2012). *Encounters Through Generations. Becoming and Being a Psychoanalyst.* London: Institute of Psychoanalysis. www.psychoanalysis.org.uk/audiovisual-generations.htm

Shedler, J. (2010). The efficacy of psychodynamic psychotherapy. *American Psychologist,* 65(2), 98–109.

Steiner, J. (1993). *Psychic Retreats. Pathological Organisations in Psychotic, Neurotic and Borderline Patients.* London and New York: Routledge

Stern, D. N. et al. (1998). Non-interpretive mechanisms in psychoanalytic therapy: The "something more" than interpretation. *International Journal of Psycho-analysis,* 79, 903–921.

Whan, M. (1987). On the nature of practice. *Spring.*

Wiener, J. (2007). Evaluating progress in training: Character or competence. *Journal of Analytical Psychology,* 52(2), 171–183.

Chapter 8

Lionel Corbett

I was born in England in the middle of the Second World War, amidst air raids, food rationing, and a general sense of danger and deprivation. I still have vivid memories of gas masks, the air raid shelter in our backyard, and a bombed-out house a few hundred yards from my own. The war colored my psyche. My father had been in a Nazi concentration camp and had lost most of his family in the Holocaust. He always refused to talk about his experiences, but they left an indelible mark on him. My father carried with him a persistent sense of sadness, hopelessness, and resignation that I felt viscerally as a child. Some of my earliest memories are of grieving refugees gathering in my home, sharing memories, sighing deeply, speaking a kind of hybrid Yiddish-German-English. The Holocaust had cast a dark shadow over our lives. My mother's father and grandparents had escaped to England from pogroms in Eastern Europe, so the Holocaust seemed to be the continuation of a long series of persecutions that were felt to have had a kind of inevitability about them. I spent a great deal of time with my grandparents, but there too was an inescapable family atmosphere of heaviness and pessimism. There was a sense that persecution might resume at any time, even in England, where anti-Semitism was cloaked in politeness but was just as prevalent as it was in other parts of Europe. It has been a lifelong task to shed my early identification with the kind of chronic melancholia that pervaded my family. My mother was a very loving but anxious woman who struggled to provide emotional support, but often felt overwhelmed by the vicissitudes of post-war life and the poverty we experienced. With this combination of overburdened parents, I grew up feeling that my own needs and feelings were trivial or unimportant in the face of the suffering I saw all around me, and I learned not to express them. I did develop a passionate desire to understand why people behave as they do, and I remember being preoccupied with this question early on.

My father repeatedly told me that it was important for me find a career that I could take with me "when" (not if) this would all happen again to my generation. Mainly for this reason I was encouraged to go to medical school, much to the

DOI: 10.4324/9781003148968-9

delight of my mother's father who had been ejected from a medical school in a Balkan country because he was Jewish. It is not surprising that I would eventually study psychiatry, which was an unconscious attempt to understand more of what had happened to the people who populated my childhood. It took many years of clinical practice and study before I was able to gather together what I have understood so far about suffering and evil, by writing books on these problems. I have learned a great deal in the process, although the mystery simply deepens as one goes into it. Jung's notion of the dark side of the Self has provided some clarity here, for which I am grateful.

I was drawn to the study of Jung through a fortunate synchronicity, which I now see as fated. In the late 1970s I was working at a research institute in Chicago, mainly concerned with the biology of schizophrenia. I had trained in England in a psychiatry program that was exclusively biologically oriented, and I had intended to spend my career doing psychopharmacology. However, I was unhappy because it was dawning on me that something was missing in this approach to psychological difficulties. One day, I happened to meet a colleague with whom I shared my misgivings. He suggested I read June Singer's *Boundaries of the Soul*, which had a gripping effect on me. It felt as if a light had dawned. In about 1978 I went into analysis with June, who had recently arrived from Zurich and started the Chicago Jung Institute. My Jungian training was scornfully interpreted by the chairman of the department of psychiatry in which I was working as my not taking my career seriously. At the Institute, I was fortunate to meet Arwind Vasavada, who had arrived from Zurich having trained with Jung. He had a major influence on me, largely because of his interest in non-dual spirituality, which has become my personal spiritual commitment in combination with Jungian psychology.

I have always had a background sense of a spiritual dimension, but as a result of the Holocaust I had developed (and still have) a deep suspicion of all forms of organized religion, which seemed to me to be largely a source of conflict and violence. I realized to my great relief that Jung provides a form of spirituality that bypasses most of the problems of the theistic traditions and provides a container for the individual's experience of spirit, without recourse to traditional doctrines, dogmas, sacred texts, and religious hierarchies. Jung's notion of the religious function of the psyche has had a profound effect on me, leading to my writing several books and chapters on this subject. I believe it is possible that Jung has laid the groundwork for a new religious form, a new myth of God, that is slowly emerging alongside our existing religious traditions. As many of us are called to do, I see my work in this area partly as an attempt to address unsolved problems that earlier generations have passed on to us. I often wonder if my ancestors would approve. I wish I could ask them.

Varieties of Numinous Experience

The Experience of the Sacred in the Therapeutic Process

Originally published in 2006, A. Casement (Ed.), *The idea of the numinous*. New York: Brunner-Routledge. Reprinted with permission

During a period of despair, a man had the following waking vision:

> The vision that came to me felt unlike any daydream. I was seeing as if my eyes had been turned backwards and I was looking at something taking place within me. A huge thick curtain slowly came down and surrounded the back walls of a large space in my mind. I was lifted up and stood on a high mountain peak with large rock outcroppings. I could not see over the edge. The space was at once open and contained. The mountain was ancient and felt volcanic. Surrounding me, sitting among the rocks, were the shadow forms of the hosts of heaven. I knew they had gathered there in order to meet me. They seemed to be expecting me and to delight in my presence. A soft white glow radiated around me and I felt a deep warmth and sense of belonging . . . for that moment in time, I was heaven's agenda.

I hardly need to mention the restorative effect of this vision. But what is the clinician to make of such an experience when it is brought into the consulting room? Was the experience defensive, or the result of an overheated imagination? In this chapter, I will make a case for my own belief that such numinous experience is an authentic experience of the sacred.[1]

Initially the onus is often on the clinician to recognize the nature of numinous experience, since the patient is often bewildered or simply unsure of its significance. This is especially so when the experience does not take a traditional Judeo-Christian form. We therefore need some kind of criteria for recognizing the presence of the numinosum, such as those of Otto (1917/1958), who describes it as mysterious, tremendous, and fascinating. The important factor is the affective quality of the experience rather than its specific content. In its grip, we feel we are facing something quite outside our usual experience, something awesome or uncanny. Sometimes the event is dreadful or terrifying, at other times profoundly peaceful or joyful. Often the experience inspires worship, or a sense of atonement or blessing. It may produce a religious conversion, or simply awaken a spiritual disposition in the soul that has so far remained dormant—an important factor if we take seriously Jung's notion that the development of a religious attitude (not necessarily based on a creed) is vital in the second part of life.

William James (1958, pp. 292–293) noted four characteristics of such experiences. (1) They are ineffable—they defy expression in ordinary conceptual language. Unless one has experienced something like it, one is incompetent to understand such experience. (2) They have a noetic or cognitive aspect, in that they produce an overwhelming sense of understanding or clarity: we know something we did not know before, such as the unity nature of reality or its ground of love. This knowledge carries with it an extraordinary sense of authority, so that the experience is self-authenticating. (3) The experience is transient, usually lasting less than half an hour and rarely more than a few hours, at which point everyday consensual reality supervenes. (4) Whether such experience is induced or spontaneous, during the experience one is passive; one's own will is in abeyance, in the grip of a superior power.

Important to the psychotherapeutic context is the fact that contact with the numinosum may have a healing effect (Jung, 1973. p. 377). In what follows, I would like to describe a variety of manifestations of the numinosum, point out some of the ways in which they are healing, and discuss the relationship of such experience to psychopathology and character structure. Finally, I will indicate some of their effects on the therapeutic relationship.

Types of Numinous Experience

Numinous experience occurs through a variety of channels, perhaps related to innate factors such as temperament or to the various ways we may experience the unconscious based on our typology. In this chapter I will describe manifestations of the numinosum within dreams and visions, in the body, in nature, within the individual's psychopathology, and induced by means of entheogens. (Hardy [1997] offers a much more elaborate classification of a large number of numinous experiences.) Regardless of the subject's personal religious and cultural background, numinous manifestations may contain imagery from any religious tradition, and often their content is entirely novel. However, they are always specifically tailored to the psychology of the individual, which makes numinous experience relevant to psychotherapeutic practice rather than solely the province of professional theologians.

The Numinosum in Dreams

The classical Jungian literature is replete with examples of numinous dreams, but these tend to be demonstrations of the positive aspects of the numinosum.

However, the numinosum may also appear in a terrifying manner, often depicting the archetypal core of a complex, or clearly linked to the dreamer's psychopathology, as the following dream illustrates:

> I'm in a maze of stairs, doors, and ramps, something like an Escher drawing. I am running from the giant, severed head of my mother. Streaming from her head are tentacles that move like snakes and allow her to chase me. I perceive her as a monster. I am afraid of and disgusted by her, and I do not want her to touch me. She is laughing, as if it is silly that I am running from her because there is no way I will ever escape. To tease me, she occasionally catches up to me and touches me with a tentacle, just to let me know that I cannot outrun her. I run to a door and slam it behind me shutting her out, but then I turn to see that there are only more ramps, stairs, and doors, to which she has as much access as I do. I am crying in frustration. She laughs.

Here the numinosum appears as the Gorgon or terrible Mother. Equally as darkly numinous is the following dream of a young man:

> I am tied to the stake at the base of a high gilded throne, on which sits a huge woman with large teeth and long flowing hair. Blood flows like a river down the steps in front of her. This is a hazy, bloody scene. I cannot talk as my energy drains: another woman is sucking blood from my neck and arm. I'm terrified, but too weak and helpless to do anything.

This dream combines the mythology of the vampire with a Kali-like[2] image. This kind of imagery led Jung to say that the experience of the archetype strikes at the core of one's being. Such dreams contribute to the individuation process, but can hardly be said to have a visibly healing effect. Yet numinous dreams clearly may do so, as the following demonstrates.

A woman lost her 21-year-old son in a drowning accident suddenly and unexpectedly. This tragedy almost destroyed her mental and physical well-being. She was filled with pain, anguish, and guilt. Although deeply religious, she could find no solace in her tradition. Nevertheless, she would pray to ask where her son was. She believes that her prayer was answered in the following dream, in which she felt as if she were fully awake:

> A magnificent panoramic view appeared before me. There was no sun, only a soft twilight glow in the atmosphere. As I looked from left to right, I saw hundreds of people of all ages settled in small groups. I felt that this must be the place where my son was located. I searched through the crowd but could not find him. I began to panic, and called out to him, "Michael, Michael, where are you?" Suddenly, out of nowhere, came a three-year-old child on a tricycle laughing out loud and riding in and out of the crowds. As he came nearer, I saw that he was Michael as he was during his childhood. My fear quickly turned to joy and thanksgiving.

As a result of this dream, she was convinced that life continues on another plane of existence. From that moment, her pain, guilt, and death anxiety were greatly alleviated. This is obviously not the kind of dream that needs much analysis if we take it at face value. It could of course be reduced to a defensive operation in the face of intolerable grief, or simply seen as the emergence of a joyful, young aspect of the dreamer. However, like all numinous encounters, this type of dream carries a sense of such authority and authenticity that I am convinced that it is a message or statement rather than a defense. I hear such dreams not uncommonly after a death has occurred, and I suspect they are fairly frequent but rarely discussed, except in the privacy of a therapeutic situation. I realize that, should they be defensive, I may be colluding, unable to tolerate the patient's pain. In practice, I find no need to maintain an artificial professional persona that insists on a quasi-scientific skepticism or a hermeneutic of suspicion. Rather, one has to rely on one's human response in such a situation and not fall back on metapsychology, a belief system that is often as metaphysical as one's commitment to spiritual realities. In fact, a spiritual commitment may be solidly based on personal experience, whereas metapsychological concepts are often based simply on hearsay. Our theories are based on abstract thought, but authentic mystical experience reveals the deep structures of reality. The very fact that numinous experience is considered to be rare, or is rarely spoken of in polite conversation, illustrates the distance between that reality and the Western ego.

The Numinosum in Visionary Experiences

Many psychotherapists and psychoanalysts, steeped in the tradition of Western science, equate visionary experience with some kind of pathology, either organic or psychogenic. The materialistic assumption underlying this tradition is that there cannot be any such thing as an authentic spiritual experience, because reality is only physical. In this view, metaphysical in its own right, a visionary experience must have a physical or psychological explanation; it cannot be an authentic experience of another realm of being.[3] Because of this cultural bias, visionary experiences are the least likely to be brought into the consulting room. The patient is often afraid that he or she will be thought to be insane, using drugs, hysterical, or just endowed with too vivid an imagination. Accordingly, we have no idea of the true incidence of visions. In an effort towards correcting this cultural bias, I would like to focus particularly on this type of numinous experience.

Prior to the following experience, a senior nursing administrator had just resigned her position as a result of "severe compassion fatigue" and a bitter power struggle with an unsupportive administrator. All her life she had been a caretaker and was very identified with professional success. Wanting to be in a helping position, she now found herself in an adversarial role rather than being a voice for patient care. In colloquial terms, she was "burnt out" and painfully obsessed with her failure to meet her own high standards. Awake one night, ruminating about her career, feeling helpless and wondering what to do with her life, she had the following experience:

> Suddenly I was aware of a pinpoint of light at the foot of the bed. I became alarmed as it expanded in size to about a six-inch oval, floating mysteriously in the dark. I was fearful and fascinated, awestruck by the weird presence of something other than me in my bedroom. I was sure I was not dreaming. The oval of light spoke wordlessly and identified itself as the Compassionate Heart (I thought of Jesus and Buddha). A loving presence filled the room and flooded me. The oval of light shot a beam of light directly to my heart. In that moment I saw myself with divinely compassionate eyes and was filled with a sense of forgiveness, unconditional love, and complete self-acceptance. I did not need to do anything, the silent voice instructed; I just needed to be as I was in this love-filled moment. My heart felt so expanded that I began to experience tremendous chest pain. I thought of calling for help but I was paralyzed. After this moment of true terror, I experienced such peace that I thought I had died. In that moment of surrender I saw the most loving moments of my life and the ones when I had constricted the impulse of love. I saw the moments when I had judged myself as lovable only because I had tried to live from a conscious standard of love and service. I surrendered to my death and remembered nothing more.

This vision initiated a process of self-discovery, during which she realized that her overwork had often been a masochistic exercise. She realized how much she was the victim of a judgmental superego, and she became clearer about the childhood origins of her need to care for others instead of herself. This experience opened up an authentic capacity to love, not based on a professional persona. Eventually she left nursing and entered the ministry.

The following vision occurred to a woman who had been severely abused in childhood. She had suffered all her life from feeling alone, unloved, and unable to love, only able to make a close connection to the family dog but not to people. Accordingly, she has an intense need for relationship, but this remains "the most elusive and difficult aspect of my life." During a particularly painful period,

> A figure appeared dressed in a long, heavy, dark, brown-hooded robe, and stood on my pelvic bones facing me. I felt her presence and saw her clearly, although she was silent and virtually weightless as she stood on my body. My heart pounded, and I was unable to move, but I did not feel afraid. I sensed her deep caring and her intention to help me. She leaned forward and with her index finger she touched the place between my breasts adjacent to my heart. As she did so, she drew up her finger and began to withdraw a heavy, rough cord from around my heart. I could feel the sensation of it unbinding my heart and felt an ease as the weight and heaviness of the rope

was drawn away. As she continued for many minutes, the heavy cord progressively diminished in size, becoming like course homespun, then a finer weave, finally emerging as a very thin, silver-white gossamer thread. As she withdrew the fiber, she was simultaneously weaving a cloth that fell to the floor and so covered a large, dark puddle that was beside me. This experience permeated me so deeply that I was profoundly touched, shaken, and moved.

She realized that the "heart" meant the ability to love and be loved, to live in relationship, and to feel a sense of belonging with others. A student of mythology, she associated the weaver with the figure of Clotho, the spinner of life in Greek mythology, one of the Fates who determined the course of human lives. Clotho opened her heart by progressively unbinding the protective barriers against love. The thread that had bound her heart was woven into a way to cross the murky waters of her chronic depression. The fact that this figure was weightless suggests that the whole experience occurred at the level of the subtle body rather than the physical body. Why should we assume that this experience is merely allegorical? All the world's esoteric traditions describe a spiritual body that cannot be seen with ordinary vision, presumably based on this kind of experience. Here one could invoke the notion of the *imaginatio* or the *mundus imaginalis*, which, as Corbin (1972, p. 7) tells us, is ontologically as real as the world of the senses and the intellect. He also points out that the noetic and cognitive power of such perception—the information that it imparts—is as real as that of the five senses and the intellect.

One of the standard critiques of mysticism in general is that mystics tend to bring the particular theology of their tradition into their experiences. I suspect that this situation is more apparent than real: unorthodox or nontraditional manifestations of the numinosum are either dismissed as demonic, reported in a way that distorts the phenomenology of the experience,[4] or simply not reported at all, in order to avoid conflict with ecclesiastical authorities. Contemporary individuals who are committed to the Christian tradition may still experience the numinosum with a Christian content, but I have spoken with many Christians who experience highly unorthodox or even heretical manifestations of the numinosum. For this reason, religious establishments do not encourage mystical experience. It is not unusual, for instance, to dream of Jesus as a woman. The following experience, which begins with a traditional Christian content, ends in a way that furthers the subject's spirituality.

I awoke with an overwhelming sense of a presence in my home. There was also a vacuous, eerie silence. I sat up in bed. Suddenly a very quiet, low, rumbling tone began. A tiny white light appeared. As the tone's volume increased, so did the size of the light, becoming a ball that increased in circumference. The tone grew so loud I could hardly tolerate it. By this time the globe of light was about five feet in diameter and difficult to look at because of its brightness. The light became a golden color, and upon it appeared a symbol I did not understand. From the center of the light I heard a voice say "Jesus" as the ball of light moved towards me, striking me with a force that gently rocked me. Then everything disappeared; the room became quiet and dark. Within a second, a second tone and dot of light appeared, which also grew in volume and brightness. Upon it was a different unknown symbol, and this time the voice said "Christ" as the light flew into me and dispersed. Following a brief moment of dark and silence, a third tone and dot of light appeared. The light grew as before, but when it flew into me it was silent. Finally, the room returned to normal, leaving me awestruck.

Intuitively, the subject realized that the third light represents that aspect of the divine that cannot be named or spoken of, taking him into a nonconceptual experience of Silence.

I occasionally hear of contemporary numinous experience that spontaneously repeats or affirms some of the world's most powerful spiritual imagery, which makes me suggest that some of our classical spiritual metaphors originally arose as visionary experiences. During an intensely lonely period of his life, the following happened to a 17-year-old boy with no knowledge of Eastern spiritual traditions. He reported the vision to me 35 years later, when it was still clear; the memory was indelible.

Out of the darkness, faintly at first then with increasing clarity, the thin strands of a web appeared. It seemed to be a huge spider's web stretching out over an unimaginable void. The silken threads reached out endlessly in all directions. There was no center to this web, or everywhere was the center. Wherever my eyes roamed, wherever my gaze settled—that was the center. The strands of the web, its warp and woof, seemed to be space and time themselves. Wherever they intersected, at every juncture, there was a single dewdrop. Each drop contained within itself a spark of Light. There was a great stillness, a pregnant expectancy. Suddenly, as if tapped into motion, the jeweled web exploded into a dazzling display of light. Each drop sparkled and flashed, piercing the darkness, every drop dancing with the colors of its own light and reflecting the dance of all the other drops. Waves of motion coursed throughout the breadth and depth of the web, each drop linked to every other through delicate strands, each drop responsive to every other, finally settling back into stillness.

Not until many years later did this man come across a description of Indra's net, a metaphorical depiction of reality from the *Avatamsaka Sutra*, the Flower Garland Sutra of Buddhism, written around the first century C.E. Here, instead of dew drops, at each connecting knot of the web lies a jewel in which can be seen the reflection of every other jewel—an image of the interdependent, mutually co-arising universe in which every part reflects the whole. What puzzled him was that Indra's net is not usually said to be in motion. Much later, he associated the movement with the idea of the music of the spheres, an archetype of Apollonian mysticism, of harmonic rhythms and relationships, which informs Western consciousness and contemporary science. This vision seems to be a profound syzygy of Eastern and Western archetypal images of reality.

The following experience, reported to me by a middle-aged ministerial student, occurred when she was a young child, but remains fresh in her memory.

> I was walking on a beach with my family, on a misty day. I had trailed behind the others, and so was running to catch up with them. Suddenly a horrible thing happened. The whole world disappeared. There was a black, shining surface that was really a vast, immeasurable void, sort of like a transparent lens over nothingness, and a vast nothing above it. This vastness was horrible; it was alive and I could feel it, but it was not like a creature or being of any kind. As I opened my mouth to scream, nothing came out. I could not make a sound. I looked below my feet and saw that I was standing on nothing. I looked at my mother, walking ahead of me with her friend; they were suspended over "the nothing," but they did not seem to realize it. They did not realize that "the nothing" was the only thing there. I ran to the tent, sobbing. My mother was angry when I tried to tell her about it, and accused me of being silly. But I believed that if you did not know about "the nothing" you were safe, because then the illusion of all the solidness in the world would keep you from seeing the emptiness, the vast, deep void. Since I knew, I stayed in the tent.

Obviously, this experience could be explained away as the result of some kind of abandonment or separation terror. However, it happens to correspond perfectly to Buddhist notions of the Void, the ultimately empty nature of all phenomena.

Another "teaching" example is provided by the following, in which a vision follows a dream with the same theme. In the relevant part of the dream, which occurred during a period of loss and desolation, a woman meets the figure of Death. He is tall and black-robed, his face covered with a long veil. When she tries to run, he follows her, and she realizes that she must not panic or he will pursue her aggressively. She thinks of lifting his veil to look directly at his face and ask him what he wants of her, but she is too afraid to do so. In the next few months she was haunted by this dream image. She often attempted active imagination with the figure, but would receive no response. Then:

> One night I awoke to a vision of veiled Death standing in the corner of my bedroom. I felt curiously calm and yet driven to know this figure more fully. In a strikingly autonomous active imagination, I approached Death to throw back his veil. As I did so, I was met with a blinding white light that receded just enough for me to make out the featureless face. Neither male nor female, Death was a shining, white-skinned fetus, unformed and yet formed, lacking any human particularity yet awesomely beautiful in its unborn potential. As I realized that Death was life ever poised between being and non-being, Death bent towards me gently and tenderly laid its cheek against mine—a gesture like a benediction. I was flooded with an overwhelming sensation of

bliss and love. My heart and brow seemed to open and teem with an exquisite energy. The experience of being touched by this figure was profound . . . it had the potential to be any being, all beings or no being. The touch of its skin was the most amazing sensation, moist and malleable and positively teeming with life, as if I could feel its cells dividing, changing, and dancing beneath the surface.

The dreamer felt that this encounter was an "intimation of immortality." I suggested to her that the experience points to the fact that birth and death are, at a deep level, aspects of the same archetypal reality or process; she agreed that this might account for the tremendous feelings of both dread and longing that were evoked. The experience alleviated some of her death anxiety.

A numinous experience may tell us something we already know cognitively, but the information is given in a way that is so powerful one cannot resist its impact. The following waking experience happened to a woman who had experienced an extremely deprived childhood.

One night, when the moon was dark and my bedroom lay in inky blackness, I sensed a presence in the corner of the room. I was afraid. The presence grew and grew, until, pulsating, it filled the entire room, throbbing within the confining walls. The whole room seemed to tilt, as if accommodating itself to another dimension. I lay in terror, with my eyes tightly closed. A voice, deep and gentle, said to me: "Love. The whole thing is love." Slowly, the energy ebbed from the room, leaving me in paralyzed terror in the darkness.

She went on to say that there had been many occasions in her life when she wanted to give up, to be "small and hard and raging." However, she said that the memory of that night "calls me back to life" and to the challenge of discovering what "love" might be. Obviously, to hear that "the whole thing is love" is not a new idea in the history of spirituality. However, that sounds like a useless platitude to a person whose character structure and developmental history do not allow love. But this intense experience opened the possibility for this individual.

The Numinosum in Nature

A further genre of numinous experience occurs to people who find the sacred within the natural world. A few traditional religionists were nature mystics, but today this sensibility is mostly found in the guise of political movements such as environmentalism. What often drives environmentalists is a profound feeling for the numinosity of nature, so that to desecrate the land is tantamount to sacrilege. One can recognize such individuals when they have this type of experience:

Hurrying to a class at the university, because I was late I had to cross an expanse of lawn. As I ran across the grass, I had the most amazing and horrible experience. I could feel that each blade of grass had a life force, that the ground had a life force, that everything was bound together in this wonderful dance. I could feel my feet crushing the blades of grass, I could hear the crunch, I could feel the pain the grass felt. From this experience of expanded consciousness and oneness—which came totally unbidden and unexpected at that moment—I realized that I was something more than this pocket of flesh and mind, wondering and searching.

Entheogens and the Numinosum

There is controversy about whether entheogens, or psychedelics, produce authentic spiritual experience or whether their effects are simply the result of a disordered brain. Based on the following type of experience, I believe that these compounds affect brain functioning in a way that allows us to experience realms of reality that are not normally accessible to us.

> Suddenly I became aware of a presence that was enormously powerful and nurturing. It/She reassured me that I could surrender to the experience. I had an odd sensation of separating from my body, and suddenly felt myself floating, exquisitely light and free. I seemed to exist as pure consciousness within brilliant light, and felt blissful peace and joy. I became aware of two beings composed almost entirely of light. We discussed my path in life, significant events, and their relevance to my life's purpose. The deep wisdom and compassion of these beings helped me understand and accept several painful life events and feel forgiveness towards people who had hurt me. I felt relief and emotional healing. Next, they led me to a golden platform that ascended seven levels, like a stepped pyramid. At the top was a blaze of brilliant, diamond light, radiantly clear, sparkling with flashes of color. I was awed, and sensed that this was a divine presence. The light coalesced into the form of a goddess with an Asian face. No words were exchanged, just unspeakable reverence and devotion on my part, and unfathomable love on hers. I knew her to be Guanyin. She smiled at me, then turned her gaze at what appeared to be the earth far below, surrounded by the darkness of space. As I looked at the planet, I saw countless drops of light, which I knew represented every living being on the earth. My heart opened as I experienced an incomparable love for all life, and the deepest compassion I have ever known. I felt unconditional love for all, including rapists and murderers, whom I loved with the sadness of one who sees their suffering. I knew them as lost souls who had forgotten their true nature, and I felt a deep desire to help guide each one towards their birthright. Looking at Guanyin, I realized that my experience was simply a reflection of her divine nature, shared with me at this moment.

Needless to say, this experience was directly relevant to the subject's developmental history. She had been raised in an abusive household and was often beaten, shamed, and ridiculed by her mother. Guanyin is the archetype of a loving, compassionate, divine mother, of the kind that she did not have as a child. The vision was therefore extremely helpful. Again, depending on the therapist's personal commitment, one could dismiss the experience as defensive, merely a fantasy released by the drug, or as a healing contact with the numinosum. I believe that the high level of spirituality revealed in this experience, together with its coherence, are evidence that it was authentic.

The Numinosum in the Body

In the West, the body is a neglected source of numinous experience because of the generally negative stance taken towards it by our religious traditions. Nevertheless, it may be a vehicle for sacred experience.

> Immediately following an intense meditation practice, I lay down to relieve pain that had developed. I experienced sensations of extraordinary energy, light, and movement in my body. I heard a voice say that this was an experience of, and an opportunity to observe, Eros and its energy. It entered from above my body through a point midway between the pubic area and the navel as a column of white light with radiating yellow/gold light at its base. The sensations of this energy were simultaneously exciting, sensual, sexual, powerful, hot, vibrant, radiating, expansive, enlivening, and frightening. It was like observing Eros in a pure and intense form, like watching electrical energy, but seeing it as an energy of the heart. My initial reaction was to jolt myself out of the experience, but recognizing its power and importance, I was able to maintain a silent, still awareness for some time. As I became self-conscious and also exhausted, the energy receded and left. Later in the retreat, I experienced an extraordinary sense of both being, and being enveloped by, a completely opened heart that was all-expansive and all-encompassing. It left me with an amazing sense of joy and peace, and a feeling of being wholly part of the cosmos.

Unfortunately, the Western religious traditions have ignored what many Eastern cultures have understood; sexuality can be an important vehicle for the expression of our spirituality. As Jung (1978, p. 105) put it, sexuality is "a genuine and incontestable experience of the divine, whose transcendent force obliterates and consumes everything individual." Sexuality can allow ecstatic union with the sacred, during which our sense of being separate individuals disappears—a brief experience of enlightenment. Following an intense night of lovemaking, a young woman described a heightened state of spiritual awareness, during which

I stood outside of time. It was as if time normally flowed in a horizontal plane, and I had somehow stepped out of this horizontal flow into a timeless state. There was absolutely no sense of the passage of time. To say there was no beginning or ending of time would seem irrelevant. There was simply no time.

(Feuerstein, 1992, p. 29)

This woman clearly transcended her ordinary personality during this experience, which is the state of mind to which so much spiritual practice is devoted.

The Effects of Numinous Experience on the Therapeutic Process

The therapist's response to a numinous encounter that is brought into psychotherapy may have a profound effect on the therapeutic process, for good or ill. We tend to describe these effects in terms of our therapeutic orientation and philosophy of treatment, but the therapist's belief system is also a crucial factor. As we have seen, the healing value of numinous experience may lie simply in its content, because the numinosum addresses a specific aspect of the patient, either a wound, a developmental difficulty, or a current problem. The therapeutic task is then to help the patient understand and integrate the experience. However, the therapist's attitude and response to the patient's experience of the numinosum is also very significant, whether or not the content of the experience can be understood. If the therapist is dismissive or reductive, the patient may be very hurt. If the therapist responds in an attuned and sensitive manner, the patient feels that his or her experience is valued and validated. This enhances the self-selfobject tie, whose healing effects are themselves numinous.

Notes

1   For the sake of space, I will not discuss the ways in which this proposition may be justified or refuted, in the latter case by insisting that such experience is simply a fantasy or a defense arising from personal levels of the unconscious that have nothing to do with transcendent reality. The argument also hinges on whether numinous experience arises from transpersonal levels of the psyche, as Jung thought, in which case the objective psyche would be responsible for what we call "God," or whether the experience is given by God in the Judeo-Christian sense, as Otto believed. For a fuller discussion of these questions, see Corbett (1996, 2000a, 2000b) and Schlamm (1994).
2   In Hindu mythology, Kali is a ferocious aspect of the Divine Mother. She is the goddess of death as transformation, necessary for the renewal of the life force.
3   For example, the experience of Saul on the road to Damascus has been attributed to temporal lobe epilepsy. The visions of Hildegard of Bingen (1098–1180) have been described as the result of migraine because they are strikingly similar to the visual auras that accompany that illness (Singer, 1958, and Sacks, 1992). However, to dismiss them as only due to migraine is to ignore the possibility that severe migraine, like any disorder of the brain, may open a window onto a spiritual dimension. A severe illness, especially one that affects brain functioning, reduces the hegemony of the ego. One function of the ego is to maintain a barrier or gate between consensual reality and the larger order

of reality. Once the ego is weakened, the veil between this reality and spiritual reality becomes much thinner. That is, Hildegard's many illnesses—not all of which were migrainous in nature—allowed her to talk to the angels rather than causing her to do so. (Sacks himself, although committed to the medical paradigm, does point out that a diagnosis of migraine does not mean that her visions did not allow authentic insight into spiritual reality.)

4 See for example Jung's (1969) description of the case of Brother Klaus, whose non-traditional experience of the numinosum that included the divine feminine had to be reinterpreted to fit trinitarian Christian theology.

References

Corbett, L. (1996). *The Religious Function of the Psyche*. London: Routledge.

Corbett, L. (2000a). A depth psychological approach to the sacred. In D. Slattery and L. Corbett (Eds.), *Depth Psychology: Meditations in the Field*. Zurich: Daimon.

Corbett, L. (2000b). Jung's approach to the phenomenology of religious experience: A view from the consulting room. In R. Brooke (Ed.), *Pathways Into the Jungian World*. New York: Routledge.

Corbin, H. (1972). Mundus Imaginalis or the imaginary and the imaginal. *Spring*, Dallas, TX.

Feuerstein, G. (1992). *Sacred Sexuality*. New York: Jeremy Tarcher.

Hardy, A. (1979/1997). *The Spiritual Nature of Man: A Study of Contemporary Religious Experience*. Oxford: Oxford University Press.

James, W. (1958). *Varieties of Religious Experience*. New York: The New American Library, a Mentor Book.

Jung, C. G. (1969). Brother Klaus. In *Psychology and Religion: West and East. C.W. 11*. Princeton: Princeton University Press.

Jung, C. G. (1973). *Letters*, Vol. 1. G. Adler and A. Jaffe (Eds.), R. F. C. Hull (Trans.). Princeton: Princeton University Press.

Jung, C. G. (1978). *Psychological Reflections*. J. Jacobi and R. F. C. Hull (Eds.). Princeton: Princeton University Press.

Otto, R. (1917/1958). *The Idea of the Holy*. New York: Oxford University Press.

Sacks, O. (1992). *Migraine: Understanding a Common Disorder*. Appendix 1, *The visions of Hildegard*. Berkeley: University of California Press.

Singer, C. (1958). *From Magic to Science: Essays on the Scientific Twilight*. New York: Dover Publications.

Chapter 9

George B. Hogenson

I have always found it very difficult to give an account of how I became involved in the study and eventual application of Jung's system of psychology. In fact, I seriously question whether a clear account of any project that becomes a lifetime's concern can be fully worked out. In most cases, when asked, I give a rather linear account of the steps that led to my original work on Jung as a graduate student in philosophy at Yale University, the publication of my book on Jung and Freud, and then on through a series of appointments in academics and the foundation world to finally training as an analyst at the C. G. Jung Institute of Chicago. This account usually starts by noting that I was not overtaken by some compulsion to study Jung after reading *Memories, Dreams, Reflections* or some other text. In fact, initially I really didn't want to work on Jung, and I spent a year after the death of my father in 1977 trying to find some other topic on which to write my dissertation. I suppose the fact that nothing came of this effort to get away from Jung says something about the necessity of doing the work, although I am deeply suspicious of notions such as destiny or fate. The turning point came in 1978, a year after my father's death, which was unexpected and violent, when I returned to Japan where I had studied the modern Japanese philosopher Nishida Kitaro for a term as an undergraduate under the guidance of Professor Masao Abe. Professor Abe had introduced me to the Jesuit scholar and mystic William Johnston, whom I visited in the mountains above Kyoto. At the time I was not aware of how deeply Johnston had studied Jung, but in the course of an afternoon of quiet conversation it became clear that I needed to return to Yale and my advisor, Rulon Wells, and begin again on Jung.

I have been very fortunate in the mentors I had in this stage of my life. By far the most important was Rulon Wells, professor of linguistics and philosophy at Yale and a legend for his vast, encyclopaedic knowledge. He originally wanted to work on *The Tibetan Book of the Dead*, but it turned out that was more an avenue to work on Jung—he had previously directed dissertations on Freud and Lacan. I had, in fact, already developed some interest in psychoanalysis by way of reading Paul Ricoeur's monumental *Freud and Philosophy*, which I bought in 1971 as I was about to leave Yale for active duty in the Air Force after one year in the Department of East Asian

DOI: 10.4324/9781003148968-10

Studies, where I was continuing my study of the history of Buddhism, begun as an undergraduate at St. Olaf College. Jung first came into the picture in a seminar on Leibniz with Professor Wells, when I stumbled on Jung's synchronicity essay and von Franz's book, *Number and Time*, while writing on Leibniz's philosophy of time. I suppose, seen in light of the majority of the writing I have done over the last 20 years, that von Franz's book resonated with me in ways that other Jungian texts did not. But my dissertation, and subsequent book, *Jung's Struggle With Freud*, did not address the issues of synchronicity and the mathematics of symbolism but rather examined the disputes that arose around the foundations of psychoanalysis.

A lack of job opportunities in philosophy in 1979 led to my joining the faculty of the Yale School of Management where my experience in the Air Force as a strategic planner allowed me to teach in the public policy program of the school and chair the faculty research seminar on international security policy. Needless to say, this was far removed from further work on Jung, but it would lead to my joining the staff of the MacArthur Foundation in 1986 and my involvement with the research recently underway on complex systems theory at the Santa Fe Institute, which the Foundation was funding. When I reflect on it now, it was at this point that my first encounter with Jung, by way of synchronicity and von Franz's speculations on the mathematics of symbolism and time, reconnected with the work I was directly involved with. Complex systems theory and the mathematics of symbolic systems would come to dominate the research and theorizing I would undertake beginning in the late 1990s, but I first had to be persuaded, by my long-time friend Bill Borden, to undertake training as a clinician, and then as an analyst.

I completed my analytic training in 1998 and set out to attend the IAAP Congress in Florence, Italy, by way of Zurich where I attended the Congress of the International Association for Adaptive Systems, the group of researchers involved in complexity theory, theoretical robotics, artificial life and related research programs. This combination of analytical psychology and the cutting-edge research in the sciences has largely defined my work since becoming an analyst—at least as far as my writing is concerned. As a clinician I think more in terms of allowing myself to inhabit the inner world of my clients in order to accompany them into the darkness and hope for some light. I suppose one could say that this is how I experience the opposites, stretched in some way between the rationality of numbers and the depths of the affective. Fortunately, I have found others in the Jungian community who live in a similar space, particularly my friends Joe Cambray and Harald Atmanspacher. I feel very fortunate to know many other remarkable individuals in the Jungian world—Murray Stein was my first analyst and remains a close friend, Tom and Jean Kirsch became close friends, although Tom could never figure out why I didn't list *Memories, Dreams, Reflections* among the books I would take to a desert island—my official list was *Moby Dick*, Kant's *Critique of Pure Reason* and the Bible. Tom Kelley is among the kindest and most supportive people I have ever met, and Jean Knox, who shared in the development of the emergence model of thinking about archetypes, is among the most careful and critical thinkers I know.

There are many others, but central to the work I have done over the last 30 some years are my wife, Kate, and our children, Peter and Katherine, who have put up with and sustained my work and life in ways I will never be able to repay.

Synchronicity and Moments of Meeting

Originally published in *Journal of Analytical Psychology*, 2009, 54, 183–197. Reprinted with permission.

Introduction

This chapter is part of a continuing effort to connect theoretical work on issues of emergence, archetypes and synchronicity, with clinical experience. An earlier approach to this topic was presented in Rome in 2005 at the gracious invitation of Massimo Giannoni and his colleagues, and a shorter version of that chapter may be found in Ann Casement's book, *Who Owns Jung?* (Hogenson, 2007). That chapter asked the question of how analysis heals and drew on the clinical and developmental theories of a group of American psychoanalysts collectively known as the Boston Process of Change Study Group (BPCSG) to provide a clinical perspective on the question. This chapter draws on them once again.

The Rome chapter focused on the role of the symbolic in analysis; this chapter will address synchronicity and the analytic process. The two chapters are intended to complement one another, but the issue in this chapter is the emergence of meaning, and what grounds we have for attributing meaning to analytic states. I take it that the notion that synchronicity is concerned with "meaningful" coincidences warrants this inquiry.

Synchronicity

Considerable attention is currently being paid to Jung's theory of synchronicity, and proposals intended to illuminate the meaning of and processes contributing to synchronicities are developing from a variety of points of view. These range from efforts to bring the new insights of complex dynamic systems theory to bear on the processes that might give rise to synchronicities (Cambray, 2002) to cultural interpretations of Jung's role in the "re-enchantment of nature" programme which began in 19th-century Germany (Main, 2004, 2007a, 2007b; Rowland, 2005). Important work has also gone on regarding the historical development of Jung's thinking on synchronicity (Gieser, 2005). Closer to what I propose to do here, in 1997 George Bright wrote an important chapter in the *Journal of Analytical Psychology* (Bright, 1997) that examined synchronicity as a guiding principle in the establishment of an analytic posture in the clinical setting. Common to all of these renderings of synchronicity—with the possible exception of the purely historical accounts—is the presupposition that when one talks about synchronicity, or synchronistic events, one is actually talking about something distinctive happening in the world. Indeed, the something happening has very particular characteristics such as a fundamental sense of the transcendence of temporal and spatial boundaries, of the meaningful or meaning-laden conjunction of psychological and material conditions, and, most importantly, of the absence of any conventional sense of causal foundations. In his chapter, Bright elaborates these characteristics by appeal to Jung's notion of the psychoid, which Bright parses as a theory Jung proposed for grounding individually meaningful states in an objective domain of meaning that influences both mind and matter. In a large measure all of these characteristics of synchronicities bottom out on Jung's theory of archetypes insofar as Jung argues that a synchronistic event marks the activation of an archetype.

Beginning with this last point, however, we can question the nature of synchronicity by asking what precisely we mean by the activation of an archetype. As Jean Knox has demonstrated, Jung has a variety of definitions of archetype, and it is difficult to determine from one place to another precisely what definition he is using. She has gone on to develop an important point of view on archetypes as emergent developmental achievements, or "image schemata" (Knox, 2003). Peter Saunders and Patricia Skar (Saunders and Skar, 2001) have argued that archetypes are emergent aggregations or classes of complexes, reversing Jung's hierarchy of psychic structures and raising important questions about the foundations of the theory of archetypes. In several chapters I have argued that one cannot say that an archetype exists "in the sense of being a discrete ontologically definable entity with a place in the genome or the cognitive arrangement of modules or schemas in the brain" (Hogenson, 2005, p. 279), but rather that they are "emergent properties of the developmental system of brain, environment and narrative" (Hogenson, 2001, p. 607). Beginning somewhat earlier, David Tresan (1996) and, to a degree, John van Eenwyk (1997) had already introduced the language of emergence and self-organization into the Jungian lexicon, and emergence has since become one of the most widely discussed candidates for explaining a number of phenomena in both the Jungian community and, as I will discuss later, the psychoanalytic community.

The question that then arises is what impact on the theory of synchronicity will follow from taking seriously the implications of these formulations? If archetypes are emergent properties of circumstances in the here and now, rather than eternal forms (Plato), *a priori* categories (Kant) or cognitive modules in the brain (Chomsky), is an alternative view of synchronicity possible or even necessary? To answer this question I will propose that we may need to view synchronicity as first a very early or primitive developmental experience, perhaps the most elementary of all, which establishes the fundamental relationship of the individual to the possibility of meaning as an emergent property of the psyche.

To further develop the argument I will examine the claims made for a specific set of clinical phenomena defined by the members of the Boston Process of Change Study Group (BPCSG). Largely under the leadership of Daniel Stern, this group of psychoanalysts has produced a series of chapters and books that provide a window into the micro-behaviours of infant interactions. This attention to micro-behaviours has since been extended into the description of processes in the analysis of adults that result in the formation of new levels of interrelational knowledge. This approach stands in contrast to the more traditional interpretative or hermeneutical understanding of the analytic process. I will attempt to show how the elements of their analysis dovetail with the emergent model of the archetype, and how our understanding of synchronicity can be incorporated in this same model.

The Elementary Model of the Archetype

Jung's first published use of the term archetype occurred, as is well known, at a joint meeting of the Aristotelian Society, the Mind Association and the British Psychological Society in 1919 (Jung, 1919). Coming shortly after the end of the Great War, it was also one of the first public presentations made by Jung following his "encounter with the unconscious." As Jungians are aware, the encounter with the unconscious involved a long process of visionary encounters, and the writing of the Black Books and the Red Book, in which Jung wrestled with his experiences. It is hardly an exaggeration to say that these experiences are close to what many people would associate with archetypal phenomena, in their profound impact on Jung and the dimensions of their imagery. Nevertheless, when Jung spoke in London these phenomena played no role in his initial definition of the archetype; Jung's simple formulation was that the archetypes were

> *a priori* inborn forms of 'intuition', namely the *archetypes* of perception and apprehension, which are the necessary *a priori* determinants of all psychic processes. Just as his instincts compel man to a specifically human mode of existence, so the archetypes force his ways of perception and apprehension into specifically human patterns.

> (Jung, 1919, para. 270)

Elsewhere Jung tends to compare his notion of the formative powers of the archetypes to the behavioural patterns of animals, such as the bowerbird, with its characteristic nest building practices. In more contemporary biological terminology these behavioural patterns are referred to as species typical action patterns, a term that I will rely on in what follows. Jung returns to the theme of the pattern of action or behaviour on a number of occasions, most notably in his discussion of the leaf cutting ant in "On the Nature of the Psyche," where he makes the important point that his conception of the "image" is in fact the totality of the situation within which an organism's "pattern of behaviour" emerges. The "image" of the leaf-cutting ant is the totality of its environment and the behavioural patterns of the ant appropriate to that environment (Jung, 1954). So what precisely would the image of the human be? If it is the case that the archetypal image involves "elementary forms of intuition" embedded in an environment to which they are specifically suited, how would we come to understand the archetypal in the human context?

Intentionality

To answer this question I need to comment briefly on Freud and the necessary foundations of any system of psychology that posits a theory of the dynamic unconscious. In his chapter on synchronicity, Bright suggests that Jung's theory should be seen as comparable in its system-building role to Freud's analysis of parapraxis. Specifically, an instance of parapraxis, such as a slip of the tongue, is interpreted by appeal to the unconscious contents that it is alleged to reveal. I want to suggest that this understanding of parapraxis, while accurate within the theoretical world of Freudian psychoanalysis, is the precise inversion of its actual theoretical significance. What is actually at stake, rather, is that certain assumptions about the nature of mind, when linked to the occurrence of parapraxis, contribute to the development of a theory of the dynamic unconscious. As a student, Freud had attended lectures given by Franz Brentano, who is best known in the history of philosophy for resuscitating the scholastic arguments for the intentionality of consciousness. Brentano was also the teacher of Edmund Husserl and thus stands as the godfather to Husserl's phenomenology, for which the theory of intentionality is foundational (Moran, 2000).

Intentionality, in Brentano's sense, is not a matter of intentions in the sense of purposes for action, but rather of the object-relatedness of consciousness—all acts of consciousness must have an object, there can be no "empty" acts of consciousness. Historically, it is not clear that Freud attended those lectures given by Brentano that dealt directly with his theory of intentionality, although Ellenberger provides some evidence that Brentano's theories did influence Freud's work (Ellenberger, 1970). Be that as it may, it is clear that once one has the theory of intentionality in hand Freud's understanding of the dynamic unconscious is far more comprehensible. Parapraxis is a case in point insofar as the argument goes that the slip has the form of an act of consciousness, but it has no discernible object—"I don't know why I said that"—which means that the object of the slip must not be available to consciousness. By an implicit appeal to a theory of intentionality Freud is able to convert seemingly meaningless acts into directed acts that reference a domain of intentional objects not available to consciousness. By attributing intentionality to parapraxes, therefore, Freud is actually proposing an argument for the existence of the dynamic unconscious, and in his case the set of objects to which parapraxis refers are repressed wishes.

We can now ask what intentionality implies for the theory of archetypes as an element in Jung's model of the dynamic unconscious. This question has important implications for our understanding of synchronicity. The heart of the matter lies in the nature of the objects associated with archetypal acts of consciousness. Jung's writings are replete with instances where he affirms that the image "can be considered archetypal when it can be shown to exist in the records of human history, in identical form and with the same meaning" (Jung, 1967). Thus, the objects of consciousness that may be called archetypal must first of all be transhistorical. There are a class of objects of consciousness, in other words, that perdure through time and space, which consciousness in its archetypal form takes as intentional objects. The archetypal object, therefore, is a particular subcategory of intentional objects generally, but, Jung argues, it is the intentional object that is addressed by the most distinctly human form of intuition and apprehension. Thus, the archetypes are first of all intentional states, that is, they are states in which the psyche references a specific set of objects. When we discuss the archetypes, or invoke their influence, we are discussing, in other words, a particular set of intentional states. And to the degree that a synchronistic event is characterized by the activation of an archetype, the image or intentional object of our consciousness of the event should possess the characteristic of an archetypal object.

Moments of Meeting

The Boston Process of Change Study Group has produced some of the most provocative and carefully worked out propositions concerning the therapeutic process in recent psychoanalytic theory. The basis of their work lies in the detailed research the members of the group have conducted on mother/infant interaction. The membership of the group includes such leading infant research figures as Daniel Stern, Louis Sander and Edward Tronick. In addition to the BPCSG's formal membership, several other researchers, most notably Beatrice Beebe and Frank Lachmann (Beebe, 2002), have contributed to the discussion of change process by appeal to infant behaviour. The key to their work has been the changes in our understanding of mother/infant interaction that have come about by way of almost microscopic analysis of videotaped interactive processes. What these analyses have revealed is that interactive processes are continuous, fine grained and developmental in nature. There is, if you will, a delicate process of negotiation between the caregiver and infant that leads to what the members of the study group refer to as "implicit relational knowing." The experiences that lead to changes in implicit relational knowing constitute the "something more than interpretation" which, the study group argues, is central to the therapeutic process in which "the *something more* has taken the form of psychological acts versus psychological words; of change in psychological structures versus undoing repression and rendering conscious; of a mutative relationship with the therapist versus mutative information for the patient" (Stern et al., 1998, p. 903; emphasis original). I want to emphasize the priority given to "psychological acts" as providing the something more of this approach to analysis. As Beebe and Lachmann (2002) summarize their interest in infant observation:

> The value of infant research for psychoanalysis is often derived from the ways in which this research can help an analyst and a patient imagine the patient's infancy . . . Despite the importance of this use, however, we are primarily interested in using infant research in a different way, that is, to illustrate organizing principles of interactions relevant for psychoanalysis.
>
> (Beebe and Lachmann, p. 33)

These patterns of interaction are, according to Beebe and Lachmann, as well as the members of the BPCSG, preverbal or non-linguistic and "describe lifelong modes of action sequences" (p. 34). The heart of their argument is that such act-based interactions are sorely neglected in adult psychoanalysis, while in fact providing the basis for the "procedural/emotional" dimension of interaction (ibid.).

Stern, in his book *The Motherhood Constellation*, is even more emphatic about the importance of action analysis and its neglect in psychoanalytic circles, which, by relying on the hermeneutical/interpretative tradition, demonstrate a "strong intellectual current against placing action at the center in understanding human behaviour" (Stern, 1995, p. 77). "[A]ctions committed by a human," Stern continues, "are assumed to have cultural concepts and language implicitly behind or within them. This may be increasingly true as development proceeds, but it is only partially so at the ages that interest us" (ibid.).

For these action-based analysts, the process of non-verbal interaction is continuous throughout the clinical process. The members of the BPCSG have devised a specific set of features that allow them to describe a series of stages in the interactive process leading to the development of new levels of implicit relational knowing that culminates in what they, following the lead of one of their members (Sander), refer to as "moments of meeting." Taken as a whole, the process they describe is referred to as moving along. This concept references the instant-by-instant continuum of the analytic process, paralleling, according to their model, the moving along of the mother/infant interaction. Moving along is punctuated, in turn, by "now moments," instances of closer approximation between the parties to the interaction. Finally, we come to moments of meeting:

> The key concept, the 'moment of meeting', is the emergent property of the 'moving along' process that alters the intersubjective environment, and thus the *implicit relational knowing*. In brief, *moving along* is comprised of a string of 'present moments', which are the subjective units marking the slight shifts in direction while proceeding forward. At times, a present moment becomes 'hot' affectively, and full of portent for the therapeutic process. These moments are called 'now moments'. When a now moment is seized, i.e. responded to with an authentic, specific, personal response from each partner, it becomes a 'moment of meeting'. This is the emergent property that alters the subjective context.
>
> (Stern, Sander et al., 1998, pp. 909–910; emphasis original)

Evolution and Patterns of Action

Stern and his colleagues provide an exquisitely fine-grained description of the action patterns of the mother/infant interaction, and derive from their work at that level a series of important and provocative suggestions for the conduct of adult psychoanalysis. But I will now argue that to fully understand the importance of these action patterns, and to connect them to synchronicity, we must address the question of where the characteristically human patterns of action come from. This is an evolutionary question. By way of example, in the 1980s Kenneth Kaye conducted very detailed studies of the nursing behaviour of human infants (Kaye and Wells, 1980; Kaye, 1982). Briefly, Kaye's work demonstrates the unique form of human infant nursing, what he characterizes as the "burst-pause-burst" pattern. No other mammal, including the higher primates, displays this pattern, and one must therefore conclude that such a unique yet fundamental action pattern derives from an equally unique set of evolutionary influences. It can be demonstrated, however, that the utility of this pattern has nothing to do with nutrition. To the contrary, until the mother and infant successfully negotiate the vicissitudes of feeding associated with this pattern, it tends to detract from successful feeding by interrupting the feed. This process of negotiation entails an important aspect of the mother's response to the infant insofar as she interprets the infant's action pattern as meaningful. The infant is, in the mind of the mother, communicating something to her, and she will respond "as if" the communication is meaningful by acting responsively, usually by jiggling the infant in an effort to restore the infant's interest in sucking. Ironically, just such jiggling prolongs the infant's pause rather than stimulating sucking, and it is the interaction between mother and infant that must be negotiated. These observations led Kaye, and following him, Horst Hendricks-Jansen (1996), to argue that this burst-pause-burst pattern of feeding is in fact an adaptation suited to bootstrapping the infant into a quite different, uniquely human, action pattern, namely taking turns in conversational settings. In other words, the feeding pattern of the human infant is in service to a pattern of action in adults that relates to distinctly human communication rather than nutrition. This leads to another important observation regarding infant action patterns, as Hendricks-Jansen argues, in that infant action patterns are not immature or preliminary forms of mature behaviours, but rather adaptations that facilitate bootstrapping the infant into the complex world of adult human behaviour. What makes the human world unique is that it is a world in which meaning is attributed to virtually all patterns of action; it is a world of intentional attribution. As Hendricks-Jansen writes, "Human beings can be said to live in a natural environment of meaning" (Hendricks-Jansen, 1996, p. xi). Similarly, as one observer has commented, "Kaye assumes that the infant initially has no social skills or consciousness; however, from the very beginning the parents act 'as if' the infant has both interests and intentions" (Brinich, 1983). This is a world in which intentional attribution is assumed to be the foundation of cognitive reality.

At the beginning of his chapter on synchronicity, Bright quotes Winnicott:

> A baby kicks in the womb; it cannot be assumed he is trying to kick his way out. A baby of a few weeks thrashes with his arms; it cannot be assumed he means to hit. A baby chews the nipple with his gums; it cannot be assumed that he is meaning to destroy or to hurt.
>
> (Bright, 1997, p. 613, citing Winnicott, 1987, p. 204)

Indeed, following Kaye and Hendricks-Jansen, it would be incorrect to make such attributions. But the mother does make these attributions, as does the traditional psychoanalyst, armed with a theory of infantile sexuality and aggression, because human behaviour patterns are assumed to be about something, they are supposed to display intentionality. The action pattern of the infant is, in a sense, identical to the parapraxis of the neurotic in the mind of the mature observer—caregiver or psychoanalyst. By extension, in analytical psychology certain action patterns have archetypal objects as their intentional foci.

Synchronicity and Moments of Meeting

What about synchronicity? A great deal has been written recently on the subject of synchronicity, much of it going a long way to illuminate Jung's objectives in proposing the theory. In the process, however, the most elementary features of the phenomenon as a phenomenon have been obscured. To make my argument, therefore, I will return to Jung's often cited, but still paradigmatic, example of an event in which there is a "simultaneous occurrence of a certain psychic state with one or more external events which appear as meaningful parallels to the momentary subjective state" (Jung, 1952, para. 850). This instance is, of course, the famous scarab beetle synchronicity. I will not repeat Jung's account of the beetle dream and the entry of the beetle into his consulting room. Rather, what I want to focus on is the larger context within which the event takes place. This context has only recently been outlined, largely by Paul Bishop (2000) and Roderick Main (2007a). The essence of the matter is not so much the patient's dream as it is Jung's own relationship to scarab imagery. As Main remarks, the "scarab incident" is not just a synchronicity for the patient, it is a synchronicity for Jung—indeed, I now want to suggest the incident was primarily a synchronicity for Jung. Main seems to miss this point, referring to Jung's experience as a "second-order synchronicity," even while he argues that it was Jung who was looking for an event that would break through his patient's "Cartesian rationality" and, most importantly, that "the scarab beetle already had considerable significance for Jung" (Main, 2007a, p. 28). Not just considerable significance, it would seem, based on the rest of Main's account. We first learn that Jung had a major scarab beetle dream in 1913, following the break with Freud, perhaps drawing on the large set of scarabs that Freud had in his collection of antiquities. Main goes on to outline how

Jung's "fascination with the problem of synchronicity" dates to the mid-1920s, when Egyptology had become fashionable following the discovery of Tutankhamen's tomb with its scarab cartouches. Finally, Main outlines the importance of the scarab in alchemical texts with which Jung was familiar, including the *Secret of the Golden Flower* and concludes with Jung's association of the scarab with the hero myth (Main, 2007a, pp. 28–33). An appreciation of Jung's own associations to the scarab imagery—which for him certainly possessed a "transhistorical" or archetypal quality, shifts the centre of gravity for our understanding of this incident, raising questions about the role the dream and the coincidental entry of the beetle into the room had for Jung's countertransference to this particular patient. There are, of course, other instances where Jung explicitly grappled with his countertransference, to the benefit of the treatment, and it is curious that in this instance there is no evidence in his own account that he recognized that there were important countertransference implications to the dream.

I have argued (Hogenson, 2005) that synchronicity, along with the complexes and archetypes, is an instance of variation in what I have called symbolic density, reflected in an analytic framework called a power law distribution. Briefly, a power law distribution is a way of representing the intensity of a phenomenon in relation to its frequency—the term "power law" derives from the use of exponents or powers of ten in the calculation of the distribution. Power laws show the relation between the frequency of small events and the rarity of large ones, providing a way of modelling events that are "statistically improbable" but nevertheless regularly occur. This system of analysis can be applied to a wide variety of phenomena, from activity in the brain to the frequency and intensity of earthquakes (Bak, 1996). One of the most important elements of power law distributions is their application to symbol systems. This application of power laws originated with Harvard linguist George Kingsley Zipf, and his particular application came to be known as Zipf's law. Zipf examined the frequency of words in texts, and argued for what he called the principle of least effort, by which he meant that, in general, successful communication tended to move toward relatively general categorization—people would prefer to talk about dogs rather than specific breeds of dog, because both the speaker and the listener would expend less effort in the communicative process. However, there would be instances when much greater precision, or much denser symbolic reference and association, was required—talking about the subtle variations between Irish and Norwegian wolfhounds, for example—despite the communicative effort entailed (Vogt, 2004). These variations, Zipf demonstrated, fall into a power law distribution. Zipf died in 1950, but his work became central to development of some of the most important mathematical constructs of the late 20th century in the form of fractal geometry, which also follows power law distributions. More recently, two theoreticians associated with the Santa Fe Institute, Ramon Ferrer i Cancho and Richard Solé, have, in an analysis of language formation, concluded that "any symbolic system will obey Zipf's Law"; that is, symbolic systems always display the features of a power law distribution (Ferrer i Cancho and Solé, 2003; Ferrer i Cancho et al., 2005). From this conclusion on the part of Ferrer i Concho and Solé, I have argued that we can look at the various instances of symbolic activity, archetypal phenomena and so on in Jung and find that they fall into a power law distribution following Zipf's original insights.

Building on this argument, I propose to use the term symbolic density as a way of thinking about the experienced associative, referential and semantic complexity of a given symbol. I now want to suggest, given the historical work of Main, Bishop and others, that Jung's paradigmatic instance of synchronicity, the scarab beetle incident, is precisely what is implied by the notion of symbolic density—but it is particularly dense for Jung. This way of looking at Jung's paradigmatic instance of synchronicity implies that while the coincidence between his patient's dream and the entry into his consulting room of a scarab-like beetle may seem unusual, the overall impact of the event on the course of treatment, and particularly the meaningfulness of the event, lies at the high end of a power law distribution, where symbolic events become very rare, but also very meaning-laden.

In the case of the theorizing of the BPCSG, a similar situation can be seen. Specifically, a reading of the group's chapters leads one to conclude that if one examined a distribution of events running from the ordinary moments of moving along, to the far less common now moments, and finally to the rare but meaning-laden moments of meeting, it is likely that a power law would be a productive analytic approach to a theoretical description. Adding to this the results of thinking about the evolutionary basis of the distinctly human patterns of action that comprise the most compelling aspects of now moments, that is, that they emerge as adaptive responses to the symbolic world of human adults, we can begin to see moments of meeting as tied to the power law structures of the symbolic, and thus as phenomena cognate to synchronicities. Indeed, I want to suggest that a close analysis of the moments of meeting of Stern et al. may well show characteristics that are startlingly close to Jung's notion of synchronicity, at least in the clinical setting.

Conclusion

With this framework in hand, I want to conclude by proposing some alternative understandings of the nature of synchronicity. In my earlier chapter I argued that synchronicity, "far from being a radically alien phenomenon, which departs decisively from the natural order, is in fact continuous with Jung's earlier observations, and indeed, with the most commonplace and familiar of human behaviours, language" (Hogenson, 2005, p. 272). What I want to suggest now is that the relationship between synchronicity and the symbolic, with the basic notion of the archetype as a foundation—that is, the uniquely human forms of intuition and apprehension, combined with the uniquely human patterns of action and their adaptation to the symbolic world—raises the possibility of viewing synchronicity as a basic, perhaps the basic, experience of early infant development. Could it be that the infant experiences his or her world as what the adult Jungian theoretician would identify as an almost continuous experience of synchronistic moments?

My second suggestion is that the clinical notion of moments of meeting, as outlined by the Boston Process of Change Study Group, may also be linked to the experience of synchronicity. This is an area where I prefer to be cautious about the work of the study group because they may not fully grasp the meaningfully or symbolically embedded evolutionary origins of the patterns of action upon which their theory rests—that is, that the patterns of action that matter most are adaptations to a symbolic environment and thus carry with them an implicit symbolic dimension. In their most recent work, however, it may be the case that they are approaching this question more comprehensively (Stern, Sander et al., 2007) insofar as they are concerned with the representational nature of mind, and the relationship between patterns of action and the development of language. This is a topic, however, for further investigation.

One consequence of the work of the group, however, that points in a provocative direction is their argument, in the same chapter, that giving action patterns pride of place inverts the traditional psychoanalytic taxonomy of the psyche. As they summarize their argument:

> The major point of this chapter has been to delineate the upside-down relationship between the supposedly 'superficial' layer of immediate interaction and the supposedly 'profound' layer of intrapsychic entities, such as conflict and defense. Traditionally, the intrapsychic entities were assumed to determine what happened at the interactive level.
>
> The interactive level was seen merely as the instantiation of deeper forces. We suggest instead that the interactive process itself is primary and generates the raw material from which we draw the generalized abstractions that we term conflicts, defenses and phantasy. From these moves as experienced in the interaction, psychoanalytic interpretations are drawn. It follows that conflicts and defenses are born and reside in the domain of interaction, and that this relational living out is the deep layer of experience, while the abstractions that we use to describe the repetitive aspects of these relational strategies, such as conflict and defense, are secondary descriptors of the deep level, but not the level itself, and exist further from the lived experience.
>
> (p. 14)

This argument calls into question our most fundamental assumptions about the nature and status of the unconscious, not only in the psychoanalytic tradition, but in analytical psychology as well. This is a conclusion that will require more consideration. But one issue does present itself, returning for a moment to the work of George Bright. In his chapter, his analysis of synchronicity brings him, particularly in his clinical discussion, to Jung's notion of the psychoid, as well as related concepts such as Winnicott's domain of absolute meaning, as necessary foundational concepts for the meaningfulness of their other theoretical constructs. Given the argument of this chapter, in conjunction with the work of the BPCSG, I believe it is unclear whether such states of affairs need to be invoked to underwrite meaning in any form. In a passage highly reminiscent of Jung's discussion of the image of the leaf-cutting ant, the developmental biologist Susan Oyama writes:

> What we are moving toward is a conception of a developmental system, not as the reading off of a preexisting code, but as a complex of interacting influences, some inside the organism's skin, some external to it, and including its ecological niche in all its spatial and temporal aspects, many of which are typically passed on in reproduction either because they are in some way tied to the organism's (or its conspecifics') activities or characteristics or because they are stable features of the general environment. It is in the ontogenetic crucible that form appears and is transformed, not because it is immanent in some interactants and nourished by others, or because some form is created by the precise activity of the system. Since even species-typical 'programmed' form is not one but a near-infinite series in transitions throughout the life cycle, each whole and functional in its own way, to refer to the type or the typical is also to refer to this series and the constant change that generates it.
>
> (Oyama, 1985, p. 39)

This point of view brings us, in conclusion, to the strong sense of meaning as an emergent property of the interactive processes of the species-typical action patterns of human behaviour and the species-typical environment of symbolic reference.

References

Bak, P. (1996). *How Nature Works: The Science of Self-Organized Criticality*. New York: Copernicus.

Beebe, B. F. L. (2002). *Infant Research and Adult Treatment: Co-Constructing Interactions*. Hillsdale, NJ: Analytic Press.

Bishop, P. (2000). *Synchronicity and Intellectual Intuition in Kant, Swedenborg, and Jung*. Lampeter, UK: Edwin Mellon Press.

Bright, G. (1997). Synchronicity as a basis of analytic attitude. *Journal of Analytical Psychology*, 42(4), 613–635.

Brinich, P. M. (1983). Review of *The Mental and Social Life of Babies: How Parents Create Persons* by Kenneth Kaye. *The International Review of Psychoanalysis*, 10, 482–484.

Cambray, J. (2002). Synchronicity and emergence. *American Imago*, 50(4), 409–430.

Ellenberger, H. F. (1970). *The Discovery of the Unconscious: The History and Evolution of Dynamic Psychiatry*. New York: Basic Books.

Ferrer i Cancho, R., Riordan, O., et al. (2005). The Consequences of Zipf's Law for Syntax and Symbolic Reference. *Proceedings of the Royal Society*, 272, 561–565.

Ferrer i Cancho, R., and Solé, R. V. (2003). Least effort and the origins of scaling in human language. *Proceedings of the National Academy of Sciences*, 100(3), 788–791.

Gieser, S. (2005). *The Innermost Kernel: Depth Psychology and Quantum Physics. Wolfgang Pauli's Dialogue with C. G. Jung*. Berlin: Springer.

Hendricks-Jansen, H. (1996). *Catching Ourselves in the Act: Situated Activity, Interactive Emergence, Evolution, and Human Thought*. Cambridge, MA: The MIT Press.

Hogenson, G. B. (2005). The self, the symbolic and synchronicity: Virtual realities and the emergence of the psyche. *Journal of Analytical Psychology*, 50, 271–284.

Hogenson, G. B. (2007). From moments of meeting to archetypal consciousness: Emergence and the fractal structure of analytic practice. In A. Casement (Ed.), *Who Owns Jung?* pp. 293–314. London: Karnac.

Jung, C. G. (1919). Instinct and the unconscious. *CW* 8, 129–138.

Jung, C. G. (1952). Synchronicity: An acausal connecting principle. *CW* 8, 419–519.

Jung, C. G. (1954). On the nature of the psyche. *CW* 8, 159–234.

Jung, C. G. (1967). The philosophical tree. *Alchemical Studies*, 13, 253–349.

Kaye, K. (1982). *The Mental and Social Life of Babies: How Parents Create Persons*. Chicago: University of Chicago Press.

Kaye, K., and Wells, A. J. (1980). Mothers' jiggling and the burst-pause pattern in neonatal feeding. *Infant Behaviour and Development*, 3, 29–46.

Knox, J. (2003). *Archetype, Attachment, Analysis: Jungian Psychology and the Emergent Mind*. Hove: Brunner-Routledge.

Main, R. (2004). *The Rupture of Time: Synchronicity and Jung's Critique of Modern Western Culture*. Hove: Brunner-Routledge.

Main, R. (2007a). *Revelations of Chance: Synchronicity a Spiritual Experience*. Albany: State University of New York.

Main, R. (2007b). Ruptured time and the re-enchantment of modernity. In A. Casement (Ed.), *Who Owns Jung?* London: Karnac.

Moran, D. (2000). *Introduction to Phenomenology*. London: Routledge.

Oyama, S. (1985). *The Ontogeny of Information: Developmental Systems and Evolution*. Cambridge: Cambridge University Press.

Rowland, S. (2005). *Jung as Writer*. London: Routledge.

Saunders, P., and Skar, P. (2001). Archetypes, complexes and self-organization. *Journal of Analytical Psychology*, 46(2), 305–323.

Stern, D. (1995). *The Motherhood Constellation: A Unified View of Parent-Infant Psychotherapy*. New York: Basic Books.

Stern, D. N., Sander, L. W. et al. (1998). Non-interpretative mechanisms in psychoanalytic therapy: The "something more" than interpretation. *International Journal of Psychoanalysis*, 79, 903–921.

Stern, D. N., Sander, L. W. et al. (2007). The foundational level of psychodynamic meaning: Implicit process in relation to conflict, defense and the dynamic unconscious. *International Journal of Psychoanalysis*, 88, 1–16.

Tresan, D. I. (1996). Jungian metapsychology and neurobiological theory. *Journal of Analytical Psychology*, 41, 399–436.

van Eenwyk, J. (1997). *Archetypes and Strange Attractors: The Chaotic World of Symbols*. Toronto: Inner City Books.

Vogt, P. (2004). Minimum cost and the emergence of the Zipf-Mandelbrot law. In *Artificial Life IX: Proceedings of the Ninth International Conference on the Simulation and Synthesis of Living Systems*. Cambridge, MA: The MIT Press.

Winnicott, D. W. (1987). Aggression in relation to emotional development. In *Through Paediatrics to Psycho-Analysis*. London: Hogarth Press.

Chapter 10

Donald E. Kalsched

In retrospect it seems ironic that in July of my 21st year I should find myself in the locked basement ward of a mental hospital reading Jung's "Introduction to the Religious and Psychological Problems of Alchemy." The place was Mendota State Hospital in Madison, Wisconsin, and on that hot July afternoon I was midway through an intensive summer program called "Clinical Pastoral Training" required by my Masters of Divinity program at Union Theological Seminary in New York City. On this particular afternoon, I was reading Jung because I was looking for the answer to a question that had plagued me all through my high school years and beyond—through four years of philosophy and religious studies at the University of Wisconsin. The question was simply: "Jesus Christ—myth or reality?"

The implications of this question seemed profound to me at the time. Was I going to complete my seminary training and enter some form of the Christian ministry? Or was I going to pursue a "secular" vocation teaching in a philosophy department at some university? One thing was clear to me. Central to whatever profession I chose must be the opportunity to pursue and hopefully understand the ineffable or "mystical" experiences I had throughout my boyhood and teenage years—numinous experiences that brought me to my knees with tears of gratitude. These inexplicable experiences almost always occurred in nature, sometimes listening to classical or religious music, sometimes hearing the poetry of Wordsworth, Keats or Shelly, sometimes reading the best of American philosophers and nature writers like Emerson or Thoreau. I knew exactly what William James meant in his *Varieties of Religious Experience* when he described the incontrovertible *experience* of spiritual conversion, and I knew what Wordsworth felt above Tintern Abbey when he confessed:

> ...And I have felt
> A presence that disturbs me with the joy
> Of elevated thoughts; a sense sublime
> Of something far more deeply interfused,
> Whose dwelling is the light of setting suns,
> And the round ocean and the living air,
> And the blue sky, and in the mind of man;

DOI: 10.4324/9781003148968-11

But I needed some sort of intellectual framework for these soulful experiences, and I didn't have one. The classical Christian creed with its literal understanding of the Gospel narrative (virgin birth, Christ's resurrection from the dead, etc.) left me cold and seemed utterly obsolete from a rational point of view—curious relics of a mythic past. But so did their desacralized "scientific" counterparts, which reduced everything mysterious to excretions of the glands or neurobiological excitations.

So one can imagine my pleasure when I read Jung's words:

> People have dwelt far too long on the fundamentally sterile question of whether the assertions of faith are true or not. Quite apart from the impossibility of ever proving or refuting the truth of a metaphysical assertion, the very existence of the assertion is a self-evident fact that needs no further proof, and when a *consensus gentium* allies itself thereto, then the validity of the statement is proved to just that extent. The only thing about it that we can understand is the psychological phenomenon, which is incommensurable with the category of objective rightness or truth. (CW 12; para 35)

I had to put the book down. Something had just cracked open, and the light of a "third" possibility between the mythic and the real was dawning on the horizon of my awareness. Jung was talking about a different kind of truth—symbolic truth—psychological truth. He was saying that if millions of people, for thousands of years, have been riveted and compelled by the Christian story, then it contained "truths" that are "self-evident." What were these "truths?" Well, that the Divine incarnates itself in an individual personality who suffered a mortal human life and died a human death—not "out there," that is, once in human history—but over and over again— in every human heart and soul. That this incarnation was an act of love, and that love was the motivating core of the "person" so created. That if we are to emulate such a person (as in the *imitatio Christi*), we will have to take seriously our dual destiny and our dual "parentage"—divine and human—and suffer the tension between these realities. That in addition to our human struggles to realize ourselves, we will have to take our "immortal longings" seriously. That in the darkness and *"prima materia"* of every life there are scintilla of light—that our names are written in heaven (Luke 10:20) and that there's a star over every cradle in a Bethlehem of our beginnings.

As I left the locked ward at Mendota State Hospital that evening, the sun had just painted the western sky red and I could hear the carillon bells ringing in a nearby church. It was one of those special moments of "vocation," when one's life makes complete sense. I knew now that between the worlds of Spirit and Matter there was a mysterious intermediate "third" and that this is where the soul lived . . . and where the heart opened and where the imagination was quickened, and where my sacred experiences found a home. This is where I was most alive and wanted to be. I had discovered the luminous, evanescent, fugitive, *reality of the psyche*, and my work was cut out for me.

I graduated from Union Seminary and entered a Ph.D. program in clinical psychology at Fordham University. I entered Jungian analysis and soon thereafter entered the training program in New York, graduating in 1978. For the ensuing 40+ years, I have been plumbing the waters of the psyche, writing about my findings. Along the way, I discovered that the human psyche will do almost anything to protect and defend that starlit soulful core of selfhood that lives between the worlds but is injured and encapsulated by childhood trauma. Often my patients' healing comes about through a painful rediscovery—mediated by a renewed capacity for authentic suffering of feelings—of the "new life" described by that ancient rabbi who stood astride the two worlds and said, "I have come so that you might have life . . . and have it more abundantly" (John 10:10).

Donald Kalsched, Ph.D. Santa Fe, New Mexico, 2020

Getting Your Own Pain

A Personal Account of Healing Dissociation with Help From the Film *War Horse*

Originally published in Hockley, L. (2018). *The Routledge International Handbook of Jungian Film Studies*. New York: Routledge. Reprinted with permission.

Introduction

In this chapter I want to describe a healing, albeit painful, personal encounter with a recent film (Stephen Spielberg's *War Horse*) that "unlocked" a long-dissociated pocket of childhood experience and helped me recover a piece of my personal story that had been lost in obscurity. In retrospect, I think of this experience (in the language of another film about dissociation, *Equus*) as "getting my own pain," that is, uncovering a lost piece of my *personal* story, lost in the *generic* story of my life as I knew it thus far. Fifteen years of Jungian analysis with three different analysts and other psychotherapists before that had never touched this unremembered all-too-personal pain, nor had the symptoms that clustered around this dissociated complex ever been satisfactorily interpreted. Thanks to the triggering effect of a powerful scene in the film *War Horse*; thanks also to my dreams that night; and thanks especially to the tender but insistent ministrations of my wife Robin (who is also an analyst), I was able to revisit this "story within a story" and feel its emotional impact for the first time. My experience illustrates how modern cinema can provide a *via regia* into dissociated contents of the unconscious, bypassing resistances and defenses that have cordoned off the relevant material for decades. This fact carries important therapeutic implications that I explore briefly at the end of the chapter.

Jung and Implicit vs. Explicit Stories

In a memorable interview with Laurens van der Post (1986, p. 15) at his Bollingen retreat, Jung once confessed that his work as a healer did not take flight until he realized that the key to the human personality was its story.

> Every human being at core, he held, had a unique story and no man could discover his greatest meaning unless he lived and, as it were, grew his own story.

Jung did not complete the telling of his own personal story until he was 83 years old when he decided to write his autobiography, *Memories, Dreams, Reflections* (Jung, 1963). It was a difficult undertaking, because he discovered that as he directed his attention inward and let the light of his consciousness illuminate the obscure darkness of certain aspects of his early childhood, feeling-experiences began to emerge that were painful to him, and he resisted the process of recovering these memories.

He described this struggle in a letter to an anonymous friend (Jung, 1975, p. 408):

Dear N,

You must bear with my peculiar mental state. While I am writing this I observe a little demon trying to abscond my words and even my thoughts and turning them over into the rapidly flowing river of images, surging from the mists of the past, portraits of a little boy, bewildered and wondering at the incomprehensibly beautiful and hideously profane and deceitful world.

This bewildered and awestruck little boy comes alive in the pages of Jung's autobiography, and much of what he recovered of this child's memories carries the mark of trauma and dissociation (see Kalsched, 2013, Chapter 8). The act of writing it was a healing act in which he gathered together some of the previously dissociated pieces of his life and wove them into a coherent narrative that made sense out of his otherwise fragmented experience. He was, in effect, "getting his own pain." In the process, Jung discovered that he had two autobiographies, not one—the first one known and familiar, made up of explicit memories and conscious experience, the other unknown and unfamiliar, made up of memories and experiences that were heretofore unconscious. Jung named these his number one and number two personalities.

In completing his actual autobiography, Jung was rediscovering in his own life, the importance of untold stories that he had earlier discovered in the lives of patients he treated as a young psychiatrist at the Burgholzli Mental Hospital in

Zurich. Looking back over many years of experience, Jung offered the following reflections:

> In many cases in psychiatry, the patient who comes to us has a story that is not told, and which as a rule no one knows of. To my mind, therapy only really begins after the investigation of that wholly personal story. It is the patient's secret, the rock against which he is shattered. If I know his secret story, I have a key to the treatment . . . but how to gain that knowledge? In most cases exploration of the conscious material is insufficient. Sometimes [projective techniques] can open the way, so can the interpretation of dreams, or long and patient human contact with the individual.
>
> (Jung, 1963, p. 117)

While films are not projective techniques in the classic sense, they are imaginal, artistic products of the human psyche, and like a collective dream, they can give us access to orphaned parts of ourselves and their "stories"—what Theodore Reik (1964) called "voices from the inaudible." We all have "secret stories." Sometimes these stories are secret because they contain "shadow" contents and feelings-parts of our experience that we're ashamed of or embarrassed by. When we get in touch with those parts of the story, we blush or change the subject, but we recognize the difficult truths they contain and eventually, if we are in a trusting environment, we learn to include their repressed contents in our overall autobiographical narrative about ourselves. That represents a major part of the psychotherapy process—filling in the gaps in our personal story . . . integrating the shadow, as Jung would say, becoming more "whole."

But then there are some stories that are so secret that they are unknown even to ourselves. In that case, they are the implicit memories that follow the kind of emotionally "shattering" experiences that Jung references. And another word for this shattering is trauma. Trauma creates unbearable pain and anxiety, and this leads to defenses that are more primitive than repression. The main such primitive defense is *dissociation*. When traumatic parts of our experience are split off from the ego by dissociation, we don't "make sense" to ourselves. We cannot tell an emotionally coherent story about our lives. We may have flashbacks or major gaps in experience—blacked-out places that frighten us. Or, strange symptoms may defy interpretation because they seem unrelated to the known places where we are injured. In short, major pieces of the puzzle remain in what neuroscientists call "implicit" memory (see Siegel, 2010, p. 148ff)—out of reach of our story-telling capacity—our "autobiographical memory." This is the reason that trauma survivors must often lead a double life, with one apparently normal story "on the surface" but inwardly haunted by another unformulated "implicit" story—an untold and untellable story, composed of the painful memories of abuse, neglect or betrayal that remain a shameful secret.

In what follows, I would like to describe how a dissociated complex of my own forgotten childhood experience was "triggered" by a sequence of dramatic scenes

I watched in the film *War Horse*. This micro-complex of dissociated material had apparently lain dormant for over 60 years, including 15 to 20 years of psycho-analytic work on myself plus almost 50 years of attention to the psyches of my patients. My story illustrates how the healing of trauma is a lifelong adventure and how the story we tell ourselves and others about our lives may have holes in them big enough to drive a truck through!

My Experience of the Film

Shortly after the film version of Steven Spielberg's *War Horse* (DreamWorks Pictures, 2011) started showing around town in Albuquerque, New Mexico, my wife Robin and I went to see it. Based on the Tony award-winning Broadway play, the film is set in the beautiful farm country of rural Great Britain before World War I and features a close friendship that develops between a young boy named Albert and a horse named Joey. Joey has been purchased from a town auction by Albert's drunken father Ted, who was supposed to bring home an inexpensive plow horse but instead spent the whole month's rent on a sleek thoroughbred. A deep bond develops between Joey and Albert, who trains the horse not only to ride, but also to accept a plow, and he and Joey set about saving the family farm, which ultimately they do. When WWI breaks out, Albert's father, drunk as usual, sells Joey to the Army to pull cannons. Albert is crushed, but himself enlists in the army and vows he'll see Joey again.

The film then follows the separate stories of Joey and Albert for several years, as they endure the horrors of the war, Joey pulling cannons and surviving only because of his strength and endurance, as well as the respect and care he evokes from his soldier caretakers on both sides. Albert meanwhile suffers the horrors of trench warfare wounded by machine-gun fire and is temporarily blinded by exploding mortar shells.

In one of the final chapters of the movie, the events of the war bring Joey and Albert together in the same front line, facing the German enemy across "no-man's land." Albert, temporarily blind and slowly recovering from his wounds behind the lines, does not know that Joey is nearby. In one dramatic scene, Joey is startled to madness by exploding shells and charges off into no-man's land crashing through stanchions of barbed wire and barricades until he collapses in coils of barbed wire, unable to rise, slowly dying, looking up with his soulful luminous brown eyes, as if imploring both sides to stop this senseless carnage. A British soldier erupts out of his trench and, heedless of danger, runs to the dying animal trying desperately to free the horse from the wire. German machine guns are trained on him and we expect that at any minute he'll be gunned down. Instead, from behind the German lines, wire cutters are thrown and several enemy soldiers come out to help free the animal. For one remarkable moment, a mini-truce is declared and the opposites are united through both sides' compassion for this innocent and beautiful animal. All through this moving scene, which results in the badly wounded horse being freed and returned to the British lines, all I can think of are Joey's eyes. They are speaking directly to me, although I don't know what they are saying. All I know is that I am convulsed with sobbing and struggle to contain my unbidden emotion in this public theater.

Slowly I got control over my emotion and sat quietly for a few moments until the next scene broke me open again . . . the "reunion" scene. Covered with mud and bleeding from his wounds, Joey is led back to the British lines. The commotion alerts Albert, who is now nearby. Albert now hears the unmistakable sounds of his beloved, long-lost and unrecognizable animal. Yet the Army veterinarian who has examined the horse's wounds orders the horse put down. Reluctantly following orders, the sergeant unholsters his pistol. Joey lowers his head as if accepting his fate. There is a deafening silence. Then, instead of the death-dealing report of the gun, we hear Albert's whistle in the near-distance—the same whistle that Joey learned from the boy as they bonded years earlier on the farm. Joey jerks his head up in recognition, as everyone is amazed and looks around. And again those beautiful eyes! This scene is repeated two more times—each time the pistol aimed and the whistle instead of the shot—now growing closer. Finally Albert comes stumbling along the trenches into the scene, his half blind eyes bandaged, his long-lost soul animal obviously overjoyed to see him again. And again I am convulsed with sobbing. This time I couldn't stop until the final scene of the movie.

This scene was filmed against a deep red-orange sunset as a lone rider appears on the horizon, approaches and dismounts. He embraces a woman and a man. Then all three embrace the horse's head. Music swells and we know that Joey and Albert have returned to the family and the farm where their relationship began. As Robin and I sat in the darkened theater, I slowly returned to a more or less regulated state. Like us, most people were deeply moved by the film and stayed in their seats until the credits ran.

Resistance to Feeling and a Final Breakthrough

We filed out of the theater hand in hand, everyone in silence. On the drive home Robin and I talked about what a good anti-war film this was—about the beauty of the "truce" scene where soldiers dedicated to killing each other paused and together freed an innocent animal. We talked about the terrible violation of innocence—man and animal—and then, for some reason (we both had previously studied theology) the question came up of "where God was in this film." I had an immediate surge of conviction and said emphatically (and probably a little arrogantly) that "God was in the luminous eyes of that horse . . . that's where God was." (I was thinking, when I said this, of a moment described by Elie Wiesel [1982] in his book *Night* that I had never forgotten, where he and other inmates at the Auschwitz concentration camp were forced to watch as three prisoners were hung on the gallows, and among them was a small child. The child did not die when the chairs were tipped over and dangled from his noose writhing in agony for half an hour as Wiesel was forced to watch. A prisoner behind him asked in agony, "So where is your God now!?" And at that moment from deep within himself, Wiesel heard a voice answer, "where is He? He's up there hanging from the gallows.")

Wiesel's horrific story and the scene of Joey dying in the mud and barbed wire, his innocent eyes looking imploringly at us before the fire went out of them, both seemed to capture the terrible paradox of the human condition described by Jung's little boy—"bewildered and wondering at the incomprehensibly beautiful and hideously profane and deceitful world" (Jung, 1975, 408). This agony, I thought to myself, is what God must have suffered in "coming down" into this world in the Christian incarnation story and also somehow what we must take on if we are to let God take up residence in the human heart.

Of course I was not conscious of all this at the moment, but my conviction that "God was in the eyes of that horse" was as close as I could get to what I felt. Robin, however, was not convinced. She was on another track. She was struck by the fact that the same patriarchal God was worshipped by both sides in WWI and it was in His name that all the killing was going on and, she wondered, "where was the feminine in all this horror?" Robin was furious about the waste of lives depicted in the film and not very sympathetic to what I considered my poetic and mystical interpretation, and it seemed to me she dismissed it out of hand. This irritated me further, and I expressed my chagrin that she was stuck in a shallow feminist argument against the patriarchy and by the time we got home we were both irritated—me fuming and agitated, she quiet and withdrawn.

Feeling misunderstood and alienated, I stormed downstairs to get away from her while she got ready for bed. I opened my computer and started writing, trying to process for myself what had just happened and why I was so upset. Was it the film? Was it the horse? Was I just in the wrong marriage? What was going on? No conclusion.

When I came back up and sullenly went about my bedtime ritual, Robin approached me and said something like, "sweetheart, I'm sorry if I hurt your feelings . . . I didn't realize you felt so strongly about this. I've been thinking about it," she continued. "Could it be that you're so moved by that scene in the movie because your Dad put a gun in your hands when you were only five years old and took you hunting animals a year later . . . do you think maybe that could be part of your reaction? You must have watched many animals die and you were so young."

I cut her off quickly. "Of course not," I said. "You don't understand the context of that early hunting!" Now I felt even more misunderstood and angry. Here were my intense vulnerable feelings—my conviction that the soul of the whole world was in the eyes of that innocent animal—all this was now being interpreted and reduced by my psychoanalyst wife to a stupid childhood experience.

I was incredibly defensive and more than a little self-righteous. I explained how my early hunting experiences were an important initiation into my own manhood . . . weekends hunting with my dad, my grandfather and my uncle in the woods of northern Wisconsin. I described how I was a crack shot by age five and how proud I was of that and what self-esteem this gave me with my father and grandfather. I described the beautiful days I had afield with them, the lunches along the logging roads in northern Wisconsin, the stories about our adventures after ruffed grouse, the late afternoons listening together to the Wisconsin Badgers football games. I explained how cool I was with other boys my age—how we never shot game we didn't eat, how my father taught me the ethics of safety and conservation . . . not just how to kill animals, but how to honor and respect them and end their suffering immediately. I went on to say how nowadays nobody knows where their meat comes from and how most of it is raised in cages and packaged in cellophane, and how it was a good thing that I learned how to kill and clean animals for the table. At least I wasn't a part of this miserable disconnected culture. And besides, I said, hunting is an archetypal experience and I turned myself over to it with enthusiasm like generations of young men before me. It was formative of my very being!

"Well I just wondered," Robin said. "I've always felt you were too young to be your Dad's hunting buddy at five years old. You told me you were five when you shot your first squirrel. You were so innocent at that age . . . this is too early for masculine initiation rituals! Some part of you would have still been identified with those animals. It might have torn you apart."

Somehow that last point reached me. I was just completing a book in which a whole chapter was devoted to innocence and how much it's been neglected in our field of therapy and how traumatic it can be for innocence to gain experience too early. I began to wonder whether this chapter could possibly have something to do with me.

So, partially reconciled, we went to bed. But I couldn't sleep. I tossed and turned and in the hypnagogic images that came up in that twilight of sleep, I started to get fragments of memories that upset me. Then it was like a secret file opened in my brain and images spilled out—painful and shame-filled memories of animals dying. The first was a dream of my father with his famous "varmit rifle" having just shot a porcupine out of a tree. There was an image of this animal with its blood and guts spilled all around, and I realized as I woke from this dream that the imagery constituted a partial memory of being dragged by my proud father to see his massacred trophy when I was only three years old. There was no feeling to the dream . . . just the image, but there was the vague memory of fainting and throwing up when I had seen this poor animal and feeling embarrassed that I had disappointed my father with this "weakness."

Then there were owls shot out of trees and a great blue heron wounded at 500 yards that I had to go and tackle and kill. I was only eight. There was the rancher's feral cat that I shot for him across the road in the sagebrush and the way that animal wailed and clawed at me and the image of its eyes before I shot it a second time . . . there was the time when at nine years old I led a gang of younger boys on a mission to climb a tree in a neighbor's yard and kill baby robins by bashing them on the ground . . . and the punishment that followed from my mother which I didn't understand. Wasn't I my father's son? Wasn't I supposed to be a hunter and a killer? Finally, I remembered the time in my 30s when, on a visit home to

Wisconsin with my two-year-old son, I was cleaning some mallard ducks that my father and I had shot on the Mississippi River. I had their gutted carcasses laid out on the basement ping-pong table and was preparing to take off their heads, wings and feet. I picked up a drake mallard and readied the scissors when my son suddenly looked upset: "Poor little fella," he said, "gone from the sky." I remember being shaken by this moment and again the familiar tears from I-knew-not-where. What I did feel was shame that I had exposed my beautiful little boy to such butchery at the age of two. I did not connect this moment to my own violated innocence, but I remember how a fleeting thought crossed my mind that maybe I should stop hunting.

By the time morning came, I felt exhausted. I needed to talk about all this with Robin who, thank God, was willing to listen. I poured out the dream images and memories that had come to me, crying intermittently the whole way through, realizing that this had truly been a trauma—one I had covered up, one I couldn't afford to feel because I loved my father so much and because I was embedded in an heroic narrative that left all this pain and grief out. Now I felt heartsick for the little boy that was me and rage at his violation, however well-meaning and unknowing it had been. This wasn't about me; it was about my father and having my adoring eyes on him and my being just like him. Why had he not honored my boyhood innocence? Was he so desperate for a hunting buddy that he had to make a child soldier out of me at age of five or six? I was furious at him for this, and also sad for him that his life was so permeated with a culture of guns and killing that it left him terribly empty at the end.

In retrospect, I realize that memories of these experiences were dissociated because they were in some ways unbearably shameful and incompatible with my story about myself—my ego-ideal—and my story about my wonderful childhood as the beloved son of a loving father. That story is not false . . . it just didn't include the underlying truth of how my sensitivities as a small child were injured and unconsciously even exploited. The surface story of my number one personality required that I divide myself in two, growing up too fast, leaving a part of my story behind in the unremembered past beyond the influence of reflective self-awareness or subsequent experience. Back there and orphaned by my precociously grown-up narrative was the young seeker of beauty in the world, the young boy linked to the mystery of animals, the lover of all life, identified with the beautiful soulful eyes of dogs and horses, torn away from his own soul by prematurely learning how to kill.

As Robin and I talked, further parts of my "forgotten" life-story came into focus. For example, as a young man, I had a bothersome "symptom" of being afraid to have my own blood drawn, and I would also get queasy in films where there was a lot of blood spilled—for example if someone was shown helplessly wounded or having cut their own wrists. This symptom worried me a good deal because I originally went to college to become a doctor and on several occasions I had fainted during various "demonstrations" for premedical students. I remembered one in particular where dogs were shaven and cut open, their hearts exposed with heart-lung machines pumping their blood through tubes. I fainted dead away and had to be carried out. This seemed to my naïve mind to spell the end of my future medical career, and I was depressed for weeks afterwards.

In my original Jungian analysis, this problem was labeled my "blood complex" and, because blood is frequently symbolic of affect and feeling, it was interpreted as my fear of strong feeling in general. That made sense to me, but it didn't really help much. My symptom continued. The only thing this interpretation did was make me feel bad that not only was I afraid of blood, I was apparently afraid of what blood represented—strong emotion! Never explored were my early child-hood experiences of traumatically violated innocence and the guilt about the blood I had spilled.

These memories remained implicit, encoded in parts of my brain that did not connect to higher cortical centers that would have allowed me to reflect on the experience and bring it back into autobiographical memory. Instead, these trau-matic memories lay in wait, ready to be triggered. This was equivalent to a flash-back, the irruption of the past into the present, not yet recognized as the past but only taken in as a "symptom." That's what my fainting episode in the surgical demonstration represented. It's like reliving an earlier injury right now without recognizing it as a past injury. The threat of helpless animals being sacrificed (no matter how justified the rationale) was one I had already seen countless times at my own hand, but never explicitly known. Such is the defense of dissociation, which cements the memories in the lower right hemisphere where they remain implicit and unprocessed by higher cortical centers. I was overwhelmed by tears looking into the eyes of the war horse, but I didn't know why. I didn't know I was looking into the eyes of my own impossible experiences. When Robin and I went through our argument together, these early implicit memories were processed in the storm and stress of relationship and became explicit, conscious for the first time.

Getting Your Own Pain

As I was preparing the manuscript of this chapter for publication, I was reminded of a scene from another film, *Equus*, which struck me as uncannily relevant to the experience I have just reported. It has to do with finding one's way to a uniquely personal—as opposed to a generic (mythic or collective)—life.

Equus, the 1977 film directed by Sidney Lumet and starring Richard Burton as the psychiatrist and Peter Firth as his young patient, is an adaptation of Peter Schaefer's award-winning 1973 play *Equus*, which I had seen in New York at a special screening for the C. G. Jung Institute where I was training to be an analyst. Remarkably enough, both the play and the film constitute a drama about the kill-ing of innocent animals (horses) by a young stable boy (Alan Strang), and about the "god" he sees reflected in the eyes of the horses, one of which (Nugget) he rides naked at night in what amounts to a Dionysian ritual of orgiastic ecstasy fol-lowed by the boy's prostrating himself before his "god" Equus.

Tragically—and unlike my own experience in *War Horse*—the "god" that Alan sees staring back at him from the horses eyes is a wrathful Deity, mocking him (in his twisted projection) for his failed lovemaking attempt with a beautiful young woman in the stable the night before. The shame he feels is so intolerable that the boy blinds the horses with a steel spike in a horrific scene, killing them, while at the same time "killing" his own consciousness of his erotic arousal, his shame about it, and his unbearable "failure" as the lover of a real woman. The unbearable personal/human story—now mixed with the crime of killing the animals he had worshiped—has been dissociated and the result is complete psychosis. The rest of the play is about the slow therapeutic abreaction of Alan's dissociated crime and the uncovering of his "true story."

While I remember being horrified by the images of the boy killing the horses (for reasons that the previous narrative makes understandable), the particular scene that riveted my attention and stayed with me for more than 40 years was a piece of dialogue between Alan, who is now in a psychiatric hospital, and his treating psychiatrist, Martin Dysart. Dysart is cast as an obsessively intellectual man living a conventional life in a loveless marriage with florid fantasies of unlived erotic and "primitive" life, which he indulges in sublimated form by reading Greek mythology. From his repressed state of sclerotic rigidity, he is mesmerized by his young patient's archetypal revelries. Alan's ritual enactments of Dionysian ecstasies have a fascination for him that parallel Jung's fascination with what he called "living one's own myth," a parallel (and confusion) I will attempt to sort out in a moment.

In the following scene, Dysart is talking to Hesther Salomon, a nurse, about the boy's suffering and about whether he has any right to take his pain away from him. In the particular dialogue that I found unforgettable, Dysart is trying to explain to Hester what it means to "get your own pain." (The following is from the text of the play *Equus*, 1974, p. 94.)

HESTHER: . . . but he's in pain Martin. He's been in pain for most of his life. That much, at least, you know.
DYSART: Possibly.
HESTHER: Possibly?! . . . That cut-off little figure you just described must have been in pain for years.
DYSART: [doggedly] Possibly.
HESTHER: And you can take it away.
DYSART: Still—possibly.
HESTHER: Then that's enough. That simply has to be enough for you, surely?
DYSART: No!
HESTHER: Why not?
DYSART: Because it's his.
HESTHER: I don't understand.
DYSART: His pain. His own. He made it.
    Pause.
    [earnestly] *Look . . . to go through life and call it yours—your life— you first have to get your own pain. Pain that's unique to you. You can't just dip into the common bin and say "that's enough!"* . . . He's done that. All right, he's sick. He's full of misery and fear. He was dangerous and could be again, though I doubt it. But that boy has

known a passion more ferocious than I have felt in any second of my life. And let me tell you something: I envy it. [Emphasis added.]

HESTHER: You can't.

DYSART: [vehemently] Don't you see? That's the Accusation! That's what his stare has been saying to me all the time *"At least I galloped! When did you?'* . . . [simply] I'm jealous, Hester. Jealous of Alan Strang.

HESTHER: That's absurd.

Hesther is not happy with Dysart's analysis and we shouldn't be either. When he says we all have to "get our own pain—pain that's unique to us," he's right. That would be equivalent to "growing our own story," as Jung suggested to Laurens van der Post (earlier). When he says, "You can't just dip into the common bin," he's right again. We can't just live a generic life, fitting in with the common bin of so-called everyday suffering as it is defined for us by the narrative about ourselves that we adopt from others and from the prevailing culture. But when he says that the boy has "done that," that is, gotten pain that's unique to him, Dysart has got it exactly backwards.

In Jungian language, Alan has been possessed by an archetypal image—that of the god Equus—and is burying his own repressed sexuality and twisted personal pain in a mythic enactment that keeps him away from the deeper unbearable story and his consciousness of it. Just as my own generic "mythic" story of myself as a heroic young hunter masked the deeper personal pain that was unique to me and would have to be discovered through the difficult process of remembering that I've described earlier.

In the same way, for Alan Strang "getting his own pain" means recovering those dissociated and shameful personal experiences lying behind his archetypal enactment—his crime of blinding the horses. This means recovering the pain of his own violently repressed and distorted sexuality and recovering this from the shaming defenses that he's projected onto the horses, whose huge eyes on him while he tried to make love in the stable are leering and mocking and preventing him from loving a real woman. It's as if he's turned his painful personal story over to an archetypal enactment, in order not to feel it. He's living a myth instead of his own life. Discovery of his painful personal story and the violent rejection of his own sexuality lies ahead of him in the film—just like it lay ahead for me, in the unbearable reality of my own childhood killing of animals. It's the difference between living a personal limited life and being lived by a generic mythic one.

As a young man studying to be a Jungian analyst when I saw Peter Shaffer's play and the later screenplay by him, I was captured by the same romantic vision of "getting your own pain" as was Dysart—surrendering oneself to archetypal affects—living out a kind of possession by one's own personal daimon. This was made even more confusing for me by the way Jung himself sometimes spoke positively about finding one's own myth—the myth that you live by—as if this was an important part of individuation.

In his autobiography, Jung even describes his envy of people who are unconsciously embedded in the archaic and the mythic. Specifically, Jung described (Jung, 1963, p. 247) his encounter with a Taos Pueblo Indian chief Ochwiay Biano, who lived inside a mythic world view in which he believed his ritual worship of the sun would actually help the fiery orb cross the sky. Jung felt that this belief—"primitive" as it was—gave his life dignity and a meaningful place in the cosmos. Jung envied him for it.

> It springs from his being a son of the sun; his life is cosmologically meaningful, for he helps the father and preserver of all life in his daily rise and descent. If we set against this our own self-justifications, the meaning of our own lives as it is formulated by our reason, we cannot help but see our poverty. Out of sheer envy we are obliged to smile at the Indians' naïveté and plume ourselves on our cleverness; for otherwise we would discover how impoverished and down at the heels we are. Knowledge does not enrich us; it removes us more and more from the mythic world in which we were once at home by right of birth.
>
> (p. 252)

Here Jung is lamenting the same impoverishment of modern life and objective "knowledge" that Dysart felt with Alan Strang. Fortunately, Jung finds his way out of his "mythological envy" with a new understanding. Dysart is not so lucky. Here's Jung's description of his envy of Ochwiay Biano and its resolution:

> I had envied him for the fullness of meaning in that belief, and had been looking about without hope for a myth of [my] own. [But] now I knew what it was, and knew even more: that man is indispensable for the completion of creation; that, in fact, he himself is the second creator of the world, who alone has given to the world its objective existence—without which, unheard, unseen, silently eating, giving birth, dying, heads nodding through hundreds of millions of years, it would have gone on in the profoundest night of non-being down to its unknown end. Human consciousness created objective existence and meaning, and man found his indispensable place in the great process of being.
>
> (p. 256)

Jung resolved his envy of his Pueblo friend's mythic embeddedness through the discovery of a new myth—the myth of consciousness, in which he could participate enthusiastically even as a modern man. He thus deepened the integration and connection between his inner symbolic life on the one hand and his personal/ professional life as a psychiatrist and scientist on the other. Dysart in Schaeffer's play and later film is unable to make this transition. Reluctantly he treats the boy and helps relieve the unbearable pain that was being enacted in (and disguised by) his archetypal symptoms. But even in the film's final farewell to Alan Strang, Dysart is full of ironic regret: "you won't gallop any more, Alan. Horses will be quite safe. . . [but] you'll be without pain. More or less completely without pain" (Equus, pp. 124–125).

Of course the playwright and his character Dysart have it backwards again. The process of recovering his traumatic memories (depicted in the last third of the film) is extremely painful for young Alan Strang, and it is precisely this that constitutes his "getting his own pain"—not galloping to a frenzy in the fields at night in an archetypal ritual that shames him and that he doesn't understand. Granted, he will not be carried away by the same volcanic affect or riveted by the same passionate obsessions, but he will be living a personal life and not a generic or mythic one. In the same way, my discovery that the archetypal and heroic rituals of hunting that had so obsessed and enthralled me as a young man had to be given up was its own form of initiation . . . initiation into my own greater consciousness, into my own personal pain and into my own individual and authentic suffering.

It is possible that we all start out living a generic life and eventually, if we're lucky, slough off our "mythological envelope," so to speak, finding our way—with help—to "getting our own personal pain." This is undoubtedly a prerequisite for what Jung meant by the "vocation" of personality and why he said (Jung, 1932, para 284), "the ultimate aim and strongest desire of all mankind is to develop that fullness of life which is called personality."

Final Thoughts

As I look back over the process of writing this story, two things occur to me. First, just as Jung got some help with a coherent autobiography by writing his story at 83 years old, with help from his dreams, I too, at age 73, have benefitted from this process of writing and integration—helped along by the memory-triggering impact of a contemporary film. I hope that this narrative of my experience in the film *War Horse* helps underscore how helpful movies can be in opening up ("triggering") early unremembered trauma and, in this way, helping us to both "get our own pain" and also our own greater consciousness.

Since this experience I have paid particular attention not only to my patients' dreams, but also to the films they find compelling and especially to the particular scenes they find themselves returning to . . . sometimes year after year for decades. I make an effort to see films that are important to my patients and we discuss them. I have found this cinematic attention rewarded many times with profound insights into their lives and a deep resonance in the transference as we have, in effect, shared a common dream.

Second, my story demonstrates that dissociation is an amazing thing. It can encapsulate a complex of memories and keep the shame associated with them out of consciousness for 60 years! This encapsulated "complex" of affects and images was like a cyst in the musculature of my psyche. While it did not dramatically hamper my overall development, it was a secret source of embarrassing symptoms during my formative years and constituted a gaping hole in any coherent personal narrative of my life. It also helped change my direction from medicine to psychology and (in retrospect) informed my interests in trauma and dissociation as well as the emphasis I have placed in my recent book (Kalsched, 2013) on violated innocence. As a so-called expert helping other people with their trauma histories, I was humbled to find this missing piece of my own forgotten personal history.

Bibliography

Jung, C. G. (1932). The development of personality. In *Collected Works, Vol. 17*. New York: Bollingen Foundation, Inc., 1954.

Jung, C. G. (1963). *Memories, Dreams, Reflections*. A. Jaffe (Ed.), R. Winston and C. Winston (Trans.). New York: Vintage Books, Random House

Jung, C. G. (1975). *Letters, Vol. 2*, 1951–1961. G. Adler (Ed.), R. F. C. Hull (Trans.). Princeton: Princeton University Press

Kalsched, D. (2013). *Trauma and the Soul: A Psycho-spiritual Approach to Human Development and its Interruption*. London: Routledge.

Reik, T. (1964). *Voices From the Inaudible: The Patients Speak*. New York: Farrar, Straus, & Co.

Schaffer, P. (1974). *Equus*. New York: Avon Books.

Siegel, D. L. (2010). *Mindsight: The New Science of Personal Transformation*. New York: Bantam Books

Van der Post, L. (1986). *Resurgence*, No. 117, July/August, pp. 14–17.

Wiesel, E. (1982). *Night*. Stella Rodway (Trans.). New York: Bantam Books.

Chapter 11

Eva Pattis Zoja

I met analytical psychology in Vienna in the seventies and without being aware of the fact that it was strange to meet Jung in Freud's homeland.

I only knew that I would not be able to expose my wounds to a traditional Freudian gaze, and so I came across the office of the only Jungian analyst—of American origin—who, even after five years in Vienna, could not speak German. My English was rudimentary.

The analysis continued on this basis and, indeed, the sharing of a linguistic obstacle allowed us to carry out more intense work on intuition and images: to understand each other, we almost had to create a language that was largely non-verbal. This meant that nothing was taken for granted or routine and, for me, the feeling that someone was listening to me with so much attention and passion was completely new.

The threads of my story are articulated around two dreams, or rather, projects for the future interrupted by historical events. The first concerns my grandfather, the second my mother.

In the spring of 1914, Rudolf Stolz, my maternal grandfather, was forty years old and a well-known painter from Bolzano, a city then under Austrian rule. He used to create interior and exterior frescoes of churches and courtyards of public and private buildings and had also made a name for himself in other regions of Austria. In April he was delivered a letter that would change his life forever: it was an invitation from the Archduke Francesco Ferdinando, heir to the Austro-Hungarian throne, to move to Vienna to paint a cycle of frescoes in his residence. For Rudolf it was the first real opportunity to abandon local provincialism and free himself from the dependence on local patrons, who were not always sensitive to his ideas. Rudolf was ready to go. But after two months, on June 28, 1914, with the assassination of the archduke and the beginning of the First World War, his dream and the lives of millions of people fell apart.

When my grandfather Rudolf returned from the war, he discovered that South Tyrol had been annexed to Italy: the great and multi-ethnic Austro-Hungarian kingdom no longer existed. Rudolf and Teresa continued to live in Bolzano, and she gave birth to seven children—my mother was the second child. At the age of

DOI: 10.4324/9781003148968-12

twenty my mother got engaged to a young man from the bourgeoisie of Bolzano. In 1940, however, that promising young man had to join the German army and take part in the expedition to Russia.

From 1940 to 1942 my mother's boyfriend did not stop sending her letters from the front in gothic letters, and she answered him just as regularly. Each letter was opened by the censors, for this reason, what was actually witnessed or what was thought never transpired. In the penultimate letter, the young soldier asked her to marry him and my mother accepted. Months of silence passed, my mother's letter went back along with all the others she wrote, only a stamp appeared that said: "Wait for the new address" followed by a swastika. He later learned that the 6th division his soldier was in was trapped in Stalingrad. But he did not give up and, for seven years, he waited in vain for his return.

In 1948 things changed and my mother decided to marry my father, a successful architect in his fifties. The night before the wedding, she typed a letter of apology addressed to that boyfriend lost in the war. We three children, born of marriage, desired and raised with dedication and care, always felt something underground and foreign, never faced. We felt that our mother's life was not exactly what she had dreamed of and that, despite having chosen an exemplary husband, it was not him she would have wanted to love. We perceived a scream beneath our lives that could not be heard because each of us, in our own way, had tried to cover it throughout our childhood.

Today I believe that that never elaborate experience influenced my decision to become a therapist. I have always wanted to go and look for those screams hidden under so-called normal lives: the failure to elaborate the traumas of war did not affect only individuals, but also the entire community of German-speaking South Tyrol.

I remember a recurring dream I had until at least thirty-five. I had to repeat the history exam in high school, but I didn't have the book with me, I had lost it or had never even bought it. There was an imminent question, or, the whole school year had already passed, I had to study the entire program and, therefore, I didn't know anything about it. It must be said by the way that I have never had difficulties in school, nor have I ever experienced the anxiety of exams. It was therefore a dream linked not so much to school, but to history, the passing of events and their memory that I did not perceive enough.

It was as if I suffered from dyslexia of historical dates, an emblematic void to understand how far the repression can go.

After ten years of psychotherapeutic work in Bolzano, in 1985 I decided to move to Milan where I opened a private practice. I stayed there for the following years, alternating a short stay in New York from 2000 to 2002 with several trips to Africa, China and Argentina to train Jungian analysts and carry out sandwork projects.

I think my patients appreciate my lack of conceptual rigidity useful for unleashing their creativity during the analysis. I often even feel a certain envy towards them; I would have loved to have myself as an analyst to encourage my creative side. This part is still neglected and in need of intervention, as is evident from one of the most harmless symptoms: every time there are no pens, pencils or markers at home, I am fine where they accumulate, but I prefer to keep quiet.

The pencil holders near the phone and on the desk are constantly empty, even if we replenish them regularly. But if I put my hand in my bag, I can take out at least fifteen coloured pencils with or without a case. The same goes for jackets and coats. Here, I really wish that all those colours and writing instruments subconsciously seized were used with more awareness.

Breathing—Physical, Symbolic, Spiritual and Social Aspects

Unpublished.

One of the installations of the exhibition *Broken Nature: Design Takes on Human Survival*,[1] consisting of a barrel filled with sandy earth, could easily have been overlooked as the steady flow of visitors pushed past it. The surface was slightly arched and dry, a few stones strewn here and there, and the scene put one in mind of a barren landscape. Was this meant to symbolise overexploitation of the soil? The artwork was unassuming, almost unattractive. But it held a surprising experience in store for whomever was curious enough to stop in front of it. While pondering on the installation's deeper meaning and fleetingly searching for a title, the domed, sandy surface almost imperceptibly lifted. Or was that imagined? Then it lowered again in the same manner, like a long sigh. There followed a brief pause, then the surface rose again as if there were an immense breathing lung in the depths beneath it. Again the brief pause, then the slow fall back down. The mechanism didn't operate entirely smoothly—sometimes the barrel jolted a little, giving the installation a somewhat homespun dimension. Nevertheless, if the sense of something large and universal was intended, it was powerfully conveyed. The spectators stood rooted to the spot, their breathing in some cases already subconsciously attuned: in and out. One sentence remained lodged in memory for days: "I saw the Earth breathe."

In the large, monotheistic religions, breath is one of the characteristic features of God. The Old Testament states, "Then the LORD God formed man of dust from the ground, and breathed into his nostrils the breath of life; and man became a living being" (Gen. 2:7).

In the Rigveda, the ancient Indian sage Vishvamitra asks the god Indra, deity of fertility and ruler over the sun, storms and rain, how he could recognise him. Indra responded, "I am breath. You are breath. All beings are breath. In breath, I permeate all spaces. Breath is life and life is breath."

In the yoga disciplines, whose origins can be traced back 5000 years, breath plays a central role: *prana*, the force of life, is tied to breath. In yoga, the aim of disciplining breath (*pranayama*) was to dissolve the accustomed flow of thoughts and to create a vacancy of mind through prolonged pauses between breaths, thereby calming and decelerating physical and mental functions. It seems that Indian yogis traditionally practised the pranayama above all as an *ars moriendi*. This aspect has faded in today's understanding of yoga, which is focused primarily on physical well-being.

Breath links the invisible inside with the visible outside world. It is not only a metaphoric connection between the inner and outer worlds; it also takes on a very concrete dimension because it is the very same air that flows from outside to in, and then back again. In both a literal and figurative sense breath is a bridge between the physical and psychic functions. Breathing rhythm and breathing volume are both strongly linked to a person's emotional state. One could even say that breath is like a seismograph for emotional fluctuation.

Countless comparable shamanic traditions have been developed over the course of human history to induce altered states of consciousness through special breathing techniques. These usually involve forced and accelerated breathing—hyperventilation, in other words—which leads to oxygen enrichment in the brain, inducing hallucinatory states, mental flashbacks and dreamlike sequences that are often intensely emotional. In the language of psychology, this is an activation of unconscious content. A shaman, on the other hand, would say that breathing has opened a door to the world of ghosts and ancestors. A number of different body-related therapeutic approaches emerged in the 1970s, such as Stanislav Grof's "Rebirthing" (2013), which is also based on hyperventilation. However, psychology's interest in breath goes back even further. As early as the 1920s, Wilhelm Reich (1969), one of the pioneers of psychoanalysis and a close associate of Freud, had begun to observe the emotional processes associated with breathing—especially the muscle obstructions related to sexuality. One of his great intuitions was to assume a self-healing tendency of the psyche through breathing. He understood breath as a sensitive organ of psychic expression and sought to use it therapeutically. Building on the work of Reich, Alexander Lowen (1976) developed the method of bioenergetics, in which targeted breathing exercises play an essential role. Breath is used, in this case, to achieve relaxation, relief and release.

Thus, the view that breath has an inherent autonomous, psychological function, aimed at lending expression to the unconscious, has faded into the background. The breath therapist Cornelis Veening[2] (1995), a practitioner who scarcely left behind any written material but referred to his encounters with C. G. Jung's analytical psychology, did follow such a path. Veening picked up the spiritual traditions of breath and studied the connection between imagination and breath. Not only did Veening see meditative breath training as physically and psychologically healing, but he also saw breath as a sensory organ for unconscious processes, that is, an epistemological instrument. For him, breath and imagination are inseparably connected and complement one another in the endeavour to experience holistic consciousness anchored in the body. With the help of breath, images can be conjured and explored. Veening (1995, p. 14) writes:

> If we want to approach our breathing in our unconscious, we must learn not to disturb it, because in it we encounter our own nature. This is why there are no exercises for breathing in this method . . . What we do in breathwork is stimulation—more precisely, spiritual stimulation! It is possible that we trigger situations and memories that we could not have anticipated, but which appear suddenly and which can only really be understood from a psychological perspective.

Concerning Veening's (1995, p. 15) work with patients, he states further:

> With a few brief words we try to attune the patient to a state where his breath is, for the moment, not consciously controlled. This is mostly achieved through a more or less passive stance, which only accompanies the breathing process. The patient discovers that there is something within him leading an almost independent life, and that he must become attuned to experience it.

One could also say that the patient learns to enter into dialogue with "something other" than his habitual consciousness.

The following clarifies what Veening (1995, p. 15) means when he refers to breath as an epistemological instrument:

> If I may offer an example here: A patient comes to me, who has no sense of feeling for himself and his momentary situation, and who only takes notice when he is shaken, which happens from time to time. Then he is violently shaken—reduced to tears—but doesn't understand why, and feels like an utterly helpless bystander. His breathing is shallow and pale and beyond his own perception, but he can breathe in and out at will. His skin is noticeably dull and his body appears uninhabited. I work with him for a few weeks and finally believe I can sense a small reaction—a slight revitalisation. I lay my hand on his stomach and ask him to continue breathing quietly. Then I vibrate my hand gently but determinedly, and ask him whether he notices—does he feel anything at all? "Yes," he says, "a distant earthquake in Japan!" I believe this clearly illustrates how far away he was compelled to place an event that had taken place in such immediate proximity—between him and myself. It was utterly impossible for him to relate this sensation to himself.

The idea of psychic and physical healing with the help of breath has taken on new forms of expression throughout the history of humankind.

What is the significance of breath in our Western civilisation? We take several breaths every minute and we eat an average of three to four times a day. Consider the comparatively major role that dietary guidelines play in present-day preventive medicine. Has anyone, by comparison, ever heard their doctor ask them after their breathing, not only their digestion? Auscultation determines the functionality of an organ, and if the lung does not present any specific illness, then the doctor assumes that it must breathe correctly. To this day there have been no systematic studies on the influence of psychic factors on the quality of breathing—the frequency and volume of breaths and the involvement of autonomic musculature. There has been some research into breathing in the fields of sports medicine, with the aim of enhancing functional performance, and in somnology, with the aim of improving sleep. Breathing as the seam between body and psyche and between inner and outer worlds, and the associated functions that maintain mental equilibrium, are not considered even in preventive medicine. Psychotherapy could take an interest in the fact that our breathing is in constant interrelation with our emotions and our imaginative capacity. But here, again, research into breathing has been neglected. Aside from body psychotherapists, who use specific exercises including breathing exercises, it is rare for a psychotherapist to work with patients to explore their breathing habits in relation to their emotional state. Those who work with imaginative methods in psychotherapy can't help but notice that often all it takes is the simple request to let a picture appear in front of the inner eye to trigger a deep, diaphragmatic breath. It would be interesting to examine whether people with pronounced imagination also breathe deeper and further and can thereby take advantage of the associated health benefits of increased oxygenation of the cells. In neurotic disorders, on the other hand, there exists the following negative interaction: emotions must be suppressed because they would cause psychological pain, and therefore imagination is also restricted along with the emotions. Since breathing is connected both with emotion and with imagination, it follows that it must remain shallow and on low flame in a neurotic person.

Even in the different schools of psychotherapy, it would be entirely possible to turn some of our attention to the breathing of our patients. After all, therapist and patient communicate with each other on many different levels during a session, and a patient's short, shallow breath—as well as posture and body language—can be transferred to the analyst and vice versa, just as a relieving sigh triggers a similarly liberating breath in the other person. Our breathing always accompanies us and responds to internal and external stimuli. Leaving aside extreme situations such as severe anxiety and panic attacks, where breathing almost stands still and a breath can be held for a very long time, breathing is involved in every eager expectation, every flight of stairs climbed, every moment of fright and every tender touch—more than that, breathing actually determines those emotions. Physical stimuli, especially on our skin, also trigger breaths: cold and warm water, being touched, a light breeze. Fear, sadness and fright lower breathing frequency and volume: this serves as a protection against pain. The extent to which sexual arousal and encounter is connected with breathing requires no special mention— indeed it is breath that enables sexual union in the first place. Likewise, it depends on breath whether the encounter becomes an act of synchronicity or whether the partners remain alone with their own arousals. Synchronous breathing also occurs between a mother and baby and, to a lesser extent, in every attentive conversation. Actors who require precise cues allow themselves to be guided by the breath of their dialogue partners. How many sighs (an involuntary breath emanating from the diaphragm) are associated with memories? *Back in the day* . . .—and already such a breath is released. Sniffing a good smell is a particularly sensitive form of breathing. This reflex, which emanates from the lower abdomen, not unlike a deep exhalation, is well known in singing lessons: singers are often encouraged to sing a note as if they were inhaling the fragrance of a flower. This causes the note to resonate throughout the body because even the autonomic musculature is relaxed in this form of breathing. Diaphragmatic breathing is the spontaneous breathing mode during rest and sleep, when the autonomic nervous system is activated. It is particularly efficient because a large volume of air can be transported to the lungs with little muscle action. Children use diaphragmatic breathing in the first years of their lives and have usually unlearnt it by school age at the latest. The diaphragm is activated in coughing, laughing, yawning and heavy crying (sobbing). Wherever emotions have to be shut out, the body almost completely abandons diaphragmatic breathing while awake, which leads to tension and fatigue. Shallow breathing has become a habit for many people, and because neither doctors nor priests habitually inquire about breathing, these individuals sacrifice a third of their lung capacity and the associated exchange of oxygen in the blood for their lifetimes.

Breath as a spiritual practice.

At this point I would like to describe an extraordinary breathing practice that is unique to Tibetan Buddhism, where until recently it was exclusively reserved for monks. It contradicts our conventional understanding of a breathing exercise, not only in the way it is performed, but above all in terms of the objective. This practice is not about personal health and well-being, but about something else.

I am referring to Tonglen meditation, and it is hardly accidental that this practice has remained relatively unknown in the West.

Tonglen is the seventh of sixty-nine guidelines of Mahayana Buddhism (literally "great vehicle"), which was widespread in India approximately five hundred years after the Buddha's death. Tong-len means to send and receive. "Tong: sending out, letting go. Len: receiving, accepting." "Sending and taking should be practised alternatively. These two should ride the breath," as it says literally in the Mahayana.

The inhalation and exhalation of breath are, however, associated with certain notions. When we inhale, we imagine everything that we loathe about ourselves; for instance, our own meanness, feelings of envy and hatred, our fears. When we exhale, by contrast, we send out everything healing and beautiful that we have thus far experienced in our life; for instance, an affectionate gesture or even a piece of chocolate. Thus, difficult and conflict-laden sentiments and memories alternate with positive and relieving ones in every breath. It requires great concentration to move from one emotional state to its opposite, and to return again, within a quarter of minute: to breathe in what disgusts us—to breathe out what does us good.

Now you might be thinking that I have confused matters in describing the mode of breathing, since your yoga teacher has always been asserting the opposite: breathe out strains and worries, and allow the light and healing powers of the universe to enter you. But in fact I have not confused matters. Tonglen is not about whether something is "beneficial" or "does us good." It is not concerned with a physiological process, but rather with an "*opus contra naturam*."

Let us consider what happens psychically when we practise Tonglen. Before we take a breath, we must try to determine what we consider evil and what good. Thus, we are sharpening our ethical and aesthetic consciousness. But this doesn't mean that we simply sweep our psychic waste out the door; on the contrary, it is about acknowledging those deeds and traits that we would preferably forget as belonging to us.

We can imagine the effect of such an exercise on a neurophysiological level: non-verbal, negative memory traces are continuously activated and then "cast aside" again. What is dark, oppressive and unjust stands directly alongside what is light, expansive and generous—and does so one breath after another. In daily life, these polarities are of course never stimulated and coupled in such rapid succession. Our breath doesn't mix them; it carries them.

Now the overall aim of such meditation is not that everything dreadful that we breathe in becomes transformed within us and is subsequently breathed out as something "released" or "redeemed." There can be no question of transformation. Nor is the Tonglen breathing practice about an inner acceptance of suffering in a Christian sense. There is no mention in Tonglen of salvation through suffering. Rather, Tonglen is rhythmic alternation: both sides appear as two aspects of the same phenomenon.

Advanced Tonglen enables a confrontation with collective matters. In this practice, which was initially practised only by monks, the meditator imagines breathing in everything obnoxious, sordid, ignorant and wicked brought forth by humanity: environmental pollution, injustice, violence, war and the unspeakable suffering of humans and animals. Not only do we breathe in these horrors, but we also absorb them through the pores of our skin. In return, we breathe out into the world every conceivable positive image and notion we have ever encountered.

Chödyam Trungpa (2005, p. 41) writes:

> Sometimes we feel terrible that we are breathing in poison which might kill us and at the same time breathing out whatever goodness we have. It seems to be completely impractical. But once we begin to break through, we realise we have even more goodness and we also have more things to breathe in.

Furthermore:

> In Tonglen we are aspiring to take on the suffering of other sentient beings. We mean that literally: we are willing to take that on. As such it can have real effects, both on the practitioner himself and on others. There is a story

about a great Kadampa teacher who was practising Tonglen and who actually did take another's pain on himself: when somebody stoned a dog outside his house, the teacher himself was bruised.

And finally:

> The basic idea of practising sending and taking is almost a rehearsal, a discipline of passionlessness, a way of overcoming territory. Overcoming territory consists of going out with the outbreath, giving away and sending out, and bringing in with your in-breath as much as you can of other people's pain and misery. You would like to become the object of that pain and misery. You want to experience it fully and thoroughly.

We can understand that Tonglen was practiced only by monks.

In the following, I would like to show that unconscious imaginations, for example dream images, can indeed manifest spontaneously, which could stem from a similar archetypal matrix to the origins of Tonglen meditation. In the case I wish to describe here, breath faltered altogether out of fright. The case pertains to a patient's dream that withstood every attempt at comprehension through its absolute horror and senselessness.

It is the dream of a young woman who grew up in one of the Baltic republics during the Soviet occupation. First, I must describe some biographical details so that the patient's individual, psychological contribution to the making of such a dream is understood. The woman experienced repeated violence during her childhood, including the humiliation of the local population at the hands of the Soviets, domestic abuse at home and destitution during her lengthy stays at her grandmother's (who lived in complete isolation in one of the restricted military zones). This young woman was also raped during puberty. This series of traumatic experiences led to an obsessive, self-destructive form of behaviour in her adult years. After six years of analysis, however, the woman had gained control over this behaviour. She was now in her mid-thirties, studying and working. She had also taken up meditation.

During the course of analysis, she had had countless dreams featuring violence in every conceivable shape and form. Little by little, however, the dream ego had begun to distance itself from the victim's role and started confronting these attacks. Her behaviour in the outer world had also changed. She refused to be exploited in personal relationships and at work.

Nevertheless, although neither perpetration nor victimisation any longer played a role in her outer life, she still suffered from regular nightmares. Let me report one of the dreams that not only unsettled her deeply for weeks, but also frightened her to such a profound extent that she considered giving up analysis: she stayed away for two months and didn't answer the telephone.

It was like being inside a mountain; I saw a vast number of cows standing, like in a large stable. But the cows had no skin. They stood there, utterly motionless, since even the slightest movement would have caused intolerable pain. Their eyes [the dreamer remembers the sweet-tempered faces of the calves in her hometown] *were lightbulbs; the animals didn't have real eyes.* [In the dream, the dreamer experienced nauseating pain. She could hardly finish her account during the session and seemed not to be breathing at all. She tried to communicate her deep compassion with the animals, but the words were drowned in tears.]

Even my own breath faltered as I listened. The dream seemed to illustrate the suffering endlessly inflicted on the animal population of the entire world. I tried to cautiously point this out to her—but it sounded rather beside the point.

Nor did the question that I repeatedly asked myself after the session help to advance matters: what was the purpose of such a dream? What function might the depiction of such brutality have? The only visible effect was renewed traumatisation. No one except her, who had been forced to survive on the edge of what was humanly tolerable, was being confronted with images of such unimaginable suffering—seemingly out of sheer mockery, and precisely at a time when, after years of analysis, she had managed to form a protective skin for the first time. It seemed that she was now being deprived of that existential foundation of trust which had saved her as a child after the adults had abdicated: a foundation in nature, especially in animals.

In the dream, her compassion had been so profound that it was as if she herself had been skinned. And the word *compassion* finally led me to think of Buddhist practice. In one of our next sessions, after she had resumed analysis but was still scared of dreaming, I asked the patient if she had heard of Tonglen meditation. She said she had not. The idea of first evoking and then breathing in the mental image of something awful bewildered her.

When I suggested the possible parallel between this practice and the drama in her nightmares, we were able to establish the possibility that some of her nightmares might be related to the practice of Tonglen. That is, we came to suppose that the psyche might have found it necessary to deal with not only the most awful personal images in her experience, but also those which are suffered by others. This supposition was supported by the fact that, at night, when the influence of the conscious ego is reduced, the dreamer is guided as if by the force of nature to practise Tonglen breathing. "If that is the case," the patient exclaimed with excitement and a great sigh of relief, "then my nightmares would make sense."

Conceivably, then, this particular case allows us to frame a theoretical perspective on the psyche's capacity—paradoxically, it seems, but actually in an integral way—to lead those who are strong enough to enlarge their capacity for suffering. One could imagine that an archetypal tendency to deal with all of humanity's horrors is expressed in the psyche of certain people who already have a particularly high potential for empathy—be it due to their disposition or their life history.

Consequently, nightmares and the Buddhist breathing practice of Tonglen would originate in the same matrix. We could further speculate that if a person afflicted with nightmares took up Tonglen, this could help alleviate the nightmares—not because their contents would dissolve, but because this tendency of the psyche would have already found an alternative channel rooted in consciousness. The person afflicted with nightmares would thus venture voluntarily into human abysses and would not need to be wakened against their will. As for my own patient, although she did not take up the practice of Tonglen, her nightmares have diminished somewhat and she now approaches them differently.

Perhaps the connection between Tonglen breathing and nightmares becomes clearer if we look at other phenomena from the perspective of Tonglen. Take a historian, for instance, who spends a lifetime researching human tragedies, or a forensic archaeologist busily recording atrocities for decades, excavating bones from mass graves and piecing them together into skeletons, even though these victims have no surviving relatives. Neither the seriousness nor solitude of such people allow for any reductive interpretations. In both cases—the historian and the forensic specialist—such people are very probably guided by an inner urge to dedicate themselves largely and in detail to human excesses. Not in order to make anything better, not to bring about any form of healing after the fact, but quite simply because they have an inclination to deal with the horrors committed by humankind and are prepared to commit their own vital energy as a counterpoint. Perhaps these people practise something akin to Tonglen without being aware of it.

In the West, we have no symbol for the rhythmic coexistence of light and dark. Coming from the East across millennia, Tonglen is a highly differentiated and accomplished expression of what analytical psychology calls the "integration of the shadow."

If this rhythmic absorption of the dark side were more widely perceived and practised, then we could become grateful for the nightmares that awaken us from sleep, leaving us soaked in sweat: what unsettles us so profoundly at night could well be an initial, unconscious breathing-in, true to the psychologically "nourishing" practice of Tonglen. The fact that breath is used as a vehicle in this practice—which, as we heard at the beginning, is linked to deity itself—makes the practice deeply intimate and radical: difficult to fathom and difficult to integrate for the Western world view.

From all that has been said so far, it becomes clear how elusive, flexible, autonomous, how easily subjugated and also how unpredictable breath can be.

Covid-19 and breath.

Let us now move on to the situation in May 2020. An illness affecting breathing has broken out, and the lungs of several million people have become hard as stone as a result of this disease. This outright alarmed the doctors when they were performing the first autopsies. It was gradually discovered that, long before a patient infected with Covid-19 complained of shortness of breath, the oxygen levels in the blood were already dangerously reduced and the lungs were hardened. Patients themselves describe the breathing difficulties of Covid-19 as a journey to hell and back: "The lungs feel as though they were made of glass; you want to breathe but everything remains inflexible; you feel like you are already dead and yet you are still alive; it is the absolute worst thing I have ever experienced," said a thirty-year-old athlete.

The pandemic caused by Covid-19, which has affected all of humanity in just a few months, has affected our breathing and—perhaps—also raised awareness for it. Without engaging in esoteric considerations, we can safely say that breath has been grossly neglected in our civilisation. We have no perception of its function as a sensory organ for emotions and for psychological and physical states. This goes hand in hand with the lack of attention and concern we pay to the quality of the air we breathe in the big cities. The 75,000 annual deaths[3] caused by environmental pollution in Europe are largely due to respiratory illnesses, even without the novel virus.

Why does breathing receive so little attention? Has it been too long since divine breath awoke us from dusty earth to living beings? Are we so confident that matter can hold itself together without breath? Are we afraid of becoming aware of our own breath because we think that something unknown might be awakened in us? Or are we afraid of having no inner world at all—no space which breath could penetrate and fill?

Or is it our fear of laughter and crying that makes our breath run shallow, because these emotions are beyond our control? Or is it the inflationary consciousness of self, typical of our modern civilised societies, which resits almost all attempts of penetration by breath for fear of sinking into an instinctive or even vegetative state of being? It is interesting to note that the social restrictions imposed by the virus have forced us, to a large extent, to relinquish our activities in the outside world. All those of us privileged enough to be able to stay at home, with few outside commitments, were obliged to rely on ourselves for company. Our breathing may have become shallower still out of fear and anxiety about the disease, but on the other hand we may also have recognised, for the first time, the importance of healthy lungs and the privilege of being able to breathe without a ventilator. Millions of people will not be able to help but pay more attention to breath in the coming years. Just like our heartbeat, our breathing is an expression of psychic vitality. Breath is connected to psychic processes on many levels, and there is still a whole world concealed within it, which Cornelis Veening and his student Ilse Middendorf (Middendorf, 1985) only began exploring.

Let us return once more to Cornelis Veening's (1995) example of one of his patients. "Distant earthquake in Japan" had been the image for this man's psychic reality. Emotionally and psychically, he was infinitely removed from himself and from other people. His breath had not only acted as a seismograph for emotions, but also for relationships.

We can engage in any number of thoughts and speculations and live our lives relatively unconsciously, and our breath will not interfere—it will do its duty and fill our lungs with oxygen up to a third of their capacity several times a minute. But the moment something "other" appears—in thought, in fantasy or even in concrete reality, from outside—breath registers this immediately. This "other" could be a person walking in the door, but it could also be no more than an "other" thought, a word, a feeling, a smell, a sudden memory. Moments like these trigger a breath: deeper, more expansive, directed towards engagement and just waiting to relate to something; as if the breath would like nothing more than to flow from something known to something unknown and back again—from the inside out, from the outside in, from the body to the psyche, as if it were in fact, in its essence, a cognisant spirit.

Notes

1 XXII International Exhibition of La Triennale di Milano 2019.
2 Veening, Cornelis: (1995) *Das Bewirkende, Texte aus Erinnerung*. Berlin: Hrsg. Waldmatter Kreis, AFA Geschäftsstelle.
3 European Environment Agency Report 2012.

Bibliography

Britannica. www.britannica.com/biography/Zhuangzi
Chögyam Trungpa, Rimpoche. (2005). *Training the Mind & Cultivating Loving Kindness*. Boston and London: Shambala Publications.
Grof, S., and Grof Ch. (2013). *Holotrophes Atmen. Eine neue Methode der Selbsterforschung und Therapie*. Solothurn: Nachtschatten Verlag.
Lowen, A. (1976). *Bioenergetics*. London: Penguin Books.
Middendorf, I. (1985). *Der erfahrbare Atem*. Paderborn: Jungermann Verlag.
Reich, W. (1969). *Die Funktion des Organsmus. Die Entdeckung des Orgons*. Köln: Kiepenheuer & Witsch.
Steiner, R. (1936). *Die Philosophie der Freiheit. Grundzüge einer modernen Weltanschauung*. Hamburg: Severus Verlag.
Veening, Cornelis. (1995). *Das Bewirkende, Texte aus Erinnerung*. Berlin: Hrsg. Waldmatter Kreis, AFA Geschäftsstelle.

Chapter 12

Andrew Samuels

Jung famously wrote that "every psychology is a personal confession," and that remark guides me here. I'd like to show why—to the best of my conscious knowledge—some of the themes in my work came to be there from a personal angle.

In 1967, at about the age of 18, I was a highly political young man, but trying to realize my political dreams through the arts—specifically, theatre. We were a radical theatre company, in those remarkable days at the end of the 1960s when you could get money from the English Arts Council for way-out theatre companies. Then, after becoming a youth worker and a counsellor working with young people, an encounter with humanistic psychology—and that was a serious option career-wise for a while—led me into analysis, and I dropped out of the political world for a decade. So, when Thatcherism came in the 1980s, there was I, former Trotskyist and student radical, busy writing Jungian books!

Gradually, the political side of my personality, and my interest in society, came back in and merged with my clinical concerns, leading to the formation in 1994 of Psychotherapists and Counsellors for Social Responsibility. Then, when I began to have children, as often seems to happen with men, a third strand came in, which we could call "spiritual." Psychotherapy, politics, and spirituality—three sides of a coin! Charles Péguy said, "everything starts in mysticism and ends in politics."

The account up to now is somewhat external and avoids my beginnings in the family. I have always struggled to find a vigorous to-and-fro in my image of my parents' marriage. I am not saying it was never there, only that I had an image of a conventional togetherness without much passion or risk-taking. They were kind to each other but never went near (in my fantasy anyway) the grotesque and divine experimentations I found a need to write my chapter on, "The image of the parents in bed."

I will talk about my mother in a moment. My father was a gentleman, and I mean this in two senses. First, that he was well educated, had been through the war (ending up in both Italian and German prisoner of war camps), and enjoyed a cultivated and comfortable lifestyle ranging from golf to classical music. But he was also, for me, what I came to call in my writings a "dry" father, not using his body to give out much erotic or aggressive playback—but a decent and polite

DOI: 10.4324/9781003148968-13

man. In fact I felt he depended on me to provide a kind of excitement and, via my rebellious, bad and rejecting behaviour, and that is what I did. His father was a self-made immigrant tycoon type, though the family business went bankrupt in the end.

My concern—even obsession—with relations between women and men stems, I believe, from this respectable but emotionally constrained background. Hence, I found it hard to buy into Jungian essentialist approaches to gender because they felt so limiting. That was why I wrote "Beyond the Feminine Principle" in 1989. And I have been strongly influenced by feminism in what I wrote over the years about the relations between women and men.

I am a competitive person, who delights in negotiation and bargaining. But over time I have become able to agree with Gerhard Adler that there is a "principle of complementarity" at work in life: some people are better than others at some things. But when it comes to other things, other people are more adept.

These four principles, stemming from my personal psychology, also lie at the heart of pluralism: competition, negotiation, bargaining, and complementarity. Pluralism gave me an opportunity to be aggressive and tolerant at the same time. Those four principles are relevant to many levels of experience.

When I wrote Jung and the post-Jungians, I was a novice analyst writing an overview of the field into which I had just arrived and it was, of course, an infla-tion. But I certainly made a name for myself. This leads me to comment a bit on my mother's influence on me. It was she who spotted, with her down-to-earth intuition and generally savvy approach to life, that writing could be a way for me to make my mark. She went on and on about this, and, unusually and amazingly, I listened even though I knew that my success was for her glory.

I have come to understand that, behind my pluralistic tendency to pop up in many fields of psychotherapy beyond the post-Jungian one (humanistic psychol-ogy, body psychotherapy, relational psychoanalysis) and in both mainstream and activist politics, there is a quest for power.

Be that as it may, I don't think it was only the need for power that motivated my controversial work on Jung and anti-Semitism from the mid-1980s until the pub-lication of *The Political Psyche* (1993). This material, and other, later discoveries, were originally published in the Journal. If there was a personal background to this project, it was simply to do with the plain fact of being Jewish in a commu-nity whose founder had written objectionable things about my people. Fred and I discussed this all the time. In addition, there was also some kind of background wish to be more accepted as a contributor to academic, psychoanalytic, and politi-cal discourses that was undermined by being seen as an adherent of that notorious anti-Semite Jung.

The reactions to my early essays into the allegations of Jung's anti-Semitism really pissed me off, though on a good day I could also empathize with them. It did feel like being in my family in which I was always the "black sheep," the Rosha—the wicked son who seeks to opt out of the Passover Seder ceremony.

In the early stages of our community's engagement with our problem, there was a closing of the Jungian ranks, a repetitious argument that Jung was merely a man of his time, and even some pathologizing of me as a Jew with a complex.

Well, Jung was not exactly a man of his time (as you can see from the detailed research I and others did), and it is those kinds of knee-jerk defences that even today sometimes represent our problem (the Jungians' problem) and not Jung's problem. Nevertheless, gradually, the Jungian community realized that some sort of acknowledgement and reparation was needed, and the informal alliance of concerned people that emerged has done a pretty good job in this regard. Of course, for those who need us as a tribal enemy, such as the psychoanalysts, the unfortunate legacy provides a marvellous base.

As I write in early 2020, similar explicatory and reparative work is beginning to be done on Jung's racial attitudes and his theories and utterances about "Africans."

Professor Andrew Samuels London March 1, 2020

The "Activist Client"

Social Responsibility, the Political Self, and Clinical Practice in Psychotherapy and Psychoanalysis

Originally published in Andrew Samuels D.H.L. (2017) The "Activist Client": Social Responsibility, the Political Self, and Clinical Practice in Psychotherapy and Psychoanalysis, *Psychoanalytic Dialogues*, 27:6, 678–693. Reprinted with permission.

The idea of the "activist client" is intended to be taken both literally and meta-phorically—applying to some extent to a wider range of clients than actual activists. The chapter develops a set of ideas about a "political turn" in psychotherapy and psychoanalysis, using the tag "the inner politician." There is a focus on working directly with political material in the session, and the pros and cos of this practice are reviewed. Wider issues such as social responsibility and social spirituality are discussed, as well as an exploration of the limits of individual responsibility. Some specific topics covered in the chapter include the political roots of depression, difficulties with the concept of the therapeutic alliance from the point of view of democratic perspectives on clinical work, and a challenge to the unquestioned valuing of empathy (based on a reading of therapy though a Brechtian lens). There are numerous clinical examples.

I rebel, therefore we are.—Camus (1951/1953, p. 111)

The main aim of this chapter is to fly the idea of the "activist client." The chapter is focused and somewhat exaggerated, to make a point. It may seem cheeky or wrongheaded to some, or as having only niche utility due to its militancy. Yet a strong single beam of light is shone across a stage, brightly illumining what is in its direct path, hence also revealing something on either glimmering side of the beam. So the chapter is not only about clients who are already activists, though it is clearly relevant to them. Other clients with other therapists may also come into the picture—for all clients and all therapists are citizens with the rights, responsibilities, burdens, hopes, and despair of citizens. I hope what I am suggesting will resonate with a wider range of clients and therapists than might seem apparently to be the case, if not with every single client at all times. With this wider applicability in mind, I suggest that the "activist client" is to be taken metaphorically as much as literally. In many ways, the linkage I am making is between two kinds of client activism—*the mobilization of political activism in society* and *the discovery of a kind of clinical activism in session.*

In general terms, the chapter is intended to contribute to the emergence of a "critical psychotherapy" (Lowenthal, 2015; Samuels, 2015a) in which psychotherapy and psychoanalysis reflect on and problematize their own practices. On an anodyne level, that is why I call citizens who want therapy "clients" rather than "patients." And their paid professional would then be a "therapist." Throughout, I have been careful with my use of the terms "therapy," "psychotherapy," and "psychoanalysis."

More specifically, the ideas in the chapter stem from the long-standing project of bringing therapy thinking to bear on politics, and political thinking to bear on therapy (Samuels, 1993, 2001, 2002, 2015b). I felt it was necessary to explore some key themes stemming from this project before introducing the "activist client" in a more direct manner. In the background lies our ever-deeper understanding that the self is a political self, that one form of psychic energy is political energy, that people have a line of political development and experience that can be elucidated and even theorized, that the unconscious is "normative" to use Layton's term (e.g. 2004). Psychoanalysis and psychotherapy generally are professional acts that cause us to discover (or maybe to rediscover) that they are by nature political. In and out of session, we are often dealing with what I call "the inner politician." Isn't the task of the therapy to facilitate people in stopping thinking like the state wants them to think, just as we try to facilitate judicious freedom from persecutory, authoritarian, and judgemental parental introjects?

Social Responsibility and Social Spirituality

A political or social focus does not remove clinical work from the psychological field. Social responsibility, freely and fully entered into, contributes to individual psychological vitality, not only in Daniel Stern's sense of "vitality affects" (e.g. 2010) but also in terms of life itself, of the principle of life itself. This piece of therapy thinking could contribute to a revitalization of our democracy: increased liveliness, energy, spirit, dynamism, passion, fire, vigour, élan, vivacity, exuberance, bounce, verve, vim, pep, brio, fizz. (These words are just a few of the synonyms one finds for "vitality.")

I think there is a variant of social vitality, which I call "social spirituality," to consider. Some clients (and probably some therapists) have never or rarely experienced this, and I think the absence is as much of a psychic problem as its opposite: a manic overinvolvement with or fetishization of politics. In social spirituality, people come together to take action in the social sphere, doing this in concert with other people. When this happens, something spiritual comes into being. Being actively engaged in a social, political, cultural, or ethical issue, together with other activists, initiates the spiritual. This is a very different perspective from one that would see social spirituality as being something done in the social domain by spiritual people. On the contrary, there is a kind of spiritual rain that can descend onto ordinary people who get involved with others in political and social issues (see Samuels, 1989, 2001). For example, the Occupy movement or the protests against global capitalism and planetary despoliation come to mind—and, sadly but inevitably, do less salubrious movements of the right—xenophobic, populist, and demagogic. Spirit has no politics as such; God has a right hand and a left hand after all!

What people are doing when they get involved in the anti-capitalist movements and the environmental and ecological movements is to participate in a general "resacralisation of culture" (Samuels, 1993). To play on the word "politicized," many activists also become "spiritualized" via their involvements and engagements. When one gets involved in idealistic politics, sometimes, not always, one gets spiritualized, and so something like the anti-capitalist movement is creating its own spirituality and, in turn, is being reflexively informed by the spirituality that it creates. Political action leads to spirituality of some kind and spirituality informs political action. Of course, eventually it may all fall to pieces; either the police wreck it or people (allegedly) "grow up," but there is a basic resacralizing tendency worth recognizing.

Now the clinical point concerns the people I mentioned who have never experienced this. When meeting a prospective client, or interviewing a prospective candidate, shouldn't we ask them about their political histories—nonjudgementally, accepting that some will not have always been on a progressive, "lefty" path? As I said, spirit is not always "good," whether we like that or not, and experiences of social spirituality are available to fascists, rednecks, and homophobes. So, too, are the services of therapists, and that is as it should be.

Nevertheless, whatever the politics of the therapist or the politics of the client, shouldn't we explore why, if there has been little engagement with public issues on the part of an individual, this has been the case? Not "Why have you been so manically political?" but "Why haven't you been involved in politics at all?" It's important to do this in the knowledge that there are no correct answers, for many reasons quiescence might exist, such as reacting to experience in a hyperpolitical family in which individual feeling was an apolitical luxury. But the point is that not to go into these areas is a truncation of what is possible in therapy.

Political Material in the Therapy Session

Yet I believe we continue to struggle to find ethical ways of working *directly*, as opposed to making symbolic interpretations, with political, social, and cultural material as it arises in the clinical encounter. Many of us seek to fully meet such material, in a responsible and relational manner. However, we still experience the psychoanalytic dead hand, the penumbra of criticism that this *Weltanschauung* is nonanalytical and that the analyst will simply foist his or her political views on the patient. When we add a "political turn" to the relational turn, it may be asserted that we are acting *ultra vires*, beyond our authority or responsibility as analysts. It is a serious and important critique that can only partially be rebutted by saying—as I and others do—that yesterday's bad or impossible practice may be the cutting edge for today's clinicians. The purposes of the present chapter include (a) the development of an adequate theoretical model to use as a basis for responsible handling of political material in the clinical session, and (b) discussion of how a supportive context for such work might be created.

Let's recognize that psychoanalysis and the psychotherapies are not alone in making a discovery or rediscovery of a latent political mission. For example, as is discussed later in the chapter, liberation theology sets out to engage with societies experienced as unjust and destructive despite criticisms from the Church establishment. So, too, have practitioners and theorists in the arts, despite criticisms from critics who regard the results as "boring" and a betrayal, nothing to do with "real" art.

Empirical research via international and multimodality questionnaires (Samuels, 2006) shows that, in many countries, clients bring political, social, and cultural material to therapy much more than they did (and, I would add, they will bring even more when they know it is "permitted" to do so, that the rules of the game allow it). Therapy becomes a place where, in dialogue, client and therapist can work out their political attitudes and engagements. This can be as psychologically transformative for each as a purely personal alchemy—and may be done even when one of them finds the political positions of the other to be horrid or reprehensible. It remains necessary to acknowledge professional fears of exerting too much influence and of "foisting" one's political views on the client. But, apparently, the risk of foisting strikes some commentators as being greater when the context and material is political than when it is sexual, aggressive, spiritual, or developmental. I am not sure this is so. The risk is there, and we should respect the history of our clinical theory about boundaries, suggestion, and neutrality. But I am not sure there truly is a special problem when it comes to politics—or, if there is, whether that should give us cause to retreat immediately into neutrality and the eschewing of the political dimensions of life.

Emergence of an Activist Client

Here is a brief example of how a client got in touch with his inner politician. An Italian man, who came to therapy because, he said, of an intense depression, dreamt of *a beautiful lake with clear deep water*. He said this represented his soul and then immediately associated to *the high level of pollution on the Italian Adriatic coast*. The image of the lake, and the association to coastal pollution, suggested, in the form of one symbol, the client's unconscious capacity for depth and his present state, of which he was all too conscious—a state of being clogged up by "algae," like the coastal waters of the Adriatic.

The client gradually became aware of the tension between the individual and the political presences of the imagery. What, the client and I asked together, is the role of pollution in the soul, or even in the world? What is the role of pollution in the achievement of psychological depth? Can the soul remain deep and clear while there is pollution in the world, in one's home waters? Did the lake, with intimations of mystery and isolation, clash with the popular, extroverted tourism of the Adriatic?

Eventually, the client's concern moved to the social level: Who owned this lake? Who should have access to such a scarce resource? Who would protect the lake from pollution? These were his associations. From wholly personal issues, such as the way his problems interfered with the flowering of his potential, we moved to political issues, such as the pollution of natural beauty, not only by industry but also by the tourism. And we also moved back again from the political level to the personal level, including transference analysis. I do not mean to foreclose on other interpretations, but rather to add in a more "political" one so that the client's unconscious political commitments can become clearer.

He subsequently made a choice to return to Italy and, in his words, to "get more involved," perhaps in environmental politics. Therapy supported what was there in him, rather than encouraging his activism. But without therapy, would this particular individuation have taken place? I remain open-minded about this question—for "spontaneous remission" is not a notion to be dismissed lightly.

"For Samuels, Politics Plays an Almost Ontological Role" (Mitchell, 2000, p. 506)

Continuing to look at clinical phenomena, we come to this rather strange section heading. But the section illustrates, I believe, that the introduction of political language and dynamics into the session requires both an adequate supportive theoretical model and also a context in which there is support for the act itself. In this section, the accent is on the context; later, in a section on a Brechtian take on therapy, I work up the theoretical aspect.

Back in 2000, this journal produced a "Jungian issue" (Vol. 10, No. 3), for which I acted as the liaison person. Seven Jungian analysts set out their stalls as clinicians and then commented on an extract from Stephen Mitchell's (1997) book *Autonomy in Psychoanalysis* (pp. 155–164). This extract concerned a piece of work with his patient, given the disguised name of "Andrew." (*En passant*, I would add that this was a marvellous project and is still the single best way to discover the range of what contemporary Jungian analysts from across the world actually do.)

The interaction and dialogue between Mitchell and me, characterized by a high degree of agreement, may bring out many of the topics and issues covered in the present chapter more convincingly than an assertive solo piece of my own could. I'd like to add as a personal note that I was working on this chapter and had a dream of a political scenario in which Stephen Mitchell played a part and in a political context. This gave me the idea to present the fragment of dialogue as part of my chapter.

In the extract, Mitchell described his work with Andrew, who had made a switch from being a music composer to being a businessman. He brought to analysis his profound sense of meaningless and of having no personal value. Andrew's father was "economically marginal." Work with Andrew led Mitchell to remember and reflect on certain experiences of his own and to evince concern that he was getting too muddled up with this patient and/or using too much suggestion.

In the book extract we were given, Mitchell was clarifying his views as opposed to those of other leading contemporary psychoanalysts. Believing the context of intellectual work to be significant, and polemic to be at the heart of advances in any field, I wondered if Mitchell was perhaps a bit too worried about getting professionally smeared for showing that relational analysts get too mixed up with their patients, work only in the positive areas, disclose their autobiography including their political histories—blah, blah, blah. (In fact, if I had a criticism at all, it was that Mitchell was too cautious in his evaluation of the marked Trickster elements in the clinical narrative.)

Whatever, the relevance of this illuminating dialogue to the current chapter are illustrated in this comment I made on some dream imagery that Mitchell (1997) reported: a prestidigitator (sleight-of-hand artist) was doing tricks with coins and there is a ring made of gold:

> The clinical material is full of economic and related imagery. The prestidigitator uses coins, the ring is of gold. Mitchell tells us that "Andrew's" father was "economically marginal." "Andrew's" corporate life is reported as lacking meaning and value. Although the principal association on the part of the analyst was not economic, it was markedly political, and in any society the economic and political reams are connected—not only in terms of results and bottom lines but also in terms of meaning and values. Hence, the economic is psychological.
>
> (p. 421)

I think that one way into Andrew's pain would have been through a psycho-economic exploration of what his job actually was and what it meant to him. Early on, I found myself wondering why the move had to be so huge, from composer to executive. It is an example of what Heraclitus called *enantiodromia*, the swing of one extreme into its opposite: the artist, all pure and high-minded, into the venal (though comfortable off) businessman.

The way I work these days (this was published in 2000), I would have engaged Andrew in what I now openly call a discussion of some of these economic and political themes. Maybe (in my fantasy) it would lead him to find a job some-where between the two extremes.

I think I would also have explored as much as possible what the relations were between his father's economic situation and his own. To what extent is he still terrified of poverty? To what extent engaged in oedipal rivalry via his economic success? If there is a rivalrous element here, then could it not be the case that, at an unconscious level, Andrew actually strives to be less successful than his father? Obviously, one cannot say what the outcome of any particular line of exploration would be, but this is what occurred to me.

I got the impression that what Andrew lacked was connection to any sense that involved *communitas*, a sense of emotional investment in his own society. I see this missing connection as imaged in the dream by the filaments that link the mov-ing coins. Andrew has yet to realize that the work he has chosen could be work that has contributed to there being no filaments in existence between him and other parts of the world (Samuels, 2000, pp. 421–422).

Mitchell (2000) replied,

> Samuels raises fascinating questions about my concerns about influence. He wonders about the intrusions of conventional morality, my fears of being smeared by my colleagues, and possible regrets about my own life choices and defenses against unconscious analytic sadism. Politics and economics play a fundamental, almost ontological role in Samuels's sense of life, so he would want to use the dream to open up questions in these areas.
>
> (p. 506)

Class and the Inner World

Mitchell's account of the work with Andrew, and the psycho-economic aspects of his relationship with his father, serves as an introduction to a brief consideration of class issues in therapy work. As Corpt (2013) wrote, in an incisive and moving account of social class in the context of psychoanalysis: "When client, analyst, and the very profession of psychoanalysis disavow the psychological complexi-ties of social class, important conflicts and injuries are inevitably over-looked and therefore are unavailable for analytic understanding" (p. 65).

The topic of economic inequality is discussed everywhere these days (e.g. Piketty, 2014), though little is done to challenge the fundamental sadism of the financial arrangements in Western polities. Thinking about inequality for a moment, it is clear that a relationship exists between *class* and the individual's *inner world*. Many people have achieved a higher socio-economic status than their parents have. Yet, in their inner worlds, encountered in therapy, in dreams perhaps, the social class they grew up in is still the social class they are in in terms of psychic reality and narrative truth.

A client who worked as a banker dreamed frequently of the coal mine where his father had worked. The (male) solidarity of the miners—for example, when there was a disaster underground—struck him as different from the atmosphere and ethos of his large Wall Street investment bank. We did of course play a little with what we were "mining" in the analysis, but the main thrust of our dialogue about these dreams was in terms of a thorough, many-layered, compassionate, and healing *comparison* of his entire situation with that of his father's. Not competition with the father. There's more to intergenerational male relating than Oedipus—and the Oedipus complex is not a politically neutral idea.

The typical move—or at least it used to be typical, it may not be so for much longer—is from working class to middle class. To the extent that a passion for social and economic justice exists (for good reasons) in the working class, you can see how destabilizing and ego-dystonic their ruthless rise to the top is for some people. I have had several clients like that. This specific point about class and the inner world applies with particular force when the client is a member of a minority ethnic community. What can't be avoided is that we may be up against a psychodynamic barrier to social mobility and economic equality. The good news is that I think, clinically and culturally, we can do something about it. (I develop these points at length in Samuels, 2014a.)

Political Roots of Depression

This chapter probes the political phenomenology of clinical work in the therapy field. It was observation and conversation with colleagues that led me to suggest that some, maybe many, clients suffer from a kind of repression of their political selves. They are cut off from the vitality of social spirituality. They are struggling to get in touch with their "inner politician." Other clients have intense political engagements—but doubt that, as an individual, they can "make a difference." Hence, their idealism goes underground and may be sometimes understood, incorrectly in my view, as political apathy or even political despair. But is it? What looks like apathy is actually a pervasive sense of powerlessness, often coupled with intensely guilty self-criticism. Sometimes apathy follows on from what is believed by the subject to be failed activism. It is a special kind of depression, with political roots.

What does it mean when people use a psychological word—depression—about a political or social issue? About a general election? If you say you feel depressed or guilty about the election, the environment, climate change, or species depletion—what are you saying? Many psychotherapists understand depression as resulting from feeling angry and destructive toward someone you basically love and need. The classic example is at a time of bereavement. The mourner may feel at some level that their bad feelings toward the dead person somehow caused the death. Or they may be angry at having been left. In either case, there is a feeling of being responsible that leads to guilt, self-reproach (often of delusional proportions), and very low spirits with a lack of emotional, cognitive, and physical energy. The capacity to act is vitiated.

That feeling of guilty responsibility interests psychotherapists who want to bring "therapy thinking" to bear on political problems. In terms of climate change, for example, we can see similar dynamics (though it's important to be careful in mapping off from individual psychology to collective psychology). We love the earth yet we can see how destructive we can be toward it. Our guilt then paralyzes us and we enter a political depression that we struggle to overcome. In order to avoid the depression, some may even deny that climate change is taking place. Hence it is reasonable to suggest that depression has social and political roots beyond revulsion at mainstream politics—and does not only have to do with parents, partners, relationships, and all the usual therapy lines. Paradoxically, political depression also has to do with commitment and activism themselves.

The question of anger comes up in therapy in relation to almost any political theme: economics, multiculturalism, war, leadership. It doesn't matter which side of a debate you are on to feel angry. In addition, you do not have to be directly affected to feel angry, though excluded and disadvantaged people are, of course, more likely to feel it. The point is that when you have political anger in a form that cannot be managed or resolved, you will find some kind of depression and guilt, and as mentioned, this works against a sense of political agency and possibility.

I recall this vividly from work with a client, called, for the purposes of this chapter, Lorraine. She was a very active feminist, undertaking spectacular public events that found their way into the media. As time passed, she began to feel it was all a waste of time and futile. She became depressed, a burned-out activist by the age of 25. I am not going to narrate that therapeutic exploration rekindled her political ardour to its former intensity and efficacy, but it did enable her to see how it was her very passion and anger, not their shameful dribbling away, that led to her intensely painful depression. She was angry with herself, her "sisters," her parents, men, the patriarchy, the corporations, and me. She had begun to feel destructive in the political sphere, and this was implicated in her depression. Gradually, Lorraine came closer to accepting that political perfection is unattainable. She discovered that if she asked of herself only that she be a good-enough citizen, she might be less mired in her sense of depressive despair. Then a small degree of political hope might reawaken, as it did in her case.

Focusing on the Client

The preceding sections of the chapter offer an essential backdrop and introduction to a consideration of the politics of being a client. What we are currently seeing in the literature, and hence we may assume is taking place in practice, is the emergence of a rather new conception of the client, a perspective that sees *the client as the motor of therapy*. This client is a heroic client, a client who knows what she needs, a client who can manage her own distress. Some clients engage less in a process of healing or cure and more in a process of ongoing personal and political enquiry. This multifaceted new client is potentially a healer of others, especially the therapist, and, in a sense, of the world.

Summarizing a mass of research findings, Norcross (2011) forced us to consider whether it truly is the therapy relationship that does the business. Is the private and highly personal therapy relationship the main thing that makes therapy work? Not really. In common with other leading researchers, such as Lambert and Wampold, Norcross summarizes that "unexplained and extra-therapeutic factors" amount to 40% of efficacy, "the client" accounts for 30%, the therapy relationship 12%, the actual "therapist" 8%, and the "school or tradition or modality" of the therapist 7%.

Of course, Norcross would be the first to admit that therapy is a melange of all of these, and I would add that the findings do not do more than behove us to reconsider our ideas about our clients. These figures are far from veridical. But let's take them as heuristic, stimulants to critical thinking about clients. Who they are, what do they want, and what point in their life journey have they reached? What stage have they reached in what Norcross calls their "trajectory of change?"

As we know, there are some clients from whom one learns great and healing lessons. My first training "case" had a dream early on in the analysis. She dreamt, "I visit a doctor who is ill in bed. He begs me to stay." Her associations to "bed" were of illness, not of sexuality. How else could we understand this dream? Was the doctor in fact me?! Or was this an assumption, intended to justify what has been called a "you mean me" interpretation (a here-and-now transference interpretation)? Was there denial here, in that she is the ill one and I am truly the doctor? Or is she in the grip of an inflation, taking herself as the one who brings life and succour, like a mother to her therapist-child?

Or was this dream, perhaps, *an accurate political perception*? I did need something from her, and not just that she sticks with me so I could get through the training. Crucially, there would be a further accurate perception in the dream: that she could in fact help/heal this doctor. This was in early 1974 and, at that time, pre-Searles (see later), it would have been difficult to think of the client as healer of the therapist. Much has changed. (I write at length about working with this client, "D," in Samuels, 1985.)

Recent thinking about the client has moved in this general direction of envisaging the client as "active." From the person-centred approach, we find Bohart and Tallman (1999) referring to the "active client." This is an important corrective to the psychoanalytic expectation that the role of the "patient" is to provide unconscious material via free association. While often very important, it is not hard to see how this perspective may reduce the value given to the client's active involvement in the work.

Rogers (1951), in the era when the discourse was of "client-centred" therapy, makes it clear that the client knows for herself what is needed, where she wants to go. Jung (1946) wrote of entropy in the client, an innate process of self-regulation. From relational psychoanalysis, we read that Hoffman (2006) regards the client as having responsibilities to the analyst and the analysis, more than just for the co-creation of the therapy relationship.

So the therapist is, in a way, adjunct to the therapy process. But she is also a contingent figure, product of a particular social circumstance. Frank (1961) suggested that what makes the therapist is not only training, techniques, wounds, but also having been socially sanctioned as a therapist, a sort of overarching placebo effect. The therapist is socially sanctioned, granted permission to be a therapist—by society, *and, I must add, by the client.* Hence it behooves us to have in mind that all the analytic creativity and innovation that we rightly applaud is an epiphenomenon of the client's having sanctioned the therapist to be so safe, smart, and related in the first place. As Paul Atkinson (personal communication, 2015) put it, "The client's gift to the therapist—firstly appearing at their door and then constantly activating the work—is the most energetic factor in therapy." This is, I think, even now a rather new version of a client: a person who does not want the therapist to be the one who knows, or even the one who is supposed to know.

This chapter began life as part of a project for a more critical psychotherapy and has the frank aim of valorizing the client's contribution. But, in true critical fashion, one needs to remain aware that active clients have the potential to ruin as well as to fashion the work. Co-creation cuts both ways, destructive as well as positive, hard as that is to take in sometimes.

Be that as it may, let's see what happens if we revision the therapy relationship with all of these thoughts about the client in mind. It has gradually dawned on me that clients sometimes do not dare to deploy their tacit knowledge and emotional literacy. We therapists are fine with this because it leaves us free to do our work. But that could and, from critical and political perspectives, maybe should change.

The "Activist Client"

These observations on the politics of the therapy relationship lead me to suggest that the new model client, the client as the motor of therapy, is increasingly a politically aware client at some level. But not all politically aware people are activists, nor are all clients. Yet the argument of the chapter is that how deeply "activist" a client may be remains something to be curious about and explicate in therapeutic dialogue. One possible outcrop of therapy might be that, during the work, the client may develop her capacity for alterity, meaning, amongst other things, an empathic concern for the other. Yes, this does mean other people—but there is a more-than-personal version of alterity to consider. For example, for a client living in a multicultural world, meeting his or her inner psychological diversity in a new and positive spirit could lead to developing an analogously positive attitude to outer diversity in society, one that had not been there before. This, in turn, might lead to active support for those discovered by the client as hitherto subject to social exclusion. The move would be from self-acceptance of previously disowned or marginalized elements in the personality to political acceptance of similar elements in culture. In general, therapy work often leads to a sharpening or awakening of various latent political "commitments," possibly entered into without full buy-in from the conscious ego.

To the idea that a client is an active client, we could now add that activist clients have the potential to be citizen-therapists for the wider world with its environmental problems, economic injustice, and ubiquitous violence. The therapy client, revisioned as a socio-political healer, may now be understood to be a socially responsible agent of *Tikkun Olam*, the drive to repair and restore the world.

Back in 1975, Searles published his chapter "The Client as Therapist of His Analyst." In summary: If part of "mental health" is to want and be able to help and heal others, then isn't this something to work on in analysis? If so, said Searles, then isn't the analyst the obvious person for the patient to practice being a healer on? In a sense, I am extending Searles's vision. His arc was the move from healing the analyst to healing other people. I extend it to embrace healing beyond specific human others, to reach out to the social and political crises of our times. This, I am saying, is good for the soul. Activism is good for the soul. Mostly. I enter this caveat because it has to be admitted, as I have done on previous occasions (e.g. Samuels, 2001, pp. 124–125), that you can't guarantee that the activism in question is one of which you approve. Sometimes what unfolds is of a prejudiced or extreme right-wing nature. Sometimes it may strike the therapist as extreme from a left-wing perspective. Whatever the therapist thinks about this, she must stay true to her task of facilitating the client in whatever direction the client has chosen to go.

But the therapist, too, may have to change direction, eschewing, possibly temporarily, what she has typically thought and done in the session. Such a change of direction in theorizing practice is the focus of the next section.

Beyond Empathy—A Brechtian Angle on the Therapy Encounter

You can call it the "alienation effect" or "distanciation" or "estrangement." In German, *Verfremdungseffekt*. Bertolt Brecht's much-studied attempts *to avoid empathic identification by the audience with the characters in a drama* seem at first sight to be utterly foreign to the values and practices of all the therapies, including psychoanalysis. Empathy is our stock in trade, isn't it? Can you imagine relationality without empathy and a degree of identification with your client? Surely "analytical distanciation" would just be a return to the bad old days of neutrality and abstinence? Let's suspend quick reactions and discuss these points for a while. I hope to persuade readers that Brecht's take on human and social dramas can be perceived as coming to the aid of the practitioner who seeks to work with the political dimensions of social experience in therapy—but may feel that there is little extant theory to act as a heuristic guide.

Brecht did not invent the idea of drama with a social conscience, but he developed the theatre as a space for social and political debate (Willett, 1959/1964). The goal was to change the status and role of the audience leading to the creation of an "active spectator," participating in an argument rather than identifying with a heroic character.

In the old theatre, the individual human being was taken for granted. But for Brecht, the characters in a play are not heroic, but ordinary persons in a social context, engaged in an episodic narrative, often expressed—paradoxically—in lyrical language. Brecht developed a raft of techniques to carry out the distanciation, including the use of placards on stage during the performance.

What does all this mean for clinical work? Earlier I was discussing the problematic of working with openly expressed political material. Now, as I suggested earlier, this is still a minefield, though it is clear that many of us want to pick our way through such dangers, sensing there is gold dust to be found.

I am proposing that Brecht's theories of theatre practice are challenging and inspiring in this context. If therapist and client think together, argue together (whether it is with one another or as political allies in relation to some opponent or crisis), then it still stays in the affective realm, still contributes to vitality.

Connection and Distanciation Function as Two Poles of the Therapy Project

The suggestion I am making is that clients, and their relationally involved therapists, start to practice "ex-volvement," a neologism that implies standing outside the play of images, affects, and bodily processes that constitute the therapeutic (or any other) relationship. So the analyzing couple might, in some circumstances (not all the time) reverse the poles of what they ordinarily do, and distance themselves from emotion. It is pretty extreme, actually, this suggestion of a depriveleging and radical reframing of the personal level. Affect, emotion, even intimacy itself—all become things to interrogate

As far as the client is concerned, for me these lessons from Brecht chime with what was referred to earlier, coming out of person-centred humanistic psychotherapy, as the "active client" (Bohart and Tallman, 1999). I've added, with a little help from Brecht, the notion of what the role of a more active or even activist therapist might be.

Here is a very brief clinical vignette of ex-volvement in the clinic. Yasmine is, let's say, Egyptian and a TV reporter on politics. I've disguised her identity. She came to analysis hoping that something might be done about her virginity at the age of almost 40. She was feeling an intense sense of failure as a woman both in terms of her background in an Arab culture and in her lived experience in a Western country. She could not comprehend how this double blow had come to pass.

Yasmine chose a Jewish male therapist on purpose. I had decidedly mixed feelings about being informed that Jewish "doctors" were legendarily smart and that the Indian general practitioner she had consulted was "useless" on account of her origins. The idealization of my Jewish background was, of course, both defensive and reactive. When the conversation turned to the Palestine–Israel situation, she was not slow to link Israel's "sadism" (her word) with the Shoah experiences of Jewish people.

It became clear that Yasmine had never really explained her sexual symptomatogy to a health professional. With the general practitioner, she had ducked the issue out of shame and embarrassment. It took a long time for her to be able to trust me with a description of her sexual experiences, and what she told me reminded me of what a girlfriend of mine had gone through almost 50 years ago. I invited Yasmine to the side of the room where the computer was located and together we Googled "hymenitis." On subsequent medical examination by an "English" gynaecologist, it turned out that there was a physical problem and the next step was to consider surgery.

All of this needs to be understood as going on against a backdrop of Yasmine's belief that, despite no actual memories, she had been sexually abused by someone in the family. There were dream images and narratives that she felt supported this hypothesis, and I considered that it was likely to have been the case. This mixture of material involved some psychological and cultural issues of great profundity and delicacy concerning femininity and the female ideal at work in Yasmine's consciousness and unconscious.

I do not think I could have worked with her through the emotional densities attached to all the apparently outer world themes if I had not practiced a kind of ex-volvement. The Brechtian place was one that provided a foundation for a series of "arguments" about ethnicity, geopolitical conflict, fertility, and sexuality, with a two-way didactic flow. Maybe neither of us used placards, but we came very close to it. To be clear, I am not saying that a therapist without the Brechtian bee in his bonnet could never have achieved a rather positive outcome. But the vignette does show, I contend, that without some kind of theory upon which to base interventions into the "real," there is a greater risk of it going wrong.

Drawing back the camera a bit, the question I am introducing based on this brief clinical summary concerns the potential deceptiveness of the personal dimension. We know this often hides and leads to a wider issue. Brecht's ideas are useful for providing a backup for the temporary avoidance of the personal and the highlighting of the political. He says to the clinician (and also to the supervisor, I think) "Follow the story, follow the argument—don't only get caught up in the human drama." Brecht might well say that empathy is itself often achieved by a suspiciously heroic effort and therapists and analysts need to see through that and question whether, in empathy, they have found their gold standard.

A Note on Some Conservative Aspects of Relational Psychoanalysis

I think there may be some institutional or even ideological obstacles to what I am putting forward, and I would like to anticipate and explore them. (A fuller account of the ideas contained in this section of the chapter may be found in Samuels, 2014b).

Have psychoanalysis and psychotherapy overdone the stress on providing a secure container within which a therapy relationship can thrive? Safety and security will always be needed at some time or other—but all the time? There may be a risk of a tilt in the direction of behavioural conformism and a corresponding moralism. This isn't going to help the activist client.

What are the disadvantages of the current stress on the frame, on boundaries, on the container? Doesn't this lose the element of surprise, the risk inherent to psychotherapy, the exposure to danger that is involved in any radical or revolutionary process of self-understanding and/or growth? Are we witnessing the deformation of psychotherapy in the relational mode into nothing more than an attuned offer of nurture, safety, and a secure parental base? Is this not therapist as parent—or, more often, therapist as mother? Could it be that when we valorize attachment and intimacy we are not aware of the political and cultural structures we have created and instead put our own conceptual needs first?

Democratic Art, Democratic Analysis, and the Therapeutic Alliance

I want to push this critique of relational work, including my own, a little further to consider whether we have created an elitist or at least nondemocratic ethos in psychotherapy and psychoanalysis. I need to pull the camera back a little to look at how an orthodox doctrine with elitist tendencies and a top-down history was tweaked so as to develop its emancipatory and inclusive potential. I am saying the same can be done with psychoanalysis.

Liberation theologians, mainly in Latin America between 1950 and 1990, reoriented the Roman Catholic Christian project in their countries. As Seligman (personal communication, 2016) put it, "They added Christian universalized charity-love to Marxism in a political activist direction." To achieve this, liberation theologians took issue with Marx. Marx considered that the lowest of the low, the lumpenproletariat, were incapable of making a revolution. Liberation theologians, such as Leonardo Boff, challenged this Marxian elitism. For Boff, it is the poorest, most downtrodden, most out-of-it, most derided and excluded who will make the revolution. Was Boff thinking of the Psalmist's image (118:22, New American Standard Bible) that "the stone which the builders rejected has become the chief corner stone [of the Temple]." Another critic of Marx's elitism, George Orwell (1949/2013), got there too: "If there is hope, it lies in the proles," thinks Winston Smith in *1984* (p. 78). Orwell wasn't concerned with Marxist theory, so by "proles" he means those of whom Boff was writing—people not considered fit to make revolutionary changes.

These thoughts about liberation theology introduce a succinct account of what I am calling "democratic art," with the aim of producing an initial sketch of what a more "democratic" and inclusive therapy might look like. One that extends beyond the conventional clinical office with the usual range of clients, and one that is truly open to all, including those clients, not all of them male, who are "hard to reach."

I am not referring, on this occasion, to the power dynamics of the therapeutic relationship and process, or to its micropolitics. Nor to analysis and therapy as social institutions with a precise place in culture, one that varies from locale to locale, era to era. Nor do I have time and space in this chapter to join in the recuperation of how it was in the past—the polyclinics, Marx–Freud projects, red therapy, and so on. All these are tremendously important topics that many colleagues have worked on. But my focus right now is a little different.

So—democratic art. In the Ice Age, 40,000 years ago, something recognizable as art gradually appeared in Europe. It was sophisticated and intentional, involving highly developed cognition and applied imagination. Curators of exhibitions (Cook, 2013) of such art asked, Why do people make art at all? Why do they shape figures to look like women and men? Why do they record their ordinary daily lives? Why do they make symbol-laden art that is not based on "reality," like the Lion Man sculpture with human body and leonine head?

Humans have needed to make art, just as they have needed to make religion or politics. My suggestion is that client and therapist alike can be inspired by the democratic realization that imagination and creativity are not reserved for the Special Ones whose culture makes it easier for them to "do" analysis. There should be no psychoanalytical equivalent of the 1% in the economic sphere!

This means that there are some significant challenges to how many of us envision the work. We value the therapeutic alliance, but could it not be said that there is a secret elitism in this core concept? Even something esoteric? The parallel is with the professionalization of art, so to speak, since the Ice Age. The therapist is the professional who belongs always already to the secret society of the therapeutic alliance. She is inviting, or, rather, hauling up the client into the alliance. We might question this exclusivity more than we usually do.

I sometimes imagine this dialogue:

> *I am the initiated analyst, ready (trained) to enter into an intense, mutual, empathic relationship and therapeutic alliance with you that, though it will benefit us both, is at your disposal, whether for relief of your symptoms, or for growth, or simply for exploration.*

But the client all too often replies, in effect: *Fuck off, you narcissist, you are so self-centred and self-important. You have put yourself up on a pedestal and you reach down to me with an outstretched hand to haul me up to your level. Big deal. Are you really and truly so much above me to start with? How can we have an "alliance" if we come from such different starting points?*

It is something I have heard from the mouths of clients who are not White, not middle-class, and not straight. But I have also heard it from the mainstream as well, and particularly from men. My imagined protest speech could be what a lot of male clients want to say and, even if I am only partially correct in this, we should be very cautious at dismissing those male traits that have been researched: the reluctance to admit that something is wrong (and this pertains to physical illness as well as psychological distress); the emphasis on quick solutions; the lack of emotional expressiveness and communicativeness. My experience, and that of others who work with men with whom I am in contact, is leading me to wonder if we have maybe underestimated men as a group when it comes to analysis and psychotherapy. Hence, holding working with men in mind, there may be a need to consider the notion that the existence of democratic art might breathe life into the hope for a democratic therapy.

Concluding Thoughts

Over the past 15 years, I have built an international practice as a political con-
sultant working with leading politicians (including during presidential or general elections), with their advisers and parties, and with activist groups. What
I have written here is grounded in these experiences. In particular, I seem to have
gravitated to work in the general area of nationalism, national identity, and nation
building—in South Africa, Brazil, Poland, and Russia (see also Samuels, 2001,
pp. 186–194).

I am not saying that every client should become an activist, only that failure
to recognize the political dimensions of personal growth is not helpful to our clients. Nor am I proposing unlimited and unending exercise of social responsibility.
There are limits to individual responsibility, and we need space to reflect upon *not*
making a difference.

What, then, is the scope of our individual responsibility for others and for the
world? What are its moral and ethical bounds? The roots of the word *responsibility* lie in *spondere*, to promise or pledge, but what happens if we promise too
much? In politics—and, I suppose, in life—there is a problem of people being too
demanding of themselves. If we cannot live up to these demands, our idealism and
energy go underground and are self-supressed. "Activist client" burnout?

Let us think about how an exaggeration and idealization of political energy and
idealism affects *Tikkun Olam*. This is, as I see it, a necessary balancing and cautionary note on which to end the chapter. If one tries to do *Tikkun* from too perfect
a self-state, it won't work, because the only possible way to approach and engage
with a broken and fractured world of which one is a part is, surely, as a broken and
fractured, stunted individual: an individual with death in mind: the "good-enough
activist." Hence, failure to make a difference in the world to the extent one had
hoped becomes something to explore in therapy, something much less shameful
so that one becomes less self-denigrating. It becomes okay to fail in politics. This
is important because shame at failure is what leads to depression and guilt and
so destroys the impulse and the capacity for action. Activists in particular need a
different attitude to their failures, particularly the failure of their political hopes,
aspirations, and projects.

References

Bohart, A., and Tallman, K. (1999). Empathy and the active client: An integrative, cog-
nitive-experiential approach. In A. Bohart and L. Greenberg (Eds.), *Empathy Recon-
sidered: New Directions in Psychotherapy,* pp. 393–415. Washington, DC: American
Psychological Association.
Camus, A. (1953). *The Rebel.* J. Laredo (Trans.). London: Hamish Hamilton. (Original
work published 1951)
Cook, J. (2013). *Ice Age Art: Arrival of the Modern Mind.* London: British Museum
Publications.

Corpt, E. (2013). Peasant in the analyst's chair: Reflections, personal and otherwise, on class and the forming of an analytic identity. *International Journal of Psychoanalytic Self Psychology*, 8(1), 52–69.

Frank, J. (1961). *Persuasion and Healing*. New York: Basic Books.

Hoffman, I. (2006). The myths of free association and the potentials of the analytical relationship. *International Journal of Psychoanalysis*, 87, 43–61.

Jung, C. G. (1946). *The Psychology of the Transference. Collected Works,* Vol. 16. London: Routledge and Kegan Paul.

Layton, L. (2004). "A fork in the royal road: On defining the unconscious and its stakes for social theory." Psychoanalysis. *Class and Society*, 9(1), 33–51.

Lowenthal, D. (Ed.). (2015). *Critical Psychotherapy, Psychoanalysis and Counselling: Implications for Practice*. London: Palgrave Macmillan.

Mitchell, S. (1997). *Influence and Autonomy in Psychoanalysis*. Hillsdale, NJ: The Analytic Press.

Mitchell, S. (2000). Response to commentaries. *Psychoanalytic Dialogues*, 10, 505–507.

Norcross, J. (2011). *Psychotherapy Relationships that Work*. Oxford, UK: Oxford University Press.

Orwell, G. (2013). *1984*. Harmondsworth, UK: Penguin. (Original work published 1949)

Piketty, T. (2014). *Capital in the Twenty-first Century*. Cambridge, MA: Belknap Press.

Rogers, C. (1951). *Client-centered Therapy*. Cambridge, MA: Riverside.

Samuels, A. (1985). *Jung and the Post-Jungians*. London: Routledge and Kegan Paul.

Samuels, A. (1989). *The Plural Psyche: Personality, Morality and the Father*. London: Routledge.

Samuels, A. (1993). *The Political Psyche*. London: Routledge.

Samuels, A. (2000). Post-Jungian dialogues. *Psychoanalytic Dialogues*, 10, 403–426.

Samuels, A. (2001). *Politics on the Couch: Citizenship and the Internal Life*. London: Karnac.

Samuels, A. (2002). The hidden politics of healing: Foreign dimensions of domestic practice. *American Imago: Studies in Psychoanalysis and Culture*, 59, 459–482.

Samuels, A. (2006). Working directly with political, social and cultural material in the therapy session. In L. Layton, N. C. Hollander, and S. Gutwill (Eds.), *Psychoanalysis, Class and Politics: Encounters in the Clinical Setting*, pp. 11–28. London: Routledge.

Samuels, A. (2014a). Economics, psychotherapy, politics. *International Review of Sociology*, 24(1), 77–90.

Samuels, A. (2014b). Shadows of the therapy relationship. In D. Lowenthal and A. Samuels (Eds.), *Relational Psychotherapy, Psychoanalysis and Counselling*, pp. 184–192. London: Routledge.

Samuels, A. (2015a). Everything you always wanted to know about therapy (but were afraid to ask): Fragments of a critical psychotherapy. In D. Lowenthal (Ed.), *Critical Psychotherapy, Psychoanalysis and Counselling: Implications for Practice*, pp. 159–174. London: Palgrave Macmillan.

Samuels, A. (2015b). *A New Therapy for Politics?* London: Karnac.

Searles, H. (1975). The patient as therapist to his analyst. In P. Giovacchini (Ed.), *Tactics and Techniques in Psychoanalytic Therapy*, Vol. II, pp. 95–151. New York: Aronson.

Stern, D. (2010). *Forms of Vitality*. Oxford, UK: Oxford University Press.

Willett, J. (1964). *The Theatre of Bertolt Brecht*. London: Shenval Press. (Original work published 1959)

Chapter 13

Pia Skogemann

When I was teenager and young in the 60s, I was heavily drawn to mysteries. Ancient civilizations and how they were, how they built the pyramids, and the wonder of the grave of Tutankhamun, how the world came to be, how humans evolved, astrology, tarot cards, I Ching, theosophy, anthroposophy, parapsychology, psychology, you name it, loads of books, but what should I become myself, maybe a painter? When old enough to go to university, I studied anthropology and prehistoric archaeology, but that wasn't really it. There was no mystery.

I didn't know what I was searching for, until one day I read an chapter about what qualities an analyst should have. I hadn't known before that it was something one could be without being a psychiatrist, but as a breathtaking revelation, I knew the description pointed straight at me like an arrow. I took a decision on the spot—I would end my university studies with a BA and get a job, because I could see that going into analysis would cost money. And that was a central part of becoming an analyst, I read.

I was always thinking that I would contact the author of the chapter in due time, but then fate interfered. At a summer course in a place I liked to come to because it dealt with all kinds of alternative things, I confessed my plans to some ladies there, who whispered to the headmaster of the school and he called me in to his office. "There is one Jungian analyst in Denmark. You should go to him." Jung! I had read the bits of Jung which were translated into Danish and had felt it was a fountain of wisdom. Was that really something one could get access to? I immediately failed the author of my initial revelation. To this day I cannot remember her name.

So I took my BA and I got a job and then I kind of waited . . . until I dreamt that I was looking out of my window, and out there was an access to another world, and it was receding, so I had to hurry to get in there. I ran down and entered that world, where one had to endure trials and overcome challenges, and I succeeded, and then I was walking back home over a bridge. A couple of large strange beings were following me from behind, and I realized that they were much stronger than I was, and if they had wanted it, they could have destroyed me. Then I heard them laughing over me among themselves and the one said to the other: "but she is just a beginner."

I mustered all my courage and called the analyst. "I would like to become an analyst," I said. "It's not something you can become just like that," the analyst answered. But he gave me an appointment.

DOI: 10.4324/9781003148968-14

That was the beginning, almost half a hundred years ago. I was 22.

As the years went on, I enjoyed my journey and I suffered for my mistakes. There were emotional ups and downs, a lot of drivenness to create and achieve this and that, intellectual and organizationally, but at the same time, for 42 years now my analytical practice was always the stable centre, of course changing over time, but always as a source of curiosity, wonder, and satisfaction.

Now, as I have turned 70, the waves have settled, and the sea is quiet. I am not full of big dreams anymore. Many of those grandiose phantasies and images from my younger years were birthed into reality, so how can one not be satisfied?

An image from the end of Tolkien's *The Lord of the Rings* comes to my mind. After the many pages of dramatic, frightful and wondrous events happening to our friends the hobbits, they return to their homeland. One morning they must go to the shores of the sea to say goodbye to their friends—Gandalf the Wizard, Galadriel the Elven queen and other high Elves who now sail away to the island of the immortal. So magic and wizardry leaves their world forever, but it has touched them and enlarged their world greatly, and changed them and left its mark on them, and is never to be forgotten.

The Daughter Archetype

Originally published in Montreal 2010. Proceedings of the XVIIIth Congress of the International Association for Analytical Psychology. Reprinted with permission.

The Daughter Archetype

I will present my concept of "the daughter archetype" and its implications for the gender discussion in analytical psychology. It was first introduced in Danish (Skogemann, 1984). While pondering on similar critiques and questions as many other female analysts in my generation have done, I have chosen another course than they have. I define the daughter archetype as a basic concept for the woman as a subject for herself, a concept for female agency that otherwise is lacking in analytical psychology. The name of the term is also chosen to differentiate it from the mother archetype. The phenomenology of the daughter archetype is represented at all levels of psychic functioning. The images range from ego-representations to goddess-like Self representations. The notion of the daughter archetype addresses the female psyche but does not define the feminine as such.

Everyday Level

By this I mean the socially recognized gender roles for young women, whose symbolic dimensions are not visible before they are looked at critically and are loosened from their absoluteness in traditional cultures. On the individual level they are often identified equally with the persona or with the projections of the anima from men. With greater social freedom in their upbringing, young women have multiple choices for their style of life, their education and profession, and their relations with other women and with men. This makes a great difference from the lack of freedom of choice of earlier generations.

Developmental Level

In the normal development of girls one can see the imagery of the daughter archetype unfolding in the plays, dreams and heroines which small girls may indulge in—from having the early pink princess fantasy to playing with Barbie dolls or listening to the story of the Swedish Pippi Longstocking. In the analysis of adults, images of the daughter archetype will often mediate aspects of the Self which should be made conscious and integrated in the female personality to serve the female individuation process. Insofar as they would tend to support the differentiation from both traditional gender roles and from identification with the anima projections from men, they support the development of ego consciousness and its growing autonomy. The differentiation between the mother archetype and the daughter archetype is very important for women, just as the differentiation of the anima from the mother archetype is for men.

The Archetypal Level

The daughter archetype is richly represented in the history of symbols as in mythology and fairy tales. Jung himself discusses one version of the archetypal daughter in his chapter "The Psychological Aspects of the Kore." Jung states that the figure of Kore belongs to the anima archetype when observed in a man and in a woman to the supraordinate personality—meaning the archetype of the Self (Jung, 1959a, para. 310). The passive, abducted Kore type, however, corresponds to a conservative gender role and/or, in my view, a poorly developed ego. In the Greek myth, the entire feminine agency is held by the mother goddess, Demeter.

The Gendered Concepts in Analytical Psychology

My notion of the daughter archetype does not question our basic concepts, but it does question the use of binary-gendered properties as a metaphorical common denominator in the following four theoretical couples:

1. Anima and animus
2. The feeling and thinking function in the psychological typology
3. Eros and Logos
4. Matriarchal and patriarchal consciousness

I see anima and animus as basically clinical tools. They refer to unconscious phenomenology, as it appears in dreams and projections, while the feeling and thinking function refers to the way the conscious mind works. It is true that a feeling-type woman often will have an animus that could be associated with thinking, but for a thinking-type woman the reverse will probably be true. In dreams I found the archetype appearing in adult women's dreams and fantasies in a way which I believe is similar to those making other analysts speak of the anima in women. However, I prefer to keep the terms anima and animus, but reserving the term anima for male fantasies about women and the feminine and animus for female fantasies about men and the masculine. Jung formulated the concept of Eros as psychic relatedness and that of Logos as objective interest (Jung, 1964, para. 255), but he nevertheless thought that woman's psychology was founded on the first and men's on the second.

This made him identify anima with Eros and animus with Logos (Jung, 1959b, para. 33) and so collapse the first three concepts into gender stereotypes. Eric Neumann's quite popular notion of matriarchal versus patriarchal consciousness implied the idea that the ego is masculine in both sexes. I find it unacceptable as a woman to think of my normal mental functions as masculine. Furthermore, Neumann's ideas of the historical development of consciousness (1954) are based on outdated archaeological and historical theories and findings.

Inanna

A presentation of the Sumerian goddess Inanna will serve as an illustration of a very different archetypal daughter-figure. Her title in the Sumerian-Akkadian era actually was "daughter of the gods." (Ishtar was her Akkadian name.) She alone among the many Sumerian gods had no divine spouse, but she was for maybe 2000 years the divine maiden, though certainly not in the virginal sense. (Actually, the Sumeric language had no word for virgin.) Only later, in the Babylonian era, was she transformed into a mother goddess. My work on Inanna (Brøgger & Skogemann, 2007) is based on the Electronic Text Corpus of Sumerian Literature (ETCS), an internet-based project of Oxford University with the latest scientific translations of about 400 Sumerian texts, among them quite a lot about Inanna. Very few people in this world are specialists in reading and understanding Sumerian clay tablets, and discoveries of new fragments have often altered older translations of a text considerably. Inanna was the daughter of the Moon god Nanna and the Moon goddess Ningal, and she was sister to the Sun god Utu. She herself in her celestial aspect was Venus. From Venus she borrowed her ever-changing nature; the horn she is associated with does not originate from the Moon, but from the sickle of Venus. Like the Moon, Venus has phases. When Venus is closest to Earth the sickle looks like the new moon, but the light is many times stronger than when Venus is full and farther away. During this conjunction Venus changes from evening to morning star, separated by few days' absence from the sky.

This is probably the astronomical background of the myth of Inanna's descent to the Underworld. Many of Inanna's attributes were such as we traditionally ascribe to men or to the masculine—she was aggressive, ambitious, assertive, autonomous and authoritative—but she was always attractive and seen as the essence of femininity, since she was the goddess of love and sexuality. Inanna is the main figure in many love songs, with Dumuzi the Shepherd (sometimes identified with the priest-king of Uruk) as her chosen spouse. Interestingly, according to Leick (1994), in the ancient Sumerian world "the phallus represented fertility [and] the vulva represented sexual potency" (p. 96), just the opposite of what we are accustomed to. Her lush gardens were a sophisticated meeting place for lovers. The garden's flowers and vegetables are often used as metaphors for the sexual organs and the erotic play itself, which is a very sophisticated thing compared with so-called primitive fertility rites. She was sexually broadminded, too: prostitutes, homosexuals, hermaphrodites and transsexuals were under her protection. Her power of creativity showed especially in all things belonging to a civilization: language, music and the song of power, in all sophisticated handcraft—and in the art of love. She was also goddess of war. She would rage wildly, if offended, and lead the battle against her enemies like a fire-spouting dragon or a wild leopard, and she would lead the king in battle and bring victory to her favourites. Her lust for expanding her power-domains was without boundaries, and as one can see in her myths, she often succeeded. When she travelled to the Underworld, it was with the intention of taking the throne of the Underworld from the goddess Ereshkigal in addition to her domains in Heaven and on Earth. But there she finally met her limit.

Madonna

I would like to amplify the archetypal imagery with an example of a modern superstar, the American Madonna, who has staged herself in an Inanna-like way, with a typical mixture of sexual and spiritual elements.

In her stage shows Madonna typically sets herself up as a fierce and aggressive dominatrix, and she often uses attributes from strip tease shows. She appeared as a sexual icon—in a book she produced herself—and repeatedly reinvented her persona. My research brought me to her biography entitled *Madonna, Queen of the World* (Thompson, 2002), very similar to one of Inanna's official titles "Queen of Heaven and Earth." Madonna's crave for fame seems to match Inanna's ever-expanding lust for power. My point here is that while these images are carrying the notion of female agency to the extreme on the grandiose side it makes no sense to term it masculine or delegate the ambition and aggression to some animus figure.

Enheduanna

We are in a position to come closer to a real woman who worshipped Inanna—as another example of female agency. A striking text called the Exaltation of Inanna

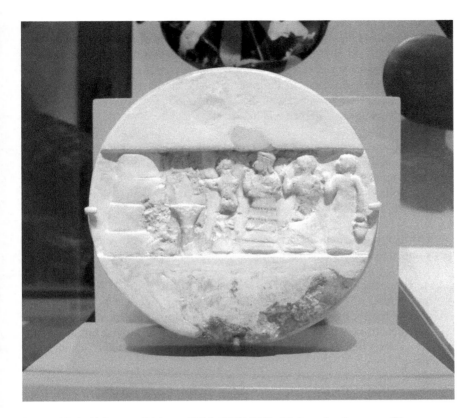

Figure 13.1 Alabaster Disk ca. 2300–2275 BCE, 25.6 cm in diameter. The reverse
side of the disk bears a cuneiform inscription that identifies Enheduanna. It reads: "Enheduanna, zirru-priestess, wife of the god Nanna,
daughter of Sargon, king of the world, in the temple of the goddess
Innana."

is authored by Enheduanna who served at the Moon god Nanna's temple in Ur
about 2250 BC. It is possible to date this text quite precisely because the narrative in the hymn describes a historical event, namely the rebellion against king
Naram-Sin led by a smaller king Lugal-Ane from Uruk.

Enheduanna's own historical existence is by chance also well documented, as
a relief alabaster stone was found in the ruins of the temple in Ur with her image
and a text identifying her as high priestess, wife of Nanna and daughter of King
Sargon, and the declaration that she made this stone as a throne for An (the god of
Heaven) in Inanna's temple in Ur—that is she had a temple for Inanna established
inside Nanna's territory. King Sargon the Great had conquered and united all the

Sumerian and Akkadian city-states a few decades earlier and made Inanna a goddess reigning over the whole empire.

Enheduanna is the earliest known example in history of an individual describing her inner mind and at the same time her Goddess-Self. Enheduanna is not praying for motherly protection or comfort, but is conjuring the daughterly goddess to take violent action. In the first 65 lines, the fiercest, most warrior-like aspects of Inanna are conjured with the aim of waking her up.

Enheduanna presents herself and her case:

> I, En-ḥedu-ana the en priestess, entered my holy ĝipar in your service. I carried the ritual basket, and intoned the song of joy. But {funeral offerings were} brought, as if I had never lived there . . . My honeyed mouth became scum. My ability to soothe moods vanished . . . I, En-ḥedu-ana, will recite a prayer to you. To you, holy Inana, I shall give free vent to my tears like sweet beer!

Enheduanna goes on to describe her complaint—how Lugal-Ane had destroyed An's sanctuary:

> In connection with the purification rites of holy An, Lugal-Ane has altered everything of his, and has stripped An of the E-ana. He has not stood in awe of the greatest deity. He has turned that temple, whose attractions were inexhaustible, whose beauty was endless, into a destroyed temple. While he entered before me as if he was a partner, really he approached out of envy.

Enheduanna further complains that Nanna—who should have been her primal divine protector—did not take care of her because Lugal-Ane had driven herself out of office and into exile:

> My good divine wild cow, drive out the man, capture the man! In the place of divine encouragement, what is my standing now? . . . My Nanna has {paid no heed to me} . . . He [Lugal-Ane] stood there in triumph and drove me out of the temple. He made me fly like a swallow from the window; I have exhausted my life-strength. He made me walk through the thorn bushes of the mountains. He stripped me of the rightful {crown} of the en priestess.

The Exaltation of Inanna

Enheduanna wants Inanna's help to change this situation. According to Zgoll (1997 p. 164), it was a completely new idea that a human being could appeal to a god in this way, and to have faith and hope against all hope. Traditionally, because Nanna had given victory to Lugal-Ane, that would have been the end of the story. But Enheduanna believes that Inanna has a higher power which she shares with

An and therefore can change fate. To ensure her assistance Enheduanna exalts Inanna above all other divinities in the next section:

> It must be known! . . . Be it known that you are lofty as the heavens! Be it known that you are broad as the earth! Be it known that you destroy the rebel lands! Be it known that you roar at the foreign lands! Be it known that you crush heads! Be it known that you devour corpses like a dog! Be it known that your gaze is terrible! Be it known that you lift your terrible gaze! Be it known that you have flashing eyes! Be it known that you are unshakeable and unyielding! Be it known that you always stand triumphant!

The Outcome

The cultic climax of the hymn takes place at midnight, when Enheduanna heaps up the coals and makes her rites to receive the Goddess or psychologically her transcendent Self. (The E-ešdam-kug shrine was a temple in the city-state Lagash, where Enheduanna probably took exile.) Out of this temporary merge between the two, the hymn was born with the cultic power to create what it named, that is, it influenced reality:

> I have heaped up the coals in the censer and prepared the purification rites. The E-ešdam-kug shrine awaits you. Might your heart not be appeased towards me? Since it was full, too full for me, great exalted lady; I have recited this song for you.

This hymn is strongly personal, indeed, but though the form is that of an intimate contact between the priestess and her goddess, it is anything but private—it is explicitly intended by Enheduanna to be sung in the temple the next day: May a singer repeat to you at noon that which was recited to you at dead of night.

This constitutes what R. J. Stark (2008) called a mystical enthymeme which involves an author, an audience and a cosmic source—in this case, Inanna herself.

Only at the very end of the hymn do we meet Inanna in her full loveliness as Venus in the sky:

> The light was sweet for her, delight extended over her; she was full of fairest beauty. Like the light of the rising moon, she exuded delight. Nanna came out to gaze at her properly and her mother Ningal blessed her.

According to Zgoll (1997, p. 158), the Sumerians believed that Enheduanna's address was effective in engaging Inanna and changing the will of the gods because king Naram-Sim managed to strike down the rebellion, and Enheduanna could return to her temple in Ur.

As far as it is possible to evaluate such a thing bridging a historical distance of more than 4000 years, it seems that Enheduanna, at the time a mature, experienced woman, used her feminine agency with integrity, sophistication and courage in order to serve her goddess in a new era.

Conclusion

I have tried to show that the notion of the daughter archetype is not limited to the postmodern gender discussion as it is also represented in ancient times in ways that transcend the classical binary way of defining feminine and masculine properties.

References

Brøgger, S., and Skogemann, P. (2007). *Inanna, Himlens og jordens dronning*. Copenhagen: Athene.

Jung, C. G. (1959a). The archetypes and the collective unconscious. *CW* 9i

Jung, C. G. (1959b). Aion. *CW* 9ii.

Jung, C. G. (1964). Civilization in transition. *CW* 10.

Leick, G. (1994). *Sex & Eroticism in Mesopotamian Literature*. London and New York: Routledge.

Neuman, E. (1954). *The Origins and History of Consciousness*. London: Routledge and Kegan Paul.

Skogemann, P. (1984). *Kvindelighed i vækst*. Copenhagen: Lindhardt og Ringhof.

Stark, Ryan J. (2008). Some aspects of Christian mystical rhetoric, philosophy, and poetry. *Philosophy and Rhetoric*, 41(3), 260–277.

The Electronic Text Corpus of the Sumerian Literature (ETCS). http://etcsl.orinst.ox.ac.uk/

Thompson, D. (2002). *Madonna, Queen of the World*. London: John Blake Publishing Ltd.

Zgoll, A. (1997). *Der Rechtsfall der En-hedu-Ana im Lied Nin-me-sara*. Münster: Ugarit-Verlag. [An English version of Zgoll's translation of the Exaltation of Inanna is included in the ETCS.]

Chapter 14

Ursula Wirtz

Born in 1946 in the Ruhr District of postwar Germany, I grew up immersed in the wartime narratives of carpet-bombings, homes engulfed in flames, ordinary people consumed by fear and hunger, and the mob fury of the Kristallnacht. My playgrounds were landscapes of rubble. The theme of violence in war and peace gave direction to my life and research into the roots of war and terror.

I understand my profession not only as a concern for individual transformation. I am also convinced that as a therapist I can contribute to a collective political, economic and social individuation. It is important for me to work on myself, expand my own consciousness, but also to contribute to the humanization of our society, to tend to the collective soul and at the same time to cultivate a responsible, committed living in solidarity.

My social, political and therapeutic engagement for justice, my caring for people who suffered from the atrocities of violence and torture led me to work as a Jungian psychotraumatologist and a clinical and anthropological psychologist in countries that have been subjected to collective trauma. I have ridden in a tank through the war-devastated cities of the former Yugoslavia, lived with female survivors of mass rapes, and worked in women's shelters and counselling centres for survivors of the Holocaust and other victims of torture. The Greek wisdom *Pathei manthanein*—learning through suffering—has guided me in these wastelands of the soul. I have deeply experienced human vulnerability and human dignity in the face of trauma and life's precariousness, as much as its beauty and preciousness.

Perhaps my birth into the house of Hades initiated me into the mystery of dying and becoming: The narrative myth is that my aging father, as he stroked my mother's heavily pregnant belly, welcoming me into life, was also in deep agony, realizing that he would never see me because he could already hear the flapping wings of his own death. He died shortly before I was born, while my mother had not yet overcome her grief and mourning of their baby boy, who had died the year before. I grew up with mother, grandmother and aunt—a very strong feminine foundation.

The paradox of the grim and yet consoling law of enantiodromia, that nothing stays the way it is, imprinted me from early on, leading me first to study philosophy and literature. In poetry and music I found access to the unspeakable in me.

DOI: 10.4324/9781003148968-15

Bach's beautiful cello sonatas, played soulfully by my beloved partner like a daily morning prayer, remain for me an infinite source of joy. The mystery of life's vicissitudes has awakened in me the "courage to be" and the respect for life as a treasure to be guarded. I love the sea and the silence of the desert; among my passions are sailing in the Mediterranean and riding horses and camels.

It was Franz Kafka who opened the door for me to Jungian psychology. I was 19 years old, writing my first seminar chapter, "Dream, Fairytale and Reality in Kafka's Short Stories." The dreamlike quality of "The Country Doctor" as well as the general atmosphere of liminality, ambiguity and paradox in all of his work enthralled me. Later I learnt about paradox as the wisdom of the spirit of the depths, and in my Zen practice I wrestled with the paradoxes of the koans. Ultimately it was my analysis and training at the C. G. Jung Institute Küsnacht that initiated me into Zen Buddhism, my second "home." Meditation deepened my analytical approach of being and doing, loving presence and critical reflection. It also assisted in the unfolding of consciousness and cleansing the doors of perception, my opening *to see things as they are—infinite* (William Blake). A connection with the transcendent dimension and analytical psychology's hermeneutics of hope has supported all of my work and helped me when confronted with questions of whence, whither, why.

In the process of aging and hopefully sage-ing, I trust in a relational mode of being that assists in the unfolding of our intrinsic capacities for love and wisdom, the logic of the heart, complementing the logic of the mind. Maybe this feminine way of being fosters a greater patience and compassionate awareness toward all that is left unresolved in myself and the world.

Traumatic Experiences and Transformation of Consciousness

Originally published in (German) "Traumatische erfahrungen und Bewusstseinstransformation. In: Spiritualität und spirituelle Krisen". Hsg. von L.Hofmann und Patrizia Heise, 2017 Schattauer Verlag, Stuttgart, S. 244-254. Reprinted with permission.

My therapeutic experiences with severely traumatized people have sensitized me to view extremely traumatizing conditions in the context of the development of new structures of consciousness. I have often observed that chaotic processes of great emotional distress can initiate painful processes of change and open a door to deeper spaces of consciousness that were previously inaccessible. In this chapter, my aim is to develop a greater openness to these phenomena of mental change and maturation in the context of traumatic shocks, in order to be able to accompany such transformations of consciousness empathically. I refer to interdisciplinary scientific research results on systemic changes and insights of wisdom traditions in dealing with suffering.

1.1 Conceptualization of Trauma

Trauma research is booming—this has led not only to a boom and an inflationary use of the concept of trauma, but also to a flood of different trauma theories and trauma constructs that have been instrumentalized both by the clinical mainstream and in the socio-political field and abused in humanities discourses (Weilnböck, 2001). David Becker has castigated this fashionable trend of trauma discourse as a "trauma business" and has even spoken of the "invention of trauma" (Becker, 2001, 2006).

Becker distinguishes three different concepts:

1. trauma as a medical, dehistoricizing concept: the complex post-traumatic stress disorder (PTSD) or disorders of extreme stress not otherwise specified (DESNOS)
2. trauma as psychological event and intrapsychic process; focus on the subjective experience of the trauma
3. trauma as a social and political process; focus on the socially relevant dimension of trauma
   I would like to propose a fourth conceptualization of trauma:
4. trauma as a transformative process of consciousness

The themes of truth, justice and reconciliation that emerge in every trauma therapy are not for me—as with Becker—located solely in the socio-political realm; I regard these questions as belonging to the spiritual dimension with its identity-forming horizon of meaning and values. In my understanding, disruptive traumatic life-events constellate an examination of spirituality, of existential questions that revolve around the loss of faith, love and hope.

In trauma the body-soul unity breaks apart; contact with body, earth and reality is lost; and the question arises in a painfully radical and unconditional way—who am I when I have lost my identity? The ego-death is like a symbolic dying and raises questions about insight and self-reflection, questions about the nature of consciousness and how the transformation of consciousness can occur.

Findings from neuroscience and modern brain research help us to better understand the profound changes in consciousness after trauma. What consciousness is, however, eludes a strict definition, because we are both the subject and the object of our investigations and circularity is inseparable from all thinking about consciousness.

1.2 Transformation of Consciousness

Per aspera ad astra—Through adversity to the stars
Through the dark to the light

Traumas are borderline experiences that influence the way inner and outer reality is perceived, that is, traumatic experiences shape our structure of consciousness.

Trauma changes the state of consciousness in many different ways, be it through numbness and constriction or through flooding and intrusion. However, not only dissociative changes in consciousness can be observed, a tunnel vision in self- and external perception, but also *achievements of overcoming* (*Überwindungsleistungen*; Petzold et al., 2002) and *non-linear developmental dynamics*. Survivors also have the ability to develop more integral perspectives on life, even in its traumatic dimensions, which become more comprehensible against the background of the theories of emergence and complexity.

Dealing with the trauma of experienced violence, the subjective perception, processing and integration into the totality of life remains a lifelong mind-altering task. Our consciousness is capable of learning, has the character of a process and reorganizes itself again and again.

Mental maturation, the process of becoming better able to cope with life and with death, is a form of unfolding of our consciousness, often initiated by the traumatic experience of our own nothingness, the insubstantiality of the personal ego and the disappearance of the subject boundaries between me and the world. In the various wisdom traditions, insight into the relativity of ego, space and time takes place through a regimen of spiritual practice. Traumatic experiences, on the other hand, thrust a person completely unprepared into such a space of consciousness, which is experienced as numinous, as terrible and incomprehensible, a *mysterium tremendum*, beyond language, space and time.

In this space the illusionary character of our experiences of ego, self and world is revealed, the dualistic world view is shattered. With the awareness of another dimension of reality, which also encompasses the transpersonal space, a leap in consciousness takes place, which affects all functions of consciousness, perception, thinking, feeling and intentional action.

Consciousness has the character of a process, is changeable and describes the totality of all experiences and states that can be experienced by a person and make him or her aware of their own identity. Reflection about oneself and the world is consciousness, that is, knowledge about one's own being.

The ability to think, to behave flexibly and adaptively and to create meaning is considered a fundamental function of consciousness. This dimension of consciousness and the human ability to transcend conscious boundaries is also effective in processing traumatic experiences.

> The only way to live a life worth living is to give it an inner meaning. And the only way to give it a meaning is to recognize and transform our spirit in order to contribute to the inner peace of everyone.
>
> (Revel and Ricard, 2003, p. 381f)

The question of the possibilities of coping with the unmanageable, of the dignity of the human despite the degradation caused by the inhumane, has occupied me with especial urgency. My approach to the transformative, mind-altering potency of trauma does not mean a denial of the destructive dimension of traumatic experience on the psyche, nor a naïve, unscientific spiritualization of clinical practice. For over 30 years I have gathered painful, intimate and enriching experiences in accompanying and supervising trauma survivors of other cultures as well, of torture survivors and refugees, displaced and sexually exploited people, Holocaust survivors and extremely traumatized men, women and children from the war in former Yugoslavia.

I am aware that quantum leaps of consciousness after traumatic experiences are context-dependent and vary according to the vulnerabilities, resources and resiliencies of those affected.

1.3 Traumatic Experience

My synopsis of traumas and changes in consciousness does not deny that traumatic experiences, especially extreme traumatization through violence, are borderline experiences of unspeakable suffering, which can overrun a person's self-protection system and individual coping mechanisms, shatter the cosmos of meaning and values and break down the psychological structure.

Traumatic experiences and crises are processes that extremely destabilize the mental system and affect all pillars of identity. The basic feeling prevails as if the whole identity were built on sand without a supporting foundation. The adaptive and integrative functions of the ego can also fail completely in the face of traumatic events that present an overwhelming threat.

The *processes of destructuring* as a possible consequence of traumatic experience make any adherence to rigid ego structures impossible and no longer allow us to cling to the old constructs of ego, self and world.

However, this state of complete destabilization and instability can be a preliminary stage to self-distance and new self-organization at a higher functional level.

Sometimes the wound, if it seems to rend body and soul, can cause the dissolution of world and ego, the emergence of the black hole of non-being, a form of death consciousness. Life then suddenly appears as a "being in death," a "dying before dying," as described in the mystical traditions.

When the familiar patterns of thought and perception dissolve in the traumatic event and we are confronted with the mystery of life and death, with total chaos and existential uncertainty, this can be experienced as a profound spiritual crisis, as a "dark night of the soul," as a loss of soul or "soul murder" (Wirtz, 1989), because in borderline situations of suffering and pain our deepest vulnerability becomes apparent, our being inescapably abandoned and at the mercy of fate.

The impossibility to communicate the extent of suffering in extreme traumatizations often leads to frightening feelings of uprootedness and alienation, which are described as a death experience, a death "that has eaten its way into life" (Le Breton, 2003, p. 38).

In this process of destructuring, the chimera of the ego evaporates and the insubstantiality of the everyday ego is revealed. This rupture in the mental order can lead to a loss of personal identity and continuity. Traumatized people then feel as if they have fallen out of the stream of time and have strayed from the course of life.

Traumas and their social destruction processes can not only shatter the primal trust in oneself and in the reliability of human bonds, but also the ability to symbolize what has been experienced often eludes linguistic expression and banishes the damaged and the silenced to a world distant from humanity. Having fallen out of the security of existence, the feelings of *disintegration* and *depersonalization* and the collapsed self-confidence and trust in the world can cause a profound *disturbance of consciousness*.

But such painful experiences of a disordered inner and outer reality can also lead to a radically new insight into the essence of reality, an inkling of what lies beyond our familiar boundaries of consciousness and has to do with wisdom-related knowledge.

As threshold experiences, traumatic shock experiences can, like an initiation, open the spiritual realm and enable an apprehension of reality that shatters the ego-perspective and perceives the meaning of the whole. Traumatized people then awaken to a consciousness of interdependence, the ultimate connection of everything with everything, a deeply spiritual experience.

I believe it is important to have a *complementary approach to the trauma sequelae*, a perspective that differs from current pathology and deficit-oriented concepts of understanding trauma and focuses on changing consciousness through expansion and opening. In my book *Trauma and Beyond. The Mystery of Transformation* (Wirtz, 2014, 2020) I refer to the potential for change inherent in extreme borderline states of desubjectivation through violence, to the *transformational power of suffering* that can become a catalyst for a reorientation in life, a breakthrough and emergence after complete collapse to new ways of seeing and being with expanded possibilities of creating and processing meaning. *Pathei manthanein*, learning through suffering, is the Greek expression, and the symbolic systems of our myths, fairy tales and religions also illustrate processes of suffering such as dismemberment, being torn apart, death and resurrection—processes in which consciousness expands instead of contracting.

Not every traumatized person experiences a revelation of the light in the darkness as Job did after his overcoming of the dark night; nor does contact with the deep always lead to a deepening of the personality; and yet destruction can have a transformative energy, as our myths testify. One of the most familiar mythological images for a possible renewal process is the phoenix, the bird that burns at the stake and transforms from the ashes to rise again into the air. "Phoenix" is therefore also the hopeful name of the discussion forum and information newsletter for the Network Spiritual Development and Crisis Accompaniment (SEN) in Germany.

1.4 The Transformative Power of Suffering

> "But where there is danger, salvation also grows."
>
> (Hölderlin, Patmos)

Ripped-open wounds demand our attention, the pain rouses us and, after thawing us out of rigor mortis, makes us aware of ourselves in a new way. In his treatise on the metaphysics of pain, the sociologist Le Breton has understood the examination of pain as a key that ultimately anchors the awareness of the value of life in us.

> Pain is sacred and wild at the same time. Why holy? By forcing man to experience his own transcendence in himself, he projects it outside of himself, reveals to him inner powers of which he had no idea. And wild he is, because he does this by bursting open the identity of the individual . . . It is up to the person to decide whether he perceives his suffering as a misfortune in which he loses himself, or at least his dignity, completely, or whether he sees it as an opportunity that allows him to experience a new dimension: that of a person who has suffered or who is still suffering, but who sees the world with open eyes.
>
> (Le Breton, 2003, 251f)

Traumatized people who have gone through suffering have been able to integrate their experiences into their life continuum and have reassembled themselves from the fragments, see the world with more open eyes. They recognize how much our suffering is determined by our spirit, and how a new state of consciousness is created through precise perception and the development of more healing states of mind.

The mystic Meister Eckhart described suffering as a power of destiny that existentially challenges man to accept the present in its Suchness and to relate to it according to the demands of the hour.

The swiftest beast that will bear you to this perfection is suffering.
(Eckhart, 1993, vol. II, pp. 458/459 quote, In Manstetten p. 32)

The sermons of the mystic Johannes Tauler (Tauler, 1979) also describe the mind-altering aspect of crises of meaning, extreme states of fear and emptiness. These mystical experiences of terror and horror, of despair and absolute forlornness in descending to the bottom of the soul, have great similarity with traumatic experiences. But Tauler also refers to the gradual ascent, the path of purification and insight leading to the acceptance of what is, the acceptance of suffering, and the awakening to becoming who you truly are.

A deepened self-reflection about the energy field of meaning and meaninglessness constellated by trauma can become a creative upheaval in the psychic structure, a reconciliation with the fateful brokenness of one's own existence, the inevitability of suffering and evil. Hofmann and Roesler also see existential suffering as a possible passage to spiritual wholeness and a deeper appreciation of life (Hofmann and Roesler, 2010).

1.5 The Paradigm of Posttraumatic Growth

The concept of *post-traumatic growth* (*PTG*) developed by Tedeschi and Calhoun (Tedeschi and Calhoun, 1995) has initiated a paradigm shift in trauma discourse. They describe far-reaching changes in self-image, triggered by the fateful compulsion to transform and refashion oneself and to expand personal competencies: greater self-distance, humour, resilience and, in relationships with others, deepened compassion, tolerance, solidarity and an awareness of the interrelatedness of all that exists. Their research (1996, 2004, 2006) points to the deepening of spiritual insights, a meaning-oriented philosophy of life, coupled with gratitude, appreciation of life and concern for creation. This *resource-oriented concept* has also been critically discussed by Becker under the aspect of denial of reality and naïve wishful thinking (Becker, 2009). Maercker and Zoellner (2004) have attempted a more differentiated criticism that is more consistent with my opinion, which does not fundamentally question the value of the concept but points out its Janus character. In contrast to PTG, Renos Papadopoulos (2007) has developed a concept that emphasizes the dynamics of development in situations of great need, *adversity-activated development* (*AAD*), a positive development that does not necessarily lead to traumatization and that can be observed already in times of peril and not only post-trauma.

Expanding the consciousness of people traumatized by torture and war testifies to the archetypal power of trauma to destroy, but also to ensoul and renew. This polarity is also evident in the naming of crisis states: positive disintegration (Dabrowski, 1964), "creative illness" (Ellenberger, 1970), shamanistic initiation illness (Eliade, 1972), "plus-healing" (Hartmut, 2008) and "blocked transformation" (von Brück, 1996). In the different conceptions an archetypal idea becomes visible that we can grow above resistances and obstacles thanks to our resilience and ability to give meaning, and that the psyche tries to heal the unbearable conflicts in a process of *metanoia* in an autonomous process of self-regulation and self-healing.

Metanoia means a reversal in thinking, feeling and perception, which leads to a changed attitude towards life, a growing beyond a previous level of consciousness. Such dynamic transformation processes can be understood as processes of *energy conversion*. The concept of energy goes back to Greek antiquity; *energeia* describes a psychic dynamic flow energy, which can be assigned to the subtle-energetic field of experience (Berner-Hürbin, 2008). These include subtle processes based on a holistic conception of man and of the world where everything is incessantly in a process of flowing, a process of constant becoming and change. Also in quantum physics, matter and reality are no longer seen as static but as something processual. Reality means potentiality, the greatest possible indeterminacy and openness.

Extreme trauma makes the fluidity of reality painfully experienced. Nothing is as it was before, but psychological destabilization is also subject to the same aspect of the ephemeral. The experience of the impermanence of all that is can turn into a restructuring, a *metamorphosis*, as described by Laing and Foudraine after psychotic episodes. Laing speaks of a

> journey within and a subsequent return (neogenesis) with an enriched and deepened sense of selfhood. One could also call it a process of death and rebirth resulting in reintegration at a higher level.
>
> (Foudraine, 1973, p. 250)

Symbolic crucifixion in suffering and overcoming it can open up a new horizon of meaning and enable greater degrees of freedom in coping with fate. I was personally very touched by how the philosopher Hans-Georg Gadamer, whose life was marked by pain after being afflicted by polio, reflected on how to deal with suffering and pain.

> In this sense, the pain . . . is perhaps the greatest chance to finally "cope" with what we are called to deal with.
>
> (Gadamer, 2003, p. 27)

Borderline experiences of pain and fear break open the shell of the persona, so that everything unimportant is lost. In the nakedness of being mortally wounded, the agonizing questions revolve around life and death, meaning and meaninglessness. In this way, every traumatic borderline experience touches the spiritual dimension of existence and challenges us to search for what holds the world together at its core.

The Hungarian Nobel Prize winner for literature, Imre Kertész, reminded us that even the greatest catastrophes can lead to insights and value orientations that can profoundly transform our consciousness, this fundamental human mode of experience:

> At the bottom of all great realizations, even if they are born of unsurpassed tragedies, there lies the greatest European value of all, the longing for liberty, which suffuses our lives with something more, a richness, making us aware of the positive fact of our existence, and the responsibility we all bear for it.
>
> (Kertész, 2002)

1.6 Transformation of Consciousness in Analytical Psychology

Analytical psychology with its *hermeneutics of hope* is about insight and reconciliation with the basic facts of our existence, that is, accepting the fact of suffering as part of the human condition. The blows of fate and trauma are seen as catalysts for changes in consciousness and personality (Hofmann and Roesler, 2010).

> Without necessity nothing budges, the human personality least of all. It is tremendously conservative, not to say torpid. Only acute necessity is able to rouse it. The developing personality obeys no caprice, no command, no insight, only brute necessity; it needs the motivating force of inner or outer blows of fate.
>
> (Carl Jung, *CW* 17, §295)

Jung is regarded as the forerunner of the psychology of consciousness. For him, self-knowledge is a spiritual obligation, responsible existence is an opening for that which seeks to become conscious, because "man's worst sin is unconsciousness" and "the sole purpose of human existence is to kindle a light in the darkness of mere being" (C. G. Jung, 1989, p. 326).

The individual and collective individuation process is a process of consciousness transformation of all dimensions of our body-soul being in the world and at the same time a spiritual mission in the sense of Rilke: "Desire transformation" ("*Wolle die Wandlung*"; Rilke, XII. Sonette an Orpheus).

Traumatic crises are related to Jung's concept of the "night sea voyage," the descent, the *nekya*, a journey into the dangerous underworld born of necessity, which Jung associated with the workings of the *transcendental function* (*CW* 7, §160). It is the ability effective deep within us, to transcend given states and mental states and often acts as a bridge between two states, that of the "now" and that of the "not yet," thus it has a *telos*, a prospective function. As a structure-changing soul energy it overcomes opposites and knows beyond an either/or paradoxical togetherness.

For Jung the Heraclitan law of *enantiodromia* was groundbreaking, that everything that happens turns into its opposite, that the living becomes dead and the dead becomes living, that destruction and becoming form an indivisible unity or whole. (Jung *CW* 6, §793).

In analytical psychology, the tension of opposites is of great importance. In trauma therapy, this tension is also important to bear until healing symbols from the unconscious spontaneously take over a bridging function to a new state of consciousness. As a relationship symbol, the bridge in a dream or in an imagination refers to the possibility of finding a new way between the conscious and the unconscious, from traumatic imprisonment in a restricted state of being to a new, more open being in the world and a complementary point of view beyond a dualistic mode, where there is no either/or.

C. G. Jung's own traumatic experiences have led to the birth of the Red Book, a testimony to a fundamental change in consciousness and a commitment to the transformative power of the symbolic dimension. At the same time, this shocking document of a traumatic crisis illustrates how dangerous such a descent into the depths of the unconscious is, what hard work on oneself is required for creative self-transcendence after traumatic destabilization.

Traumatic crises and catastrophes are forces of fate, nodal points of transformation and self-transcendence, which can trigger a reversal and a turning towards the transcendental realm, the birth of a new "courage to be" (Mut zum Sein) (Tillich, 1991).

Perhaps this new way of being can be seen as a form of the art of living based on values familiar from spiritual practice: Opening of the heart, open mindedness, capacity for love, patience, gratitude, ability to deal with life's paradoxes and to endure uncertainty. Ultimately, the capacity for wisdom becomes visible in posttraumatic narratives and new creative life plans.

The *dialectics of being and becoming* and the dynamics of change transcending the trauma are not to be understood reductively as stabilizing defence or dissociative separation. On the contrary, due to the increased vulnerability, a greater openness and permeability for areas of experience and consciousness can occur simultaneously, which transcend the everyday conscious waking state, for example the greater readiness of traumatized people to experience the phenomena of synchronicity. These emergent synchronistic phenomena can also be felt in the intersubjective field of therapy and have an effect on the therapist's consciousness in their symbolic power, provided there is a willingness to open up to the subtle-energetic level.

Nor can such developments in the tension between the possible and the impossible be denigrated as trendy "respiritualization"; rather, they testify to an expansion of consciousness for the dimension of the Invisible, a dimension which, as Paracelsus once said, has no name but nevertheless has an effect and ultimately remains a mystery.

Every development of consciousness requires sacrifice. In his teleological orientation Jung has dealt very intensively with the *transformative character of the victim archetype*. I, too, have asked myself what has to be sacrificed after traumatization in order to bring stagnated life processes back into flow and to "overgrow" traumata. Jung understands this "overgrowth" in the sense of a "raising of the level of consciousness" (*CW* 13, §17), a more fluid, reflective consciousness. For this, paradoxically functioning defence mechanisms must be sacrificed, which, although they protect superficially and serve survival (dissociation, depersonalization, a feigned "playing dead" reflex), in the long term prevent the transcending of trauma and block the flow of vital energy. The victim-perpetrator dialectic also has great significance for the individual and collective development of consciousness. There is no transformation of consciousness without dealing with shame, guilt and shadow in the horizon of traumatic events.

1.7. Transcendence of Trauma

The notion of *dynamic self-organization* in nonlinear open systems is helpful to better understand how states of imbalance caused by trauma can be stabilized and transformed into higher orders. When a system collapses due to information overload, it tends to reorganize and restructure itself on a new, higher level after chaotic inability to act. For networks and living systems, the more often they collapse and renew themselves, the more robust they become. Even traumatized people can be regarded as a living, intelligent network in which chaos and order enter into a fruitful coexistence. Dee Hock coined the neologism "chaord" for this purpose and explained that order only emerges at the edges of chaos and that the *chaordic principle* is valid for all living organisms (Dee Hock, 2013).

Nietzsche expressed this poetically:

One must still have chaos in oneself to give birth to a dancing star.
(Nietzsche, 1995, *Zarathustra,* p. 5)

The research branch of *neurobiology and the findings of modern brain research* confirm the high degree of adaptability and flexibility of human behaviour and explain this with the self-organizing capacity of the brain. Our central nervous system has structurally defined circuit patterns which are continuously transformed and reshaped by the process of their use. The plasticity of neuronal circuits gives rise to the hope that even after trauma, the brain as a dynamic system is capable of forming new nerve cells and building new neuronal circuits that open up ways of thinking and behaving to which there was no access before the traumatic experience. This creative ability to recode, reinterpret and reformulate supports processes of an expansion of awareness.

Reconstruction in thinking, feeling and acting are made possible by the erasure and destabilization of patterns that have become unusable. Gerald Hüther (1996) has pointed out that the destabilization of neuronal circuit patterns in limbic and cortical brain regions triggered by neuroendocrine reactions can lead to reorganization processes that either lead to fundamentally positive changes in thinking, feeling and acting or to irretrievable losses and reduction of capabilities.

Maturana and Varela call *autopoiesis* the property of living systems to constantly renew themselves without losing the integrity of their structure. The overturning of the system into a new structure, the emergence, corresponds to the change from chaotic states into a new order. In the framework of consciousness studies, "transcendence competence," an inner growth dynamic and potential for transcendent experience that arises after existential crises, has been explored by Mitschke-Collande (2012).

According to the gestalt psychology principle, the tendency is inherent in any gestalt to overcome contradictions, disharmonies and imperfections, and when they have become imbalanced beyond the critical point—the "bifurcation point" (Hogenson, 2005)—to transform themselves into higher complex forms of organization.

Transcending the ego's perspective is a basic human capacity. In the borderlands of the soul, faced with the realization that human beings have survived broken worlds without becoming broken themselves, we must go beyond seeking to understand; rather, we must allow ourselves to be deeply moved. It remains a mystery how in the darkness of inhumanity some people retain the capacity for goodness.

1.8 Trauma Therapy as the Unfolding of Consciousness

Processes of change in traumatic experiences of soul murder require a *container*, the protective, secure *temenos* of the healing relationship. Eros powers of connection and compassion must be constellated in the intersubjective field in order to confront suffering, to endure pain, so that scope for new options for thought and behaviour can be created and horizons of meaning can be sounded out. Descending into one's own abyss is a challenge to gain access to the essential and to reinvent one's self, restoring identity integration through interpretation and reinterpretation of the incomprehensible.

> My aim is to bring about a psychic state in which my patient begins to experiment with his own nature. A state of fluidity change and growth, where nothing is eternally fixed and hopelessly petrified.
>
> (C. G. Jung, *CW* 16, §99)

Essential for trauma therapy is the existential basic polarity of differentiation and integration, the restoration of *wholeness* amid the *broken*ness. Eros forces of connection are needed after the traumatizing forces of splitting. Survivors must reassemble themselves from the fragments in order to become a whole person again after traumatic self-dissolution and desubjectification.

In alchemy this process was described with the principles *solve et coagula*, with "dissolving and binding." These therapeutic intervention strategies were already regarded in Hippocratic medicine and Socratic psychotherapy as core elements for reaching other levels of consciousness (Berner-Hürbin, 2008). They are cleansing and dissolving processes of fixed entanglements in order to bring the mentally dead back to life. Sometimes the trauma is experienced as a catharsis, as an extremely disturbing process of purification of perception.

In the Buddhist tradition, *deidentification processes* help to dissolve ingrained habits of thinking and perception and support the process of becoming conscious, because a clear awareness of the present moment prevents fixations on fears and negative feelings. In the therapeutic process, a traumatized person practices taking an observer's position to mindfully observe the various post-traumatic strategies, thought and behaviour patterns. This conscious *process of disidentification* controls self-regulation and helps to realize that we are not identical with our patterns and strategies, that we are always more than this pain, this hatred, this despair. At the same time an awareness is growing that our mind is the master builder of the world ("mind over matter"), that the way we think and the imprints of traumatic experiences on our perception and feelings create reality. In this insight lies the chance to deal with suffering in a different way and to develop more wholesome, life-promoting patterns of thinking and feeling.

The ability of conscious dissociation from what is happening, the compassionate observation of mental processes, should not be confused with dissociation, since contact with feelings is not lost, and the mind observes how consciousness operates, constructs meaning and meaninglessness and constantly recreates realities. In this "witness consciousness" (Wilber, 1984) emotions and thoughts are perceived as transient in their coming and going. With the help of *imaginative distancing techniques*, shelters are created that protect against retraumatizing flooding. In creative work with symbols the reality of suffering is reinterpreted, and with the knowledge that our thinking can control our behaviour and our feelings, a new more reconciliatory attitude towards life with its suffering, its joys and contradictions can be worked out. Taoism teaches that the fabric of reality consists of 10,000 sufferings and 10,000 joys. Trauma therapy as a form of work to achieve greater consciousness promotes insight into the experience of the paradoxical structure of reality, a component of all wisdom traditions and spiritual paths, and the insight into one's own being and the essence of the Whole.

The experience with the paradox of *koans* makes it clear how the ego can plunge to the point of disintegration into uncertainty, despair and hopelessness when it is searching for the correct answer to an unsolvable, deeply puzzling question. Spiritual awakening, a state of maximal clarity and insight, then represents a form of *metanoia*. Even after traumatic borderline experiences, the gruelling search for the "why," where there is no "why," can lead to such a sudden transition. As a therapist, my presence is then essential, my being grounded, centred and fully there.

The conscious handling of one's own consciousness, as taught in spiritual traditions, has found its way into trauma therapy through the concept of *mindfulness*. Being aware and compassionate about what is felt in the here and now of the therapeutic situation, being aware of the breath, physical sensations, thoughts, feelings, fantasies and inner images, giving them nonjudgemental space and the right to exist, even if only for short moments, changes the experience. The identification of cognitive evaluations and emotional patterns helps to achieve more clarity and acceptance of what is real, and of how I process it in my head. The conscious concentration and opening of the heart in a moment-to-moment awareness counteracts automated dissociative processes and the generalized feeling of helplessness; it relativizes the meaning of the past by focusing on the present and takes away the life-determining and life-denying quality of traumatic experiences.

Mindful training of consciousness helps to perceive what is, to accept the fateful brokenness of existence without remaining fixated on suffering and renouncing the love of life. Trauma therapy can become a place of loving recognition, a space that releases from traumatic darkening of the soul, liberates to greater openness, deeper compassion and wiser relating to oneself and the world.

Bibliography

Anderssen-Reuster, U., Meibert, P., and Meck, S. (Hrsg.). (2013). *Psychotherapie und buddhistisches Geistestraining. Methoden einer achtsamen Bewusstseinskultur*. Stuttgart: Schattauer Verlag.

Becker, D. (2001). Trauma, Traumabehandlung, Traumageschäft. In Catherine Moser, Doris Nyfeler, and Martine Verwey (Hrsg.), *Traumatisierungen von Flüchtlingen und Asyl Suchenden*. Zürich: Seismo Verlag.

Becker, D. (2006). *Die Erfindung des Traumas- Verflochtene Geschichten*. Berlin: Freitag.

Becker, D. (2009). Extremes Leid und die Perspektive posttraumatischen Wachstums: Realitätsverleugnung, naives Wunschdenken oder doch ein Stück wissenschaftliche Erkenntnis? In Zeitschrift für Psychotraumatologie, Psychotherapiewissenschaft, *Psychologische Medizin*, Jg. 7, Nr. 1, 21–34.

Berner-Hürbin, A. (2008). *Energie, und Ekstasen: Sokratische Psychotherapie und aktuelle Bewusstseinsforschung*. Frauenfeld: Huber Verlag.

Calhoun, Lawrence G., and Tedeschi, Richard G. (Eds.). (2006). *Handbook of Posttraumatic Growth: Research and Practice*. Mahwah, NJ: Lawrence Erlbaum Associates.

Dabrowski, K. (1964). *Positive Disintegration*. Boston, MA: Little, Brown and Company.

Dee Hock. (2013). *Die Chaordan Organization*. Stuttgart: Schäffer-Poeschel Publishing House.

Eckhart, Meister. (1993). *Werke in zwei Bänden*. Frankfurt a. Main: Deutscher Klassiker Verlag.

Eliade, Mircea. (1972). *Shamanism: Archaic Techniques of Ecstasy*. Willard R. Trask (Trans.). Princeton: Princeton University Press.

Ellenberger, H. F. (1970). *The Discovery of the Unconscious: The History and Evolution of Dynamic Psychiatry*. New York: Basic Books.

Foudraine, J. (1973). *Wer ist aus Holz?* Munich: Piper

Gadamer, H.-G. (2003). *Schmerz. Einschätzungen aus medizinischer, philosophischer und therapeutischer Sicht*. Heidelberg: Universitätsverlag Winter.

Hartmut, Kraft. (2008). *PlusHeilung: Die Chancen der großen Krisen*. Stuttgart: Kreuz Verlag.

Hofmann, L., and Roesler, Ch. (2010). Der Archetyp des verwundeten Heilers. *Transpersonale Psychologie und Psychotherapie*, 1, 75–90.

Hogenson, G. (2005). The Self, the symbolic and synchronicity: Virtual realities and the emergence of the psyche. *Journal of Analytical Psychology*, 50(3), 271–284.

Hüther, G. (1996). The Central Adaptation Syndrome: Psychosocial stress as a trigger for adaptive modification of brain structure and brain function. *Progress in Neurobiology*, 48, 569–612.

Jung, C. G. (1989). *Memories, Dreams, Reflections*. A. Jaffé (Ed.), R. and C. Winston (Trans.). London: Vintage Books.

Kertész, Imre. (2002). "Eureka!" 2002 Nobel Prize speech. Suhrkamp, Frankfurt/M.

Le Breton, D. (2003). *Schmerz. übers. v. M. Muhle, T. Obergöker, S. Schulz*. Zürich, Berlin: diaphanes.

Maercker, A., and Zoellner, T. (2004). The Janus face of self-perceived growth: Toward a two-component model of post-traumatic growth. *Psychological Inquiry*, 15(1), 41–48.

Manstetten, R. (2007). Gelassenheit. Selbstwahrnehmung und Achtsamkeit bei Meister Eckart. In U. Anderssen-Reuter (Hrsg), *Achtsamkeit in Psychotherapie und Psychosomatik. Haltung und Methode*, S. 16–36. Stuttgart: Schattauer.

Nietzsche, F. (1995). *Thus spoke Zarathustra*. W. Kaufmann (Trans.). New York: Modern Library.

Papadopoulos, Renos K. (2007). Refugees, trauma and adversity-activated development. *European Journal of Psychotherapy and Counselling, September,* 9(3), 301–312

Petzold, H. G., Wolf, H-U., Landgrebe, B., and Josic, Z. (2002). *Das Trauma überwinden. Integrative Modelle der Trauma therapie*. Paderborn: Junfermann Verlag.

Revel, J-F., and Ricard, M. (2003). *Der Mönch und der Philosoph. Buddhismus und Abendland. Ein Dialog zwischen Vater und Sohn*. Köln: Kiepenheuer& Witsch.

Tauler, Johannes. (1979). *Predigten, übertragen und herausgegeben von Georg Hofmann, Freiburg i.Br. 1961, Neudruck in 2 Bänden, 3.* Auflage: Johannes Verlag, Einsiedeln.

Tedeschi, Richard G., and Calhoun, Lawrence G. (1995). *Trauma and Transformation. Growing in the Aftermath of Suffering*. London: Sage Publications.

Tedeschi, Richard G., and Calhoun, Lawrence G. (1996). The posttraumatic growth inventory: Measuring the positive legacy of trauma. *Journal of Traumatic Stress*, 9(3), 455–471.

Tedeschi, Richard G., and Calhoun, Lawrence G. (2004). Posttraumatic growth: Conceptual foundations and empirical evidence. *Psychological Inquiry,* 15(1), 1–18

Tedeschi, Richard G., Park, Crystal L., and Calhoun, Lawrence G. (Eds.). (1998). *Posttraumatic Growth: Positive Changes in the Aftermath of Crisis*. Mahwah, NJ: Lawrence Erlbaum Associates.

Tillich, Paul. (1991). *Der Mut zum Sein*. New York Berlin: de Gruyter.

von Brück, M. (1996). *Buddha und Jesus. Psychische Identität und spirituelle Transformation*. Vortrag am Kongress des Netzwerks Spirituelle Entwicklung und Krisenbegleitung (SEN), Deutschland, Todtmoos, September 1996.

von Mitschke-Collande, C. (2012). Gestärkt durch die Krise. In: Bewusstseinswissenschaften. *Transpersonale Psychologie und Psychotherapie*, 1, 65–77.

Weilnböck, H. (2001). Psychotraumatologie. Über ein neues Paradigma für Psychotherapie und Kulturwissenschaften. *Literaturkritik.de.Rezensionsforum*, Nr. 10, Jag 3

Wilber, Ken. (1984). *Wege zum Selbst*. München: Kösel.

Wirtz, U. (1989). *Seelenmord*. Stuttgart: Kreuz Verlag.

Wirtz, U. (2014). *Trauma and Beyond. The Mystery of Transformation*. New Orleans: Spring Journal Books, now Routledge 2020.

Chapter 15

Polly Young-Eisendrath

A Brief Biography in Seven Ho-Hum Haiku: Polly Young-Eisendrath

- A working-class child

  Polly in fear and awe of life
  Mute at age seven.

- Her question: Why war?

  No teacher could answer
  She left Akron to find out.

- Study, study, seek

  Present-moment awareness
  Sit, making sense Zen.

- Marry, children, seek

  Jung, teaching, writing, finding
  Couple therapy.

- Couples fight, like war

  Polarize, disgust, hate, rage
  At edge, non-hate wins.

- Embracing your own

  Non-hate for enemies, love
  Your life, it's made for you.

- Polly in mountains,

  Now content present-moment
  Respecting all conflicts.

DOI: 10.4324/9781003148968-16

Projective Identification in a Famous Zen Case

Implications for Relationships With Spiritual Masters

Parts of this chapter are from the following publication in Polly Young-Eisendrath (2020) Therapeutic Impasse in a Famous Zen Case: Memorial Tribute for Jeremy Safran, *Psychoanalytic Inquiry*, 40:5, 360–366, DOI: 10.1080/07351690.2020.1766328.

Whether or not you are familiar with the term *projective identification*, you have been affected by the experience of projective identification. Projective identification is not abstract. It is a direct experience that all of us have. In this chapter, the term refers principally to interactions with others in which you seem to be captured or kidnapped by their emotions or emotional meanings and then carried into a kind of "script" or "tape" in a way that you had not intended. The projector and the receiver of this unconscious communication may be interacting in a variety of ways (as I explain later), but as the receiver you will feel emotionally shaken or threatened or thrown. You may feel as though you have no choice except to react in a particular way. Often, you will notice this kind of unconscious communication when a partner, a therapy client, a close friend, or a mentor "rocks your boat"—and then, for example, you forget something obvious about the person just after they tell you how sensitive they are about such forgetting or you say something to them that is overly personal that you did not intend to say. Even in passing relationships we are affected by projective identification, but in close personal relationships, a chronic and repetitive projective identification can create polarization and undermine trust. In this chapter, I will analyze a famous Zen case in terms of projective identification, in order to try to understand one aspect (idealization/splitting) of the multiple ethical, sexual, and financial scandals that have come to light involving Buddhist teachers in the past decade or so in Western Buddhist communities.

In projective identification, one person projects or perceives a fantasy about the other in a way that evokes feelings or other expressions in the recipient, which seem congruent with what is felt or projected by the sender. Projective identification is a psychological process that includes or consists of any or all of the following: a type of defense, a mode of communication, a form of relating to another person emotionally, and an opening to psychological change (Ogden, 1991). Across these modes, projective identification may be a communication of something *with* someone; an expelling or externalizing of something *into* someone; an attempted control *of* someone; or an emotional assault *on* someone (e. g., Caper, 2000). Within the drama of projective identifications, many kinds of interactions may be taking place, used for different purposes that may be subconscious, partly conscious, or wholly unconscious.

For example, in the initial meeting in the form of couple therapy called dialogue therapy (see Young-Eisendrath, 1993, 2019), when the couple enters the room and sits down, the therapist says something like this, inviting them to talk together: "I'd like to hear the two of you talk together about your reasons for being here. You don't need to worry about giving me the background, because each of you will be interviewed for that. Just talk together now, as naturally as you can, about why you are here and what you hope to get from this experience." At least 80 percent of the time, one person says, "Why don't you begin?" or "Do you want to begin?" Of course, that person *has already begun*! And if the statement seems insistent that the *other* person speak first, then the first person is taking control of the interaction, saying that the other person *should* speak first. The recipient of the message may feel a pressure to comply and typically does begin to speak. This is a quick and apparently simple moment of projective identification in which one person embodies the *puppeteer* and the other becomes the *puppet*—the first person is taking *control of* the second. This is an example of a quick interaction through projective identification.

Brief History of the Term

In 1946, British psychoanalyst Melanie Klein described in her chapter, "Notes on Some Schizoid Mechanisms" (Klein, 1946/1955), a phenomenon that she had seen in young children with whom she was working in psychoanalysis. It consisted of the children describing unconscious fantasies of expelling unbearable parts of their minds into others and incorporating parts of others' minds into their own, taking a defensive position of getting rid of aspects of their own minds and identifying with others' minds. This balance of projection and introjection Klein eventually called "projective identification" (Klein, 1955). She claimed that this function both resulted from and supported the fantasy that one's mind was not separate or discrete from other minds, thereby showing evidence of a preverbal synchronizing of minds through influence and contact in both imagining and projecting. Projective identification, Klein discovered, eventually evolves into the child's attempts to perceive, organize, and manage experiences in order to communicate with others on whom the child depends. Of course, infants are very complex and extremely helpless and are faced with a barrage of complicated and frightening stimuli that need to be organized and shaped through interactions in order to survive and thrive.

Through projective identification with its caregivers, the child gradually develops the ability to keep painful, dangerous, and frightening experiences sorted separately from comforting, soothing, and calming ones. This kind of "splitting" of the "bad" from the "good," pain from pleasure, is an early development of a psychological defense to keep the "bad things" or painful experiences "outside" oneself while holding the "good" ones inside.

Psychological stability takes time to form in infancy. The mothering one(s) play an important role in that they have to be empathic in picking up accurate emotional signals from the infant and helping the infant sort out the meanings. The infant uses projective identification as a mode of fantasy and communication that serves both a defensive and a developmental function. Projective identification is the means by which the infant gets the mother(s) to feel what the infant is feeling, or, alternatively, cannot bear to feel, and so it has to be expelled. Also, this serves as a way in which the infant may feel unified with, or unseparated from, its caregivers. Because of the fantasy of non-separation, projective identification is a *transitional* or *transactional* communication in which one feels both controlled by and in control of others, and these experiences may alternate back and forth between parties. Of course, these fantasies of non-separation and control continue through childhood and adolescence, into adult life and relationships.

Melanie Klein introduced projective identification in 1946 and discussed it in only one other chapter, titled "On Identification" (1955). But her protégé Wilfred Bion (1959) elaborated on the term and expanded its usage in demonstrating it to be the most important interactive or communicative function between patient and therapist in individual therapy and the most powerful kind of unconscious communication in groups and couples. As Bion notably said, "The analyst feels that he is being manipulated so as to be playing a part, no matter how difficult to recognize, in somebody else's phantasy" (p. 149).

Bion believed and stated that projective identification expresses the desire to bring another person *under one's control*. This process typically goes back and forth, although it may also be one-sided. Bion believed that projective identification is often accompanied by behavior designed to elicit in another *in reality* what the sender is, in fact, expelling or projecting. For example, one person may project one's rage or rejection into another and then behave in such a way toward the other to provoke such a state of rage or rejection in that other person. This is called *realistic projective identification* and is evidence of the early function of parents to act safely and regularly as "containers" of their infants' painful states of mind while also experiencing their own states of mind. A good-enough parent will not retaliate in receiving a destructive or painful state of mind from the infant, but instead will "digest" the infant's or child's experience and perhaps speak it back to them, as in, "You are really upset about that, aren't you?"

Beyond Klein and Bion, other psychoanalysts who have used and developed projective identification as a clinical term and method of investigation include both Ogden (e.g., 1991) and Winnicott as well as Herbert Rosenfeld, Michael Balint, Harold Searles, Robert Caper, James Grotstein, and Polly Young-Eisendrath. These analysts have applied it variously to their clinical understanding of early development, psychotic process, unconscious communication, and couple or other close adult interpersonal and intersubjective relationships.

Before Klein coined the term for preverbal communication between infant and mother, Carl Jung (1921/1971) came up with a similar idea in his book *Psychological Types*. Jung used the French term *participation mystique* (borrowed from the French ethnologist Lucien Levy-Bruhl) to denote a kind of collective psychological state or frame of mind in which the individual seems unable to keep the boundaries of individuality, but feels in partial identification with another or others. Jung used the term especially in regard to falling in love when one person feels convinced that they can experience exactly what the other is feeling and thinking—a conviction of a kind of emotional telepathy. Like Bion, Jung thought this kind of identification with another or others played a strong role in group psychology.

In the developments and applications of the theory of projective identification, clinicians and theorists emphasize all or some of the following phenomena: direct communication 'deeper' than words" (Caper, 2019) that involves our capacity to evoke emotional states in others and communicate our states of mind; the splitting of good/bad, life/death, internal/external, and ideal/devalued, which happens quickly and implicitly in this kind of communication; the potential manipulation of another's psyche; and implicit expressions and experiences of inexplicable danger, destruction, inflation, intoxication, or omnipotence. Truly, then, we can reference everything from falling in love to being terrified of a stranger, to being swept away with tears of gratitude with a spiritual teacher (even though you might not understand the words or language being spoken), to being taken in by the "magic" of a despot. The clinical theory of projective identification maps a powerful communication that originates in our infancy and extends into our adult relations, especially in couples and groups.

A Spiritual Problem and a Famous Zen Case

The famous Zen case in which I find the problem of projective identification is the so-called meeting (not historically verifiable, but very significant in the history of Zen Buddhism) of the Chinese emperor Wu and the Zen master Bodhidharma. I will tell the story of the case later, but first I would like to introduce the problem of splitting and projective identification that occurs in some spiritual groups and settings. The problem, I believe, originates from seeking a "perfect master" who is pure and wise and can lead one from the confusions of human suffering and ignorance into the clarity of liberation. The terms *suffering* and *ignorance* have specific meanings within the teachings of Buddhism (of which I am a lifetime practitioner and student). Suffering refers to the universal quality of stress, off-centeredness, and imperfectability of human life within our ordinary consensual world. Ignorance refers to our ignorance of the radical interdependence of a life in which we are contextualized, and which we can neither control nor fully understand. Many people begin their spiritual practice, Buddhist or otherwise, wanting to find the "right" teacher or at least a "good match" because they want to move as quickly as possible from their discomfort and confusion into greater ease and clarity. This is a little like trying to find the "right partner" for love and life. The longing to find someone with whom one has an ease and comfort "too deep for words" probably exists in all of us. For Buddhists, the right teacher might be described as "pure" or "perfect."

There is nothing inherently wrong about seeking a perfect teacher as long as one becomes conscious of the fantasy motivating the desire. The same thing happens within psychotherapy: people seek a "perfect therapist" or may idealize their therapist or analyst, at the beginning of therapy, leading to envy of the therapist or a kind of childish dependence on the therapist. This kind of situation will eventually become part of the therapeutic inquiry in an effective psychotherapy. In Buddhist practice, and perhaps in other spiritual practices as well, the dynamics of splitting and idealization are typically not a part of the conversations or teachings.

A problematic alliance may then develop between a naïve seeker, who projects wisdom and purity, and a teacher who desires to be idealized (usually unconsciously, but sometimes subconsciously). On the student's side, the student wants to find a powerful master who can help the student become "liberated" as quickly as possible. On the teacher's side of that equation, there may be a problem in the teacher's unknown and/or unacknowledged emotional needs to be put on a pedestal, or seen in a fanciful way as having no aggressive, sexual, narcissistic, or self-centered motivations, but instead to be motivated *only* by wisdom or compassion. Without getting into technicalities about whether said teacher is "enlightened," the important issue is the teacher's reputation as *wise*, *awake*, or *flawless* in her/his approach to teaching, guiding, and inspiring students and others.

The teacher's reputation, and the student's desire to believe in it, set into motion a chronic idealizing projective identification between teacher and student in which they both seem to crave a "perfect" person, with one of them promoting that belief in her/his own perfection (wisdom or compassion) and the other one imagining this perfection as *belonging to the teacher*. In other words, the full range of human emotions and motivations is not allowed to be in the teacher; the teacher is imagined to have *transcended* greed, hostility, and ignorance, as well as self-protection and self-promotion. What remains dissociated or repressed in the midst of such idealizing are disavowed individual motives in both parties, including but not limited to specialness, power, aggression, vulnerability, and sexual desire.

In a long-term psychotherapy, idealization and splitting often bring about a "therapeutic impasse" in which the patient may accuse the therapist of "not providing what was promised" or "trying to control the outcome" or "not caring about" their emotional relationship. Or the patient may fall in love with the therapist and feel terribly controlled by this experience, no longer free to be in therapy, but simply bound by sexual or passionate fantasies about the therapist. It can seem as though the patient is in the therapy to "develop erotic *needs* for the therapist," while the therapist has *no needs* for the patient. In other words, the dynamics of *puppet* and *puppeteer* enter into their relationship and must then be interpreted and understood, in order for the therapy to move forward. Within a psychoanalytic context, the two parties begin to investigate this projective identification and usually discover a therapeutic richness in that process of inquiry. In spiritual situations, instead of investigating what is emerging in such a projective identification, the two individuals and their relationship become rigidified and defensive, a situation that can lead to feelings of humiliation and rage, or an enactment of some kind of misconduct.

Sexual and Financial Scandals in Buddhist Groups as Impasses

Are the scandals of sexual misconduct, financial misconduct, or other ethical failures that disrupt or destroy spiritual practice in Buddhist groups examples of "therapeutic impasses" between teacher(s) and student(s)? I believe they are. In the remainder of this chapter, I will be speaking about Buddhist teachers and context, although I think my analysis applies to other spiritual groups as well: those in which there is an idealized figure or master or elder who rises above the ordinary human being and may be seen as flawless.

The term *therapeutic impasse* can be used to describe a number of situations in which therapy stops making progress and one or both parties seem unable to explore the difficulties between them. It can occur in the form of a disagreement between the parties about unacknowledged ongoing issues, or a stagnation in the therapy. The most important symptom of an impasse is that the therapy itself takes a turn so that the parties are *not* able to *proceed with the usual process* and the client may quit or threaten to quit, as a result.

From a psychoanalytic perspective, these kinds of disruptions are not only expectable, but are also assumed to create richly troubling dynamics that allow the two parties to examine what is going on between them, as a part of therapy. There is "no blame" for the conundrum they find themselves in because it is an emergent aspect of their particular relationship and it is explored and mined for its hidden treasures (such as the unknown motivations for power, control, or specialness of one or both parties). Of course, unethical *enactments* of sexual or financial betrayals are not impasses but *violations* that break the trust necessary for the therapy to continue. When impasses lead to undermining trust, then the therapy is over and cannot be rectified.

On the other hand, impasses that are considered "grist for the mill" give the therapist a signal that something needs to be inquired into and that "business as usual" needs to slow down and be opened up into deeper consideration. The important clinical feature of therapeutic impasses, as Safran's (e.g., Safran and Kraus, 2014) research demonstrated, is that they provide a window into understanding dynamics that are disavowed or hidden in both parties. They allow us to stop and include in our conscious awareness what has been unknowingly dissoci-ated, projected, or identified with.

In my view, all therapeutic impasses, whether in spiritual development or psy-chotherapy, stem from chronic projective identification in which the interactions between the parties are distorted, frozen, repetitive, and rigidified in a way that brings about polarization and/or is defended against by repression or dissociation.

Ongoing projective identifications threaten our conscious sense of ourselves and the trust we place in therapy or spiritual practice. I regard projective identifi-cation as a kind of "internal theater" in which the projector is unconsciously evok-ing and orchestrating responses from the recipient of the projection. The recipient is also often also projecting and orchestrating. Such entangled projections and identifications may lead to the experience of being in a distorted *hall of mirrors* in which it's impossible to know who is doing what to whom.

The unintended meanings of what is projected and what is evoked in the other may or may not be similar (for the two) or fully understandable to either party, even after seeing and interpreting them. But the inquiry becomes meaningful and clears the way for more inquiry into the dynamics between the individuals. Projective identification is an ordinary part of everyday affective communication between people and only becomes pathological or anxiety provoking when it is chronic, repetitive, and polarized.

Relational Scandals in the Buddhist World

From what I have seen in my three-plus decades of being an analyst, therapist, and couple therapist for Buddhist practitioners (I live and work in a "Buddhist ghetto" in central Vermont) and teachers, there is a paucity of relational wisdom in the Buddhist community about the *emotional dynamics* of *unconscious interaction* between people. I have seen both individuals and couples who are long-term Bud-dhist practitioners in psychotherapy and analysis. Of course, I see clients who are not Buddhist as well, but most of my clients now claim to practice mindfulness, even if they are not formal practitioners.

I have been a practicing Buddhist myself since 1971; my two long-term teach-ers are Roshi Philip Kapleau and Shinzen Young. I have also practiced Phowa under the direction of Ayang Rinpoche and Anyen Rinpoche. I now also practice Zen under the guidance of Henry Shukman. I am deeply grateful for the wisdom of Buddhist teachings and practices. Buddhist practice has been the mainstay of my individuation and life on many levels. I feel nothing but gratitude for my own teachers who have always presented themselves (to me) with their failures and vulnerabilities. And so, what I write here is offered as a corrective or as a kind of feedback, and not as a major critique of the practice or teachings.

What I have noticed in doing therapy with Buddhists, and participating in study and practice groups, both in America and abroad, is that there is little under-standing of how unconscious communication works *between* people, as I men-tioned earlier, even though many ceremonies and practices depend on this kind of communication, especially on idealization of the teacher. I think some of the lack of understanding is due to the models of mind in Buddhism. Despite the fact that these models are complex and sophisticated and include maps of a vast study of unconscious dynamics, they do not include the entanglements of intersubjectivities that stem from (m)other-infant communication and continue throughout life. I have written about some differences and similarities in psychoanalytic and Buddhist ideas, particularly in the second edition of the *Cambridge Companion to Jung* (Young-Eisendrath and Dawson, 2008), which I edited with Terence Dawson, and in *Awakening and Insight: Zen Buddhism and Psychotherapy* (Young-Eisendrath and Muramoto, 2002).

In those and other places (for example, in my newest book *Love Between Equals: Relationship as a Spiritual Path*, 2019), I believe I have done due diligence grappling with the particulars of the different theories. But I can also get distracted by theoretical perspectives on the human mind because the models are abstract and do not immediately show the impact of our emotional and mental habits on our relationships.

Some Important Differences Between Psychoanalysis and Buddhism

And so, I have now shifted more towards examining, in an almost clinical way, how it is that there are so many scandals in the Buddhist world among very accomplished teachers and masters. How can a thoughtful adult practitioner of Buddhism *not* be interested in the fact that accomplished teachers create destructive and repetitive interpersonal and ethical problems?

Plunging into my perplexity, I decided to study with William Waldron, Ph.D., Professor of Buddhist Studies at Middlebury College. He is a scholar and translator/interpreter of the Buddhist theory of the unconscious. He is also a practitioner of Tibetan Buddhism. His scholarly specialty in Indian Buddhism is Yogacara (roughly third to fifth century CE). Dr. Waldron is a recognized expert on the *alayavijnana* or storehouse consciousness, also known as "home" consciousness, the model of the "unconscious mind" in Buddhism. While this mind works unconsciously in and on us, it is recognized, in Buddhism, as being *conscious itself*: we are not conscious of it, but it is conscious. (That's a nuance that psychoanalysts might want to contemplate, as we tend to call our theory of repressed and instinctual unconscious motivations "the unconscious," but also recognize that this "unconscious" has desires and intentions of its own.) Dr. Waldron and I eventually taught a seminar together on the unconscious in Buddhism and psychoanalysis.

As Dr. Waldron pointed out when we started teaching together, there is one important difference between Buddhism and psychoanalysis, which should be highlighted in comparing/contrasting them, in regard to the unconscious mind. Significantly, the Buddhist mind *wants to be enlightened*, but the psychoanalytic mind is *ambivalent* about enlightenment (see, for example, Waldron, 2003). When an individual begins to awaken to the nature of emptiness and impermanence from a Buddhist perspective, that person *feels* the pleasure of a newfound freedom and wants more. While this Buddhist mind can also be motivated by complicated entanglements with karmic urges, it has the nature to want to be awake; its only true enemy is the "ego," which is described more like a tricky criminal (like a Tony Soprano) than like an unconscious tendency to become entangled with others' desires and projections. There is also an end-point to the battle against the ego: when the ego is driven out of one's personality (one's "home"), then one's motivations and perceptions become generally pure, wise, and compassionate. Enlightenment should be the end of self-promotion and self-protection. In this way, students should not have to "worry" about a realized master in terms of that person's egotistical motivations.

In psychoanalysis, however, the mind, even when awakened, remains divided, conflicted, and somewhat unconscious of its own motivations, and so even a master would have blind spots about their own desires, motivations, and self-promotion. One reason that psychoanalysts, even when they are finished with their own training analysis, may go back into psychoanalysis with another analyst is that they assume they may find more ways to see/hear/feel their blind spots in a different relationship. In psychoanalysis, our practice is *dyadic, not individual*. We study what arises *between* two people when they project into each other. When our patients finish their therapy or analysis, they are *still conflicted*, both within themselves and between us; in fact, they may feel *more* conflicted than when they began. They recognize, at the end, how/why I "rock their boat" and how they rock mine, or want to rock it. But they also have a sense of humor about all that, are interested in how their conflicts change in different relationships and circumstances, have a knowledge of their emotional and mental habits, and have a sense of responsibility for their own darker motivations and desires.

Most Buddhist practices ask us to investigate our subjective world *solo* and then to report on it and/or to demonstrate what we discover. Although there is a strong theory of radical interdependence in Buddhism, the theory does not get mapped specifically onto a two-person relationship, such as one has in marriage or in a student-teacher dyad. Asian cultures, in which Buddhism originally developed and evolved over centuries, have not generally been interested in the two-person relationship. This kind of relationship was not valorized or emphasized, as it was in the West through the ideals of romantic love.

In most Buddhist stories and accounts, the Buddhist master is fascinating, but the student is not. The master is in a different existential register than the student—not quite human and certainly not encumbered by self-promotion and self-protection. The very assumption of being set apart and extraordinary invites a projective identification: the master is "realized" and the student is not and they both agree on this.

Within the dynamic of projective identification, the disavowed "bad" (always present in our lives as humans) aspect of the master's personality must be projected outwards; what is disavowed may be projected into the student or outside their dyad. Also, the "unenlightened" student needs the enlightened teacher, but the teacher does not need the student. The teacher can freely count on the student's dependence while the teacher is assumed to be free of dependence on the student. All of this is built into the system, not to be questioned. There are, of course, ethical precepts. And yet, if the teacher is recognized as "enlightened" or if the teacher is validated as a master, then it is possible for a teacher to reinterpret the spirit of a precept and adapt it to the needs of teaching in whatever way the teacher sees fit. In analytic lingo, this is a "one-person" model of teaching and influence: awakening is a one-way street.

The Zen Case of Bodhidharma and Emperor Wu

I would like now to examine the famous Zen case of Bodhidharma's meeting with Emperor Wu, in light of what I have been saying about projective identification and the one-way street of influence in the teacher-student relationship. Technically, in this case, the therapeutic impasse led to a "failure of treatment" because they had only one brief meeting and they never met again. And yet, the case is iconic in Zen training and serves as a model for teacher-student relating.

According to Zen tradition, (see, for example, Aitken, 1991), the legendary Bodhidharma was the first patriarch of Chinese Zen, although it's historically unclear, in fact, whether someone named Bodhidharma factually existed. In the story, he was a fierce but simple monk who traveled from India to China to bring a fundamentally new form of Buddhist practice to China, one that depends almost exclusively on sitting meditation—a mostly solitary exploration. In the most famous story about him, Bodhidharma was invited by Emperor Wu of Liang province to his court, around the year 520. Bodhidharma had been meditating in a cave and he was admired and respected for the powers he had developed.

Emperor Wu had been a faithful supporter of Buddhism in China where it already existed, in a more scholarly form. The emperor had heard about a hermit monk who was practicing this new form of meditation and the emperor was curious and invited Bodhidharma to his court. Significantly, the emperor began the conversation, saying he had built temples and given financial support to the Buddhist monastic community—a common practice for a dedicated patron. Then he asked Bodhidharma how much merit, how much spiritual credit, he had gained for these actions. Bodhidharma replied forcefully, "*None* whatsoever!" Perplexed by this, the emperor then asked, "What is the meaning of your holy truth?" to which Bodhidharma instantly replied, "Empty. *Nothing* holy about it!" Now, even more confused, the emperor queried, "Who stands before me?" Bodhidharma replied, "I don't know."

This story was originally told to me in a way that illustrated the uncompromising approach of Zen practice, grounded in emptiness and experience, eschewing dogma and devotion. Moreover, the "I don't know" was meant to be chewed on and mulled over. When I first heard the story in 1970 as a young Zen student, I was transformed by it. I loved the way the simple monk cut through the presumptions, assumptions, and defenses of the powerful emperor. I loved the ways that power and conscious self-promotion were unrewarded in Bodhidharma's response to the emperor. And of course, I simply adored the poetry of the monk's replies. For endless hours, I reflected on "I don't know." I learned a lot from the story.

And yet, over the decades, as I engaged in my own therapy and became a psychologist, then a psychoanalyst, I found I began to hear the story with a different ear. I became sympathetic, even empathic, with poor old Emperor Wu. After all, he was approaching the master naïvely and he wanted *help*. Even though he was boasting, Wu wasn't coming from a position of power. He was coming from a position of vulnerability and need. Wasn't Bodhidharma really the one who *was* actually showing off with all of his special talk? Wasn't he *missing* what Emperor Wu was asking for? Wasn't this a projective identification about their competitive needs for power and prowess, in which Bodhidharma apparently "won" and Wu was humiliated?

I began to imagine the encounter as a first meeting of psychoanalytic psychotherapy, in which the patient is Emperor Wu. In his initial meeting with Dr. Bodhidharma, Emperor Wu begins, "I have been reading recently about developments in relational psychoanalysis, and I have attended many psychoanalytic lectures over the years. Do you think these things could be helpful to my therapy?" Dr. B: "Not *at all!*" Emperor Wu: "Oh dear! I hoped it would be a little helpful. Well, what is this therapy about?" Dr. Bodhidharma: "NOTHING that can be explained!" Emperor Wu: "*Who* do *you think* you are? What gives you the right to talk to me like this?" Dr. B: "I have no idea!"

Now, unless this analyst were already well known and very idealized, someone like the notorious Jacques Lacan, he could never be so dismissive in the first meeting. The patient would quit. There would not be any therapy. And that is what happened: there was only this kind of showing off from Dr. B and the taste of humiliation in the mouth of the emperor—and probably a hopeless confusion about ever getting help from the method Bodhidharma was teaching. According to the story, Emperor Wu never again invited Bodhidharma to the court.

If this encounter had become a true therapeutic impasse—as grist for the mill—Dr. B would want to know why the patient wanted to impress him. Dr. B might feel the impact of the patient's need with some empathy. The patient idealizes Dr. B and is trying to impress him "in advance," so to speak. Dr. B might have been curious, even if a little put off, by the patient's attempts to get control of the treatment and about how he himself (Dr. B) personally *felt* in the midst of the emperor's wealth and generosity to the monastics. The effective analyst would want to know about the patient, about his defenses, and about his personality. The effective analyst would also examine his or her own reactions to the patient's personality and the patient's wealth.

The effective Zen teacher might not be interested in any of this. Whereas the effective analytic relationship is typically considered to be mutual—a two-person relationship for studying unconscious dynamics—the effective Zen relationship in this paradigm is a one-way awakening of wisdom. Dr. B's responses imply, "I'll show *you that you can't control things with your wealth and merit-making!*"

The differences in methods and models of mind create rich distinctions between these two liberation practices. Buddhist teaching tends to focus on emptiness, impermanence, and the wisdom that evolves from seeing deeply into these universal realities. But it has not been interested in examining the emotionally charged intersubjective relationship of a teacher and a student. It's not interested in examining either what might be left over in the teacher's desires for influence, power, or sexual favors after an awakening or how teachers actually need students in order for teachers to grow and develop. Psychoanalysis focuses our attention on waking up to the unconscious motivations we all share. Psychoanalysts assume that you can never become wholly conscious of everything you are doing because your mind is conflicted about becoming wholly conscious.

Looked at through the lens of these differences, we can see more clearly that teachers and students in Zen practice, following in the footsteps of this famous case, could be encouraged not to focus their attention on exactly what happens *between* them when they meet. In fact, there might be thought to be a wisdom in ignoring the specifics of need, desire, meaning, and power between them. The fixed position of "teacher" and "student" might be considered inviolable. Even if the teacher adamantly refuses to be idealized when the student continues to idealize (because that is built into the roles of the two), there may be no exploration of what that means.

From this brief illustration, it is not hard to see how both teacher and student, in the Zen situation, might miss the significance of thoughts and feelings that fall outside of the prescribed narrative of awakening. From my point of view, I think it's a short distance between believing that someone is flawless or fully awakened and assuming their motives are pure, no matter what those motives evoke or communicate.

I think, however, that Buddhist teachers (even those awakened Dr. B types) can learn from the model of projective identification, and that Dr. B would have learned a lot from sticking it out with old Emperor Wu. Dr. B might have learned about his own power motives, his longing to be in charge, and his competition with the emperor's wealth—as well as his compassion and loving kindness in the face of all that. Now that Buddhist practice has come to the West, students here don't want to overlook teachers' power motives and desires, even if the teacher is an awakened master. That fact might make Buddhist teaching in the West a bit more challenging, but it also opens the door to including more interpersonal skill in Buddhist practices. Examining the case of Emperor Wu and Bodhidharma illustrates something important about projective identification: we need to keep it squarely in mind when we engage in spiritual practices and ongoing relationships with our teachers.

References

Aitken, Robert. (1991). *The Gateless Barrier: The Wu-Men Kuan.* New York: North Point Press.

Bion, Wilfred. (1959). *Experiences in Groups.* New York: Basic Books.

Caper, Robert. (2000). *Immaterial Facts: Freud's Discovery of Psychic Reality and Klein's Development of His Work*. London: Routledge.

Caper, Robert. (2019). *Bion and Thoughts too Deep for Words*. London: Routledge.

Jung, Carl. (1921/1971). *Psychological Types: Collected Works, Vol. 6*. Princeton: Princeton University Press.

Klein, Melanie. (1946/1955). Notes on some schizoid mechanism. In *Envy and Gratitude and other Works, 1946–1963*, pp. 1–24. New York: Delacorte Press.

Klein, Melanie. (1955). On identification. In *Envy and Gratitude and other Works, 1946–1963*, pp. 141–175. New York: Delacorte Press.

Ogden, Thomas. (1991). *Projective Identification & Psychotherapeutic Technique*. Northvale, NJ: Jason Aronson.

Safran, Jeremy, and Kraus, Jessica. (2014). Alliance ruptures, impasses, and enactments: A relational perspective. *Psychotherapy*, 51(3), 381–387.

Waldron, William. (2003). *The Buddhist Unconscious*. London: Routledge.

Young-Eisendrath, P. (1993). *You're Not What Expected: Learning to Love the Opposite Sex*. New York: William Morrow.

Young-Eisendrath, P. (2019). *Love Between Equals: Relationship as a Spiritual Path*. Boulder, CO: Shambhala.

Young-Eisendrath, P., and Dawson, T. (Eds.). (2008). *The Cambridge Companion to Jung*, 2nd ed. Cambridge, England: Cambridge University Press.

Young-Eisendrath, P., and Muramoto, S. (Eds.). (2002). *Awakening and Insight: Zen Buddhism and Psychotherapy*. London and New York: Brunner-Routledge.

Contributors

John Beebe, M.D., is a North American Jungian analyst and author in practice in San Francisco, USA. He received degrees from Harvard College and the University of Chicago medical school. He is a past president of the C. G. Jung Institute of San Francisco, where he is currently on the teaching faculty. He is a Distinguished Life Fellow of the American Psychiatric Association.

Astrid Berg, MBChB (Pret), FFPsych (SA), MPhil (Child & Adolescent Psychiatry), is a psychiatrist, child and adolescent psychiatrist as well as a Jungian analyst. She is Emerita A/Professor at the University of Cape Town and A/Professor Extraordinary at the Stellenbosch University. She was one of the founding members of the Southern African Association of Jungian Analysts and its president from 1998 to 2003. She was a member of the Executive Committee of the IAAP and vice president from 1997 to 2007.

Patricia (Pat) Berry, Ph.D., received her diploma in analytical psychology from the C. G. Jung Institute Zurich in 1974. She was one of the early contributors to what came to be called, by James Hillman, archetypal psychology. She earned her Ph.D. in 1984 (University of Dallas). Many of Pat's earlier talks and chapters are collected in *Echo's Subtle Body: A Contribution to Archetypal Psychology*. Later chapters, published in various places, focus on a wide range of phenomena such as multiple personality disorder, child abuse, the orphan, film and aesthetics. She has been professionally active with Jungian educational institutions, serving as director of training and president of both the Inter-Regional Society of Jungian Analysts and the C. G. Jung Institute of Boston.

Fanny Brewster, Ph.D., is a Jungian analyst and Professor of Depth Psychology at Pacifica Graduate Institute. She is a writer of nonfiction including *African Americans and Jungian Psychology: Leaving the Shadows* (Routledge, 2017), *Archetypal Grief: Slavery's Legacy of Intergenerational Child Loss* (Routledge, 2018) and *The Racial Complex: A Jungian Perspective on Culture and Race* (Routledge, 2019). Fanny is a lecturer and workshop presenter on Jungian-related topics that address dream work, American culture and creativity. She is a faculty member at the New York C. G. Jung Foundation and an analyst member with the Philadelphia Association of Jungian Analysts.

Joseph Cambray, Ph.D., is a Jungian analyst, CEO-President, and Provost at Pacifica Graduate Institute. He is also past President of the International Association for Analytical Psychology; he served as the U.S. editor for the *Journal of Analytical Psychology* and is currently on the editorial boards of the *Journal of Analytical Psychology*, *The Jung Journal: Culture and Psyche* and I*srael Annual of Psychoanalytic Theory, Research and Practice*. He has been a faculty member at Harvard Medical School in the Department of Psychiatry at Massachusetts General Hospital, Center for Psychoanalytic Studies; adjunct faculty at Pacifica Graduate Institute. His numerous publications include the book based on his Fay Lectures: *Synchronicity: Nature and Psyche in an Interconnected Universe* and a volume edited with Linda Carter, *Analytical Psychology: Contemporary Perspectives in Jungian Psychology*.

Joan Chodorow, Ph.D., Jungian analyst, author of *Dance Therapy and Depth Psychology* and *Jung on Active Imagination*, is well known to us in Australia as the keynote speaker for the DTAA's Dance Therapy Conference in Melbourne in February 2000. Deeply involved in dance and dance therapy, with interests in early development and active imagination, Joan lectures and teaches both nationally and internationally.

Warren Colman, Ph.D., is a training and supervising analyst of the Society of Analytical Psychology in London. He is former Editor-in-Chief of the *Journal of Analytical Psychology* and currently serves on the journal's editorial board. He lectures, teaches and supervises internationally, has worked on the IAAP "router" training of Jungian analysts in Russia and Eastern Europe for many years and is the IAAP Liaison person for the developing group in Hungary. His publications include chapters on couple interaction, sexuality, the self, analytic practice, imagination and the symbolic process. His book *Act and Image: The Emergence of Symbolic Imagination* (2016) draws on cognitive philosophy, archaeology and anthropology to trace the evolution of the human psyche via the use of symbolic communication.

Lionel Corbett, M.D., trained in medicine and psychiatry in England and as a Jungian analyst at the C.G. Jung Institute of Chicago. Lionel is a professor of depth psychology at Pacifica Graduate Institute, in Santa Barbara, California, where he teaches depth psychology. His primary interests are the religious function of the psyche, especially the way in which personal religious experience is relevant to individual psychology; the development of psychotherapy as a spiritual practice; and the interface of Jungian psychology and contemporary psychoanalytic thought. He is the author of numerous professional chapters and five books: *Psyche and the Sacred*; *The Religious Function of the Psyche*; *The Sacred Cauldron: Psychotherapy as a Spiritual Practice*; *The Soul in Anguish: Psychotherapeutic Approaches to Suffering*; and *Understanding Evil: A Guide for Psychotherapists*.

George B. Hogenson, Ph.D., is a North American Jungian analyst. He received his Ph.D. in philosophy from Yale University and his M.A. in clinical social work from the University of Chicago. He is a diplomate Jungian analyst in private practice in Chicago, where he works primarily with adults dealing with life transitions, dream work and trauma. He serves on the editorial board of the *Journal of Analytical Psychology*, was the vice president of the International Association for Analytical Psychology and is the author of *Jung's Struggle With Freud* (1983) as well as numerous chapters on archetypal theory, synchronicity and the nature of symbols.

Donald E. Kalsched, Ph.D., is a clinical psychologist and Jungian psychoanalyst in private practice in Santa Fe, New Mexico. He is a senior training analyst with the Inter-Regional Society of Jungian Analysts, where he teaches and supervises. He is the author of many journal chapters, book chapters, interviews and two major books in the field of depth psychology: *The Inner World of Trauma: Archetypal Defences of the Personal Spirit* (1996), and *Trauma and the Soul: A Psycho-Spiritual Approach to Human Development and Its Interruption* (2013).

Andrew Samuels is recognized internationally as a leading contributor to psychotherapy, counselling, analysis and depth psychology. Andrew is a training analyst of the Society of Analytical Psychology, is in private practice in London and was for many years Professor of Analytical Psychology at the University of Essex. He was Chair of the UK Council for Psychotherapy and (with Judy Ryde) founded Psychotherapists and Counsellors for Social Responsibility. His many books include (among others): *Jung and the Post-Jungians* (1985); *The Plural Psyche* (1989); *The Political Psyche* (1993); and *Politics on the Couch* (2001). His latest books are *A New Therapy for Politics?* (2016) and *Analysis and Activism: Social and Political Contributions of Jungian Analysis* (edited with Emilija Kiehl and Mark Saban, 2016).

Pia Skogemann's academic background is in archaeology and comparative religion. She co-founded the C.G. Jung Institute Copenhagen in 1980. She is active as a teacher, supervisor and currently (again) director of training. Pia joined the International Association for Analytical Psychology (IAAP) as an individual member in 1985. She was also a member of the IAAP executive committee 2001–07 (involved with the developing groups, especially with the Router's exams; recently teaching at a supervisor course in Romania). Her chapters and books have been translated in English and German: *Chuang Tzu and The Butterfly Dream* (1986); *Weiblichkeit und Selbstverwirklichung. Die Individuation der Frau heute* (1988); *Karolines Buch* (1989); *Where the Shadows Lie: A Jungian Interpretation of Tolkien's* The Lord of the Rings (2009); and *The Daughter Archetype* (2012);

Ursula Wirtz, Ph.D., holds a doctorate in philosophy and German studies at the University of Munich in 1971 and taught internationally. She obtained a Lic. Phil. in clinical and anthropological psychology from the University of Zurich and a diploma in analytical psychology from the C.G. Jung Institute. She is a full member of the Swiss and international societies for analytical psychology (SGAP, IAAP, AGAP). She lives and works in Zurich, also as a supervisor with individuals and teams with a focus on psychotraumatology. She is a lecturer, training analyst and supervisor at ISAP Zurich and a trainer for Jungian psychology in Eastern Europe. She researches and publishes on the topics of sexual violence, trauma, ethics and the connection between psychotherapy and spirituality.

Polly Young-Eisendrath, Ph.D., is a psychologist, writer, speaker and Jungian analyst who has published 18 books (translated into 20 languages) including *Love Between Equals: Relationship as a Spiritual Path, The Self-Esteem Trap: Raising Confident and Compassionate Kids in an Age of Self-Importance, The Cambridge Companion to Jung* and *The Present Heart: A Memoir of Love, Loss and Discovery.* She maintains a clinical practice in Central Vermont and hosts the podcast *Enemies: From War to Wisdom* that provides a fresh look at human hostilities and what to do about them. She is a lifelong Buddhist practitioner and a mindfulness teacher.

Eva Pattis Zoja is a clinical psychologist and Jungian psychoanalyst (ÖGAP, AGAP, CIPA, NYAAP). She holds a diploma in sandplay from ISST. She teaches at the C. G. Jung Institute (Zürich), C. G. Jung Foundation (New York) and ÖGAP (Vienna). Her books include *Abortion. Loss and Renewal in the Search for Identity* (Routledge, 1997); *Sandplay Therapy: The Treatment of Psychopathologies* (2002); *Sandplay Therapy in Vulnerable Communities* (2019); and *Where Soul Meets Matter* (2019).

Index

Page numbers in *italics* indicate figures.

Ingram Content Group UK Ltd.
Milton Keynes UK
UKHW020033170323
418718UK00007B/48

9 780367 710170